METHODS IN MOLECULAR BIOLOGY

For further volumes:
http://www.springer.com/series/7651

For over 35 years, biological scientists have come to rely on the research protocols and methodologies in the critically acclaimed *Methods in Molecular Biology* series. The series was the first to introduce the step-by-step protocols approach that has become the standard in all biomedical protocol publishing. Each protocol is provided in readily-reproducible step-by-step fashion, opening with an introductory overview, a list of the materials and reagents needed to complete the experiment, and followed by a detailed procedure that is supported with a helpful notes section offering tips and tricks of the trade as well as troubleshooting advice. These hallmark features were introduced by series editor Dr. John Walker and constitute the key ingredient in each and every volume of the *Methods in Molecular Biology* series. Tested and trusted, comprehensive and reliable, all protocols from the series are indexed in PubMed.

Diabetic Nephropathy

Methods and Protocols

Edited by

Luigi Gnudi

Faculty of Life Sciences & Medicine, School of Cardiovascular Medicine & Sciences, British Heart Foundation Centre of Research Excellence, King's College London, London, UK

David A. Long

Developmental Biology and Cancer Programme, UCL Great Ormond Street Institute of Child Health, University College London, London, UK

Humana Press

Editors
Luigi Gnudi
Faculty of Life Sciences & Medicine
School of Cardiovascular Medicine
& Sciences, British Heart Foundation
Centre of Research Excellence
King's College London
London, UK

David A. Long
Developmental Biology and Cancer Programme
UCL Great Ormond Street Institute of Child Health
University College London
London, UK

ISSN 1064-3745 ISSN 1940-6029 (electronic)
Methods in Molecular Biology
ISBN 978-1-4939-9840-1 ISBN 978-1-4939-9841-8 (eBook)
https://doi.org/10.1007/978-1-4939-9841-8

This Humana imprint is published by the registered company Springer Science+Business Media, LLC, part of Springer Nature.
The registered company address is: 233 Spring Street, New York, NY 10013, U.S.A.

Preface

Diabetic nephropathy represents the leading cause of end-stage renal failure in the Western world. New treatments to either prevent this condition or delay its relentless progression are urgently needed. In this book, we have put together a toolkit of novel research approaches for investigators to study diabetic nephropathy. We hope that this will foster new research directions and inspire ideas to enhance our understanding of diabetic nephropathy and to develop treatments for this condition.

Experimental models are critical for basic science studies in the field of diabetic nephropathy, and our book describes a wide range of current models from the fly to the fish, cells in culture, and in vivo mammalian approaches. Successful studies in the field of diabetic nephropathy also require powerful techniques to image the kidney. This is an area where technological advances are rapidly occurring. Our book reflects this, and we describe not only traditional histological techniques to visualize diabetic kidneys but also innovative new approaches in electron, confocal, and two-photon microscopy. The pathophysiology of the diabetic kidney is complex, and we describe a range of techniques that can unravel these processes by examining changes in the properties of cells that make up the kidney filtration barrier, assess endoplasmic reticulum stress, apoptosis, and cell–cell interactions. The last decade has also seen major advances in techniques which take a global approach to assessing microRNAs, genes, proteins, and metabolites in disease conditions, and these are described in relation to diabetic nephropathy. Finally, advances in the renal field in gene editing and regenerative medicine are described. Although these have not been used extensively in diabetic kidney disease to-date, they provide great promise for the future.

We are grateful to all that have contributed to this book and whose aim is to help patients with diabetic kidney disease. We hope this book will support the reader in their research and help researchers to develop innovative experimental approaches in the field of diabetic nephropathy.

London, UK

Luigi Gnudi
David A. Long

Contents

Contributors

MAURO ABBATE • *Istituto di Ricerche Farmacologiche Mario Negri IRCCS, Bergamo, Italy*
LINDA AHONEN • *Steno Diabetes Center Copenhagen, Gentofte, Denmark*
KERRY ANDERSON • *Centre for Public Health, Queen's University Belfast, Northern Ireland, UK*
IOANNIS BANTOUNAS • *Division of Cell Matrix Biology and Regenerative Medicine, Faculty of Biology, Medicine and Health, University of Manchester, Manchester Academic Health Science Centre, Manchester, UK*
KARINA BARREIRO • *Finnish Institute of Molecular Medicine, University of Helsinki, Helsinki, Finland*
TIMOTHY BOWEN • *Wales Kidney Research Unit, Heath Park Campus, Cardiff, UK*
CAROLYNN CAIRNS • *Centre for Cardiovascular Science, University of Edinburgh, Edinburgh, UK*
MARISA CANADAS-GARRE • *Centre for Public Health, Queen's University Belfast, Northern Ireland, UK*
CAMILLO CARRARA • *Istituto di Ricerche Farmacologiche Mario Negri IRCCS, Bergamo, Italy*
SARA CONTI • *Istituto di Ricerche Farmacologiche Mario Negri IRCCS, Bergamo, Italy*
BRYAN CONWAY • *Centre for Cardiovascular Science, University of Edinburgh, Edinburgh, UK*
RICHARD J. COWARD • *Bristol Royal Hospital for Sick Children & University of Bristol, Bristol Medical School, Bristol, UK; Bristol Renal, Translational Health Sciences, Bristol Medical School, University of Bristol, Bristol, UK*
CRISTINA DANIELE • *Medical Faculty Mannheim, Medical Research Center, University of Heidelberg, Mannheim, Germany*
SEAMUS DUFFY • *Centre for Public Health, Queen's University Belfast, Northern Ireland, UK*
MARIA FRANTZI • *Mosaiques Diagnostics GmbH, Hannover, Germany*
DONALD FRASER • *Wales Kidney Research Unit, Heath Park Campus, Cardiff, UK*
GRACE FREKE • *Genetics and Genomic Medicine Programmes, Great Ormond Street Institute of Child Health, University College London, London, UK*
SANCHITA GHOSH • *Institute of Clinical Chemistry and Pathobiochemistry, Otto-von-Guericke-University, Magdeburg, Germany*
LUIGI GNUDI • *Faculty of Life Sciences & Medicine, School of Cardiovascular Medicine & Sciences, British Heart Foundation Centre of Research Excellence, King's College London, London, UK*
NORBERT GRETZ • *Medical Faculty Mannheim, Medical Research Center, University of Heidelberg, Mannheim, Germany*
PAUL S. HARTLEY • *Department of Life and Environmental Science, Bournemouth University, Poole, Dorset, UK*
CLAIRE E. HILLS • *School of Life Sciences, University of Lincoln, Lincoln, UK*
HARRY HOLTHOFER • *Finnish Institute of Molecular Medicine, University of Helsinki, Helsinki, Finland; Department of Medicine, University Medical Center Hamburg-Eppendorf, Hamburg, Germany*

Tobias B. Huber • *Department of Medicine, University Medical Center Hamburg-Eppendorf, Hamburg, Germany*

Berend Isermann • *Institute of Clinical Chemistry and Pathobiochemistry, Otto-von-Guericke-University, Magdeburg, Germany*

Daniyal J. Jafree • *Developmental Biology and Cancer Programme, UCL Great Ormond Street Institute of Child Health, University College London, London, UK; MB/PhD Programme, Faculty of Medical Sciences, University College London, London, UK*

Dagan Jenkins • *Genetics and Genomic Medicine Programmes, Great Ormond Street Institute of Child Health, University College London, London, UK*

Katie Kerr • *Centre for Public Health, Queen's University Belfast, Northern Ireland, UK*

Arif ul Maula Khan • *Medical Faculty Mannheim, Medical Research Center, University of Heidelberg, Mannheim, Germany*

Jill Kilner • *Centre for Public Health, Queen's University Belfast, Northern Ireland, UK*

Susan J. Kimber • *Division of Cell Matrix Biology and Regenerative Medicine, Faculty of Biology, Medicine and Health, University of Manchester, Manchester Academic Health Science Centre, Manchester, UK*

Maria Kolatsi-Joannou • *Developmental Biology and Cancer Programme, UCL Great Ormond Street Institute of Child Health, London, UK*

Abigail C. Lay • *Bristol Renal, Translational Health Sciences, Bristol Medical School, University of Bristol, Bristol, UK*

Kuo-Kang Liu • *School of Engineering, University of Warwick, Warwick, UK*

David A. Long • *Developmental Biology and Cancer Programme, UCL Great Ormond Street Institute of Child Health, University College London, London, UK*

Pedro Magalhães • *Mosaiques Diagnostics GmbH, Hannover, Germany; Department of Pediatric Nephrology, Hannover Medical School, Hannover, Germany*

Gianfranco Marchetti • *Unit of Nephrology, Azienda Socio-Sanitaria Territoriale Papa Giovanni XXIII, Bergamo, Italy*

Akash Mathew • *Institute of Clinical Chemistry and Pathobiochemistry, Otto-von-Guericke-University, Magdeburg, Germany*

Amy Jayne McKnight • *Centre for Public Health, Queen's University Belfast, Northern Ireland, UK*

Dale Moulding • *Developmental Biology and Cancer Programme, UCL Great Ormond Street Institute of Child Health, University College London, London, UK; Light Microscopy Core Facility, UCL Great Ormond Street Institute of Child Health, University College London, London, UK*

Daniela Nardozi • *Medical Faculty Mannheim, Medical Research Center, University of Heidelberg, Mannheim, Germany*

Lucy Jade Newbury • *Wales Kidney Research Unit, Heath Park Campus, Cardiff, UK*

Daniel Osborn • *Genetics Research Centre, St George's University of London, London, UK*

Nuria Perretta-Tejedor • *Developmental Biology and Cancer, Great Ormond Street Institute of Child Health, University College London, London, UK*

Raina D. Ramnath • *Bristol Renal, Translational Health Sciences, Bristol Medical School, University of Bristol, Bristol, UK*

Paola Rizzo • *Istituto di Ricerche Farmacologiche Mario Negri IRCCS, Bergamo, Italy*

Peter Rossing • *Steno Diabetes Center Copenhagen, Gentofte, Denmark; Department of Clinical Medicine, University of Copenhagen, Copenhagen, Denmark*

Daniela Rottoli • *Istituto di Ricerche Farmacologiche Mario Negri IRCCS, Bergamo, Italy*

Manpreet K. Sagoo • *Faculty of Life Sciences & Medicine, School of Cardiovascular Medicine & Sciences, British Heart Foundation Centre of Research Excellence, King's College London, London, UK*

Simon C. Satchell • *Bristol Renal, Translational Health Sciences, Bristol Medical School, University of Bristol, Bristol, UK*

Peter J. Scambler • *Developmental Biology and Cancer Programme, UCL Great Ormond Street Institute of Child Health, University College London, London, UK*

Marian Seda • *Genetics and Genomic Medicine Programmes, Great Ormond Street Institute of Child Health, University College London, London, UK*

Khurrum Shahzad • *Institute of Clinical Chemistry and Pathobiochemistry, Otto-von-Guericke-University, Magdeburg, Germany; Department of Biotechnology, University of Sargodha, Sargodha, Pakistan*

Eleftherios Siamantouras • *School of Life Sciences, University of Lincoln, Lincoln, UK*

Edina Silajdžić • *Division of Cell Matrix Biology and Regenerative Medicine, Faculty of Biology, Medicine and Health, University of Manchester, Manchester Academic Health Science Centre, Manchester, UK*

Kate Simpson • *Wales Kidney Research Unit, Heath Park Campus, Cardiff, UK*

Justyna Siwy • *Mosaiques Diagnostics GmbH, Hannover, Germany*

Laura J. Smyth • *Centre for Public Health, Queen's University Belfast, Northern Ireland, UK*

Paul E. Squires • *School of Life Sciences, University of Lincoln, Lincoln, UK*

Angelo Torelli • *Medical Faculty Mannheim, Medical Research Center, University of Heidelberg, Mannheim, Germany; Mannheim University of Applied Sciences, Mannheim, Germany*

Elisavet Vasilopoulou • *Medway School of Pharmacy, University of Kent, Chatham, Kent, UK; Developmental Biology and Cancer, UCL GOS Institute of Child Health, London, UK*

Kathryn E. White • *EM Research Services, Faculty of Medical Sciences, Newcastle University, Newcastle upon Tyne, UK*

Alexa Wonnacott • *Wales Kidney Research Unit, Heath Park Campus, Cardiff, UK*

Adrian S. Woolf • *Division of Cell Matrix Biology and Regenerative Medicine, Faculty of Biology, Medicine and Health, University of Manchester, Manchester Academic Health Science Centre, Manchester, UK; Royal Manchester Children's Hospital, Manchester, UK*

Part I

Introduction

Chapter 1

Diabetic Nephropathy: An Overview

Manpreet K. Sagoo and Luigi Gnudi

Abstract

Diabetic nephropathy (DN) is one of the most feared diabetic chronic microvascular complications and the major cause of end-stage renal disease (ESRD). The classical presentation of DN is characterized by hyperfiltration and albuminuria in the early phases which is then followed by a progressive renal function decline. The presentation of diabetic kidney disease (DKD) can vary especially in patients with T2DM where concomitant presence of other glomerular/tubular pathologies and severe peripheral vascular disease can become important confounders. All-cause mortality in individuals with DKD is approximately 30 times higher than that in diabetic patients without nephropathy and a great majority of patients with DKD will die from cardiovascular disease before they reach ESRD. The management of metabolic and hemodynamic perturbations for the prevention and for the delay of progression of DKD is very important. DKD is a global challenge and a significant social and economic burden; research should aim at developing new ideas to tackle this devastating condition.

Key words Diabetes mellitus, Diabetic kidney disease, Epidemiology, Management, Pathogenesis

1 Introduction to Diabetes Mellitus

Diabetes mellitus (DM) is a common and serious metabolic condition which presents a major challenge in twenty-first-century healthcare. The global prevalence of DM has dramatically increased from 108 million in 1980 to 451 million in 2017 and this number continues to rapidly rise [1]. Estimated figures from the International Diabetes Federation predict that 693 million people will be living with diabetes worldwide by 2045 [2] (http://www.diabetesatlas.org). At present, diabetes is the seventh leading cause of mortality worldwide and thus the diabetes epidemic requires immediate action [3].

Diabetes is characterized by chronic hyperglycemia and glucose intolerance due to impaired insulin action and/or secretion. Micro- and macro-diabetic chronic vascular complications affect the majority of patients with diabetes in both developed and developing countries. The microvascular complications include diabetic nephropathy, retinopathy, and neuropathy, and are responsible for

Luigi Gnudi and David A. Long (eds.), *Diabetic Nephropathy: Methods and Protocols*, Methods in Molecular Biology, vol. 2067, https://doi.org/10.1007/978-1-4939-9841-8_1,

significant morbidity in this patient group. The macrovascular complications include accelerated coronary heart disease, ischemic stroke, and peripheral vascular disease, and represent the most common cause of mortality in diabetic patients.

1.1 Classification of Diabetes Mellitus

Based on the American Diabetes Association classification system, the two major forms of diabetes are type 1 diabetes mellitus (T1DM), an autoimmune disorder characterized by the destruction of the insulin-producing β-cells in the islets of Langerhans which accounts for 5–10% of cases, and type 2 diabetes mellitus (T2DM), a more common form of DM which accounts for up to 90% of cases and is due to diminished insulin action. With the increasing incidence of obesity worldwide, a pronounced increase in T2DM has been noted, compared to T1DM, which now typically affects a younger and increasingly obese patient group [4]. Recently subgroups of patients have been proposed based on six variables (glutamate decarboxylase antibodies, age at diagnosis, body mass index, glycated hemoglobin, and homoeostatic model assessment 2 estimates of β-cell function and insulin resistance). The resulting groups retain a diverse disease progression and risk of diabetic chronic complications [5].

2 Overview of Diabetic Nephropathy

Diabetic nephropathy (DN) is a morbid and deeply feared complication of diabetes. A striking 45% of T1DM and T2DM diabetics are affected by this microvascular complication [6]. At present, diabetes is the single leading cause of end-stage renal disease (ESRD) in the Western world and the principal cause for patients requiring renal replacement therapy worldwide [7]. However, due to the strong association between DN and cardiovascular disease, a large majority of patients with DN will die even before progression to ESRD, as a result of cardiovascular related events [7].

2.1 Epidemiology of Diabetic Nephropathy

DN is a chronic, progressive disease of the kidney that develops over time, with a peak incidence after 10–20 years of diabetes. The severity and incidence of DN are influenced by ethnicity, as African Americans, Asians, and Native Americans are more commonly affected and typically subject to a more aggressive disease course, compared to White Caucasians [8]. In a small proportion of patients with minimal diabetes-induced renal damage, DN can remain clinically silent for their entire lifetime [9]. The incidence of DN has substantiality increased over recent years; however, data now suggests that the incidence of ESRD is beginning to plateau [10]. The cumulative risk of developing ESRD in both T1DM and T2DM, following 5 years of consistent proteinuria, stands at an estimate of 40% [11].

2.2 Pathogenesis of Diabetic Nephropathy

Persistent exposure to elevated blood glucose levels leads to damage and disruption of the renal cellular architecture and microvasculature in patients with diabetes. A number of complex pathways mediate these effects and are grouped into four main categories: metabolic, hemodynamic, intracellular, and growth factors/cytokines. As a result, unique ultrastructural changes occur in the kidney nephron, at the level of the glomerulus. The glomerular filtration barrier (GFB) is a complex structure, made of four key components: the mesangium, glomerular basement membrane (GBM), fenestrated glomerular endothelial cells, and podocytes. In DN, hallmark pathological changes occur in the GFB, including GBM thickening, mesangial sclerosis, endothelial dysfunction with glycocalyx damage, podocyte foot process effacement and detachment, and decreased podocyte number [12, 13]. Similar insults affect the renal tubular compartment resulting in progressive deposition of extracellular matrix and secondary tubular interstitial fibrosis.

2.3 Clinical Assessment of Diabetic Nephropathy

Clinically, DN is classically characterized by progressive increases in urinary albumin excretion (UAE), paralleled by an increase in blood pressure and cardiovascular risk. This is accompanied by a gradual decline in glomerular filtration rate (GFR) and eventual progression to ESRD. Defects at the level of the GFB leads toward increased urinary protein known as albuminuria, one of the earliest signs of DN and systemic vascular dysfunction [14]. The degree of albuminuria and proteinuria correlates with and is also an important clinical predictor of the rate of kidney disease progression (at the macroproteinuria stage) [15]. Estimation of GFR is an important clinical investigation utilized to monitor renal function decline. Routine annual surveillance is recommended for all diabetic patients to monitor the progression and rate of decline of renal function.

Traditionally, DN has five identified stages based on UAE and GFR: glomerular hyperfiltration, a silent stage, incipient nephropathy with microalbuminuria (the first clinically detectable sign), overt nephropathy, and, finally, ESRD (Table 1) [7].

2.4 Management of Diabetic Nephropathy

Current management of DN relies on multifactorial intervention and primarily targets concurrent glycemic, blood pressure, and lipid control, in addition to lifestyle changes. This is heavily influenced by the findings of major landmark clinical trials. The Diabetes Control and Complications Trial (DCCT) highlighted the major benefits of intensive glycemic control in T1DM in preventing GFR decline and the development and progression of proteinuria [16]. Furthermore, in patients with T2DM, the United Kingdom Prospective Diabetes Study (UKPDS) found a significant reduction in the incidence of microalbuminuria in T2DM patients with better diabetes and blood pressure control [17, 18]. Thus, glycated

Table 1
Clinical description of current stages of diabetic nephropathy

Stage of diabetic nephropathy	GFR	UAE	Blood pressure	Additional comments
Stage 1: glomerular hyperfiltration	Normal >90 mL/min/1.73 m^2 or increased	<30 mg/day	Normotensive	Renal hyperfunction and hypertrophy
Stage 2: silent stage	Normal >90 mL/min/1.73 m^2	<30 mg/day	± Hypertensive	Thickening of basement membrane and mesangial proliferation
Stage 3: incipient nephropathy	<60 mL/min/1.73 m^2	Microalbuminuria: 30–300 mg/day	± Hypertensive	First clinical signs of kidney disease
Stage 4: overt nephropathy	<30 mL/min/1.73 m^2	Macroalbuminuria: >300 mg/day	Hypertensive	Significant loss of kidney function
Stage 5: end-stage renal disease	<15 mL/min/1.73 m^2	Macroalbuminuria: >300 mg/day	Hypertensive	Major loss of kidney function. Usually requires RRT (dialysis or transplantation)

hemoglobin and blood pressure measurements are routinely monitored in these patients. Recommended lifestyle changes include smoking cessation, optimization of body mass index, and dietary modifications to reduce sodium and alcohol intake.

The main therapeutic target is a blockade of the renin-angiotensin system, through angiotensin-converting enzyme inhibitors or angiotensin II receptor blockers, which have renoprotective, anti-proteinuric, and antihypertensive effects and have been shown to slow down the progression of ESRD [19, 20]. However, current treatment strategies have had limited clinical benefit and many patients will still go on to develop ESRD. Nevertheless, recently the use of inhibitors of the energy-dependent sodium/glucose cotransporter-2 (mainly expressed in the proximal kidney tubule) has been suggested as a novel therapy for DN (https://www.janssen.com/phase-3-credence-renal-outcomes-trial-invokanar-canagliflozin-being-stopped-early-positive-efficacy) [21].

3 Conclusions

Ultimately, despite major advances in our knowledge base, DN remains a substantial clinical challenge and burden to twenty-first-century healthcare worldwide. Based on this premise, it is evident that further understanding of the pathogenic mechanisms underlying DN is still urgently needed to prevent disease progression and drive the development of novel, effective, and efficient therapeutic strategies for this devastating disease.

References

1. Collaboration NCDRF (2016) Worldwide trends in diabetes since 1980: a pooled analysis of 751 population-based studies with 4.4 million participants. Lancet 387 (10027):1513–1530
2. Federation ID (2018) IDF diabetes atlas, Brussels
3. Organization WH (2018) Global Health Estimates 2016: Deaths by Cause, Age, Sex, by Country and by Region, 2000–2016. Switzerland, Geneva
4. American Diabetes A (2016) 2. Classification and diagnosis of diabetes. Diabetes Care 39 (Suppl 1):S13–S22
5. Ahlqvist E, Storm P, Karajamaki A, Martinell M, Dorkhan M, Carlsson A et al (2018) Novel subgroups of adult-onset diabetes and their association with outcomes: a data-driven cluster analysis of six variables. Lancet Diabetes Endocrinol 6(5):361–369
6. Hovind P, Rossing P, Tarnow L, Smidt UM, Parving HH (2001) Progression of diabetic nephropathy. Kidney Int 59(2):702–709
7. Gnudi L, Gentile G, Ruggenenti P (2016) The patient with diabetes mellitus. In: Turner N, Lamiere N, Goldsmith DJ, Winearls CG, Himmelfarb J, Remuzzi G (eds) Oxford textbook of clinical nephrology, vol 2. Oxford University Press, Oxford, pp 1199–1247
8. Young BA, Maynard C, Boyko EJ (2003) Racial differences in diabetic nephropathy, cardiovascular disease, and mortality in a national population of veterans. Diabetes Care 26 (8):2392–2399
9. Gnudi L, Thomas SM, Viberti G (2007) Mechanical forces in diabetic kidney disease: a trigger for impaired glucose metabolism. J Am Soc Nephrol 18(8):2226–2232
10. Saran R, Robinson B, Abbott KC, Agodoa LY, Albertus P, Ayanian J et al (2017) US Renal Data System 2016 Annual Data Report: Epidemiology of Kidney Disease in the United States. Am J Kidney Dis 69(3 Suppl 1):A7–A8
11. Gross JL, de Azevedo MJ, Silveiro SP, Canani LH, Caramori ML, Zelmanovitz T (2005) Diabetic nephropathy: diagnosis, prevention, and treatment. Diabetes Care 28(1):164–176
12. Haraldsson B, Nystrom J, Deen WM (2008) Properties of the glomerular barrier and mechanisms of proteinuria. Physiol Rev 88 (2):451–487
13. Gnudi L, Coward RJ, Long DA (2016) Diabetic nephropathy: perspective on novel molecular mechanisms. Trends Endocrinol Metab 27 (11):820–830
14. Deckert T, Feldt-Rasmussen B, Borch-Johnsen K, Jensen T, Kofoed-Enevoldsen A (1989) Albuminuria reflects widespread vascular damage. The Steno hypothesis. Diabetologia 32(4):219–226
15. Berhane AM, Weil EJ, Knowler WC, Nelson RG, Hanson RL (2011) Albuminuria and estimated glomerular filtration rate as predictors of diabetic end-stage renal disease and death. Clin J Am Soc Nephrol 6(10):2444–2451
16. de Boer IH, Sun W, Cleary PA, Lachin JM, Molitch ME, Steffes MW et al (2011) Intensive diabetes therapy and glomerular filtration rate in type 1 diabetes. N Engl J Med 365 (25):2366–2376
17. UK Prospective Diabetes Study (UKPDS) Group (1998) Intensive blood-glucose control with sulphonylureas or insulin compared with conventional treatment and risk of complications in patients with type 2 diabetes (UKPDS 33). Lancet 352(9131):837–853
18. UK Prospective Diabetes Study Group (1998) Tight blood pressure control and risk of macrovascular and microvascular complications in type 2 diabetes: UKPDS 38. BMJ 317 (7160):703–713
19. Lewis EJ, Hunsicker LG, Clarke WR, Berl T, Pohl MA, Lewis JB et al (2001) Renoprotective effect of the angiotensin-receptor antagonist irbesartan in patients with nephropathy due to type 2 diabetes. N Engl J Med 345 (12):851–860
20. Brenner BM, Cooper ME, de Zeeuw D, Keane WF, Mitch WE, Parving HH et al (2001) Effects of losartan on renal and cardiovascular outcomes in patients with type 2 diabetes and nephropathy. N Engl J Med 345(12):861–869
21. Perkovic V, Jardine MJ, Neal B, Bompoint S, Heerspink HJL, Charytan DM, et al. (2019) Canagliflozin and renal outcomes in type 2 diabetes and nephropathy. N Engl J Med 13;380 (24):2295–2306

Part II

Experimental Models to Study Diabetic Nephropathy

Chapter 2

Modeling Podocyte Biology Using *Drosophila* Nephrocytes

Paul S. Hartley and Richard J. Coward

Abstract

Vertebrate podocytes are kidney glomerular cells critically required for normal renal filtration. To fulfill their role, podocytes form molecular sieves known as slit diaphragms that contribute to the glomerular filtration barrier. The disruption of podocyte biology or slit diaphragm formation in humans is a precursor to albuminuria, renal failure, and cardiovascular morbidity. Due to genetic and functional similarities, the nephrocytes of *Drosophila* are increasingly used to model the genetic and metabolic basis of human podocyte biology. They have the advantage that they are a much quicker system to study compared to other murine transgenic models. In this chapter we present methods to modulate and study *Drosophila* nephrocyte function and diaphragm formation.

Key words Kidney, Podocyte, Nephropathy, *Drosophila*, Nephrocyte, Slit diaphragm

1 Introduction

The nephrocytes of insects are genetically similar to podocytes [1, 2]. They are large filtration cells that contribute to cardiorenal homeostasis by clearing from the circulation unwanted proteins [3]. Due to the genetic tractability of *Drosophila melanogaster*, the insect nephrocyte is increasingly used to model podocyte genetics and slit diaphragm biology (reviewed in [4]). *Drosophila* diaphragms appear as linear arrays at the nephrocyte surface and can be imaged using antisera to dumbfounded (duf) and sticks and stone (sns; orthologs of human KIRREL1 and NEPHRIN, respectively) [1]. *Drosophila* genetics allows for cell and temporally restricted gene modulation in a range of contexts including studies of development, metabolism, and ageing. Modulation of gene expression in nephrocytes can be achieved using a nephrocyte-restricted driver based on the *Drosophila Krüppel-like factor 15* (*dKlf15*) enhancer region [5]. The *dKlf15* gene's expression is restricted to nephrocytes and required for their development to maturity and sustained function in adulthood. The enhancer sequence of *dKlf15* has been engineered upstream of the yeast *Gal4* gene, allowing use in the

Luigi Gnudi and David A. Long (eds.), *Diabetic Nephropathy: Methods and Protocols*, Methods in Molecular Biology, vol. 2067,
https://doi.org/10.1007/978-1-4939-9841-8_2,

bipartite *Gal4-UAS* gene transactivation system. The *Gal4-UAS* system is based on yeast genetics where the Gal4 transcription factor binds specifically to a well-characterized DNA sequence (the upstream activation sequence). The UAS sequence has been engineered into the enhancers of thousands of *Drosophila* genes, whereas the *Gal4* sequence has been engineered downstream of endogenous enhancer sequences. By combining the two alleles it is possible to drive *Gal4*-dependent expression of genes downstream of the UAS [6].

2 Materials

2.1 Food for Routine Propagation of Drosophila

Although diets vary between labs they typically consist of agar to make the food solid, a carbohydrate source (sucrose), protein (yeast or yeast extract), and food preservatives (methylparaben/nipagin and propionic acid). We use a version of a "cornmeal-yeast-agar" diet (1.4 L of H_2O, 15 g agar, 110 g sucrose, 35 g live yeast, 100 g maize, 7 mL propionic acid, and 3.8 g nipagin mixed with 38.0 mL ethanol).

2.2 Useful Transgenic Drosophila Lines

1. *dKlf15-Gal4* (Hartley Lab, described in [5]): This drives the expression of genes of interest specifically in pericardial nephrocytes and garland cell nephrocytes. It shows a more restricted expression pattern than *Dorothy-Gal4* (which expresses in the gut as well as nephrocytes).
2. *Dorothy-Gal4* (available from Bloomington Drosophila Stock Center (BDSC)), described by Kimbrell et al. [7]: Although expression is not as restricted as *dKlf15-Gal4*, this driver seems stronger and can drive more severe phenotypes in nephrocytes.
3. *UAS-GCaMP6* (ultrasensitive, genetically encoded calcium reporters available from BDSC [8]): These reporters have slow, medium, and fast kinetics with regard to calcium binding and dissociation. We have used all three types and given the timeframe they are used over (seconds rather than milliseconds) all three provide excellent signals. Users should define their own requirements when choosing the reporter (for example, the fast system is used in the lab for imaging calcium transients in cardiomyocytes).

2.3 Dissection

1. Triethylamine solution (anesthetic), made up at the following ratio: 50% triethylamine:25% ethanol:25% water. A 7 mL bijou containing 5 mL will last for several weeks depending on usage. A small volume is preferable because of the solution's pungent odor.
2. Empty *Drosophila* vial, with cotton stopper.
3. 30 mm diameter polycarbonate petri dishes.

4. Vacuum grease or petroleum jelly.
5. Hanks balanced salt solution.
6. 1 M Stock of calcium chloride.
7. 1 M Stock of magnesium chloride.
8. Two pairs of No. 5 Dumont forceps.
9. 3 mm Curved Vannas scissors.
10. Benchtop aspirator.
11. Paper towels.

2.4 Vital Staining/Endocytosis

1. 10 kDa Dextran.
2. Albumin.
3. Lysotracker.
4. Wheat germ agglutinin.
5. pHrodo.

2.5 Slit Diaphragm Imaging

1. 38% Formaldehyde stock solution.
2. Phosphate-buffered saline (PBS).
3. Goat anti-sticks and stones (sns) primary antisera.
4. Rabbit anti-dumbfounded (duf) primary antisera.
5. Wheat germ agglutinin.
6. Secondary anti-goat antisera.
7. Secondary anti-rabbit antisera.
8. 25% Triton X-100 stock solution made with distilled water.

2.6 Solid Food Ingestion Assay (SOFI)

1. 7 mL Plastic bijou tubes with caps.
2. 1% Agar made with distilled water.
3. 5% or 25% w/v molten *Drosophila* food made with sucrose, for low- and high-sugar diets, respectively.
4. 25 gauge needles.
5. Benchtop heat block at 60 °C.
6. Microbalance capable of measuring in the sub-milligram range.
7. Bijou tube racks (or polystyrene 15 mL centrifuge tube packaging molds).

2.7 Ex Vivo Culture of Nephrocytes

1. Schneider's medium.
2. Penicillin and streptomycin solution ×100.
3. Fetal calf serum.

2.8 Calcium Imaging

1. 1 M $CaCl_2$ stock solution.
2. 1 mM Calcium ionophore A23187 in DMSO, positive control.

3. Calcium- and magnesium-free Hanks basic saline solution.
4. High frame rate capable of at least 25 frames per second.
5. Water dipping objective (preferably 10×).
6. ImageJ software.

3 Methods

3.1 Drosophila *Propagation and Ageing*

Fly stocks are routinely maintained in incubators at 18 °C and then moved to 25 °C for experimental crossing, collection of virgin females, and ageing. Flies are maintained under 12-h:12-h light-dark cycles with constant humidity. Experimental crosses are typically set up using five virgin females and three males. For ageing, flies are collected within 1–4 days of eclosion, maintained at a density of approximately 15 flies per vial and transferred to new food at least once a week for approximately 7–10 weeks depending on the strain.

3.2 Dissecting Adult Flies to Reveal Pericardial Nephrocytes

It is preferable to routinely use females for dissection because they are larger and easier to dissect and manipulate onto slides for imaging. Males should also be examined but consideration should be given to sexual dimorphism when measuring cells (avoid pooling data from the two sexes). Dissection, once mastered (typically an afternoon's practice), takes a few seconds per fly and 20–30 flies can be prepared easily within an hour. Ambient temperatures are used and there is no need for aseptic techniques. All dissections are done using a standard dissecting microscope, using two pairs of No. 5 Dumont forceps, as well as 3 mm curved Vannas scissors. It is useful to have a small paper towel in hand so that instruments can be wiped clean of tissue as dissection proceeds.

1. Use 30 mm diameter petri dishes; these are large enough for 20–30 flies to be dissected and stained at the same time. One petri dish accommodates 3 mL of any solution; this completely submerges dissected abdomen preparations.
2. Prepare the dish by smearing vacuum grease or petroleum jelly onto the surface of the dish, deep enough to lightly embed an anesthetized fly but not too thick to impede dissection.
3. Dissection is done at ambient temperature, with age-matched flies and Hanks balanced saline solution supplemented with 2 mM $CaCl_2$ and 4 mM $MgCl_2$ (HBSS).
4. Flies are transferred from their food vial to an empty 95 mm long vial and a 20 μL aliquot of triethylamine solution is added to the innermost surface of the vial's cotton stopper. Flies are fully anesthetized within 60–120 s and remain so for up to 20 min (*see* **Note 1**).

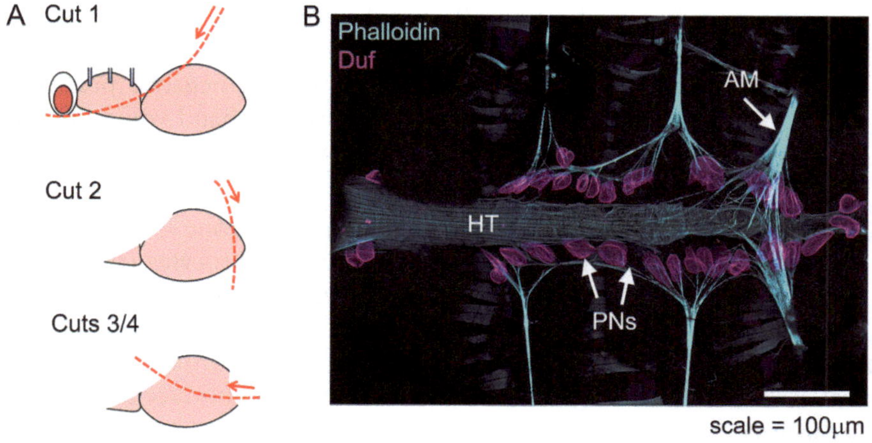

Fig. 1 (**a**) Schematic of adult *Drosophila* dissection showing the cuts required to open the abdomen and visualize the heart and pericardial nephrocytes. (**b**) The adult *Drosophila* heart stained with phalloidin to visualize filamentous actin (which is brightest at the alary muscles (AM) and heart tube (HT)), and antisera to Duf (localized to the pericardial nephrocytes, PNs)

5. Flies are then gently placed on their backs into the vacuum grease, with wings outstretched so that the abdomen is in direct contact with the grease (otherwise preparations can float off).
6. Flies are arranged in rows according to genotype (*see* **Note 2**), as this aids in visualization and subsequent processing.
7. Typically a "four-cut" preparation is performed in order to expose pericardial nephrocytes (Fig. 1a). The first two cuts are done "dry"; the subsequent cuts are done with flies under HBSS. Firstly, with the curvature of the Vannas scissors facing upwards the anterior abdomen is cut to remove most of the thorax, head, and legs. The second cut is best done with the Vannas scissors facing downwards and is done to remove the final (A8) abdominal section. This allows scissors to make the cuts on either side of the abdomen, allowing access to the abdominal cavity. The intestinal and reproductive tissues are then removed by pulling them away with forceps. This will reveal a beating dorsal vessel and adjacent pericardial nephrocytes (a stained heart, showing wild-type architecture, is presented in Fig. 1b).
8. The dish is rinsed with HBSS to remove residual tissues floating in the buffer and the dissections are "tidied" with forceps to remove any extraneous tissues accidentally embedded in grease.
9. Due to the natural curvature of the abdomen, the preparation is gently flattened into the grease so that solutions have free access to the heart and nephrocytes.
10. Finally, it is sometimes necessary to remove excess fat body and trachea that would otherwise obscure the view of the

nephrocytes. This is best done by aspiration with a 10 mL syringe attached to a small bore tube and pulled glass pipette with a narrow aperture. Gentle negative pressure from the syringe can be applied with one hand while the other guides the tip with the other, when looking down the dissecting scope.

11. It is imperative that aspiration is done so as not to damage the heart or remove pericardial nephrocytes (the former is more easily done than the latter; *see* **Note 3**).

3.3 Analysis of Pericardial Nephrocyte Endocytic Function and Preparing Flies for Imaging

1. The endocytic function of pericardial nephrocytes can be imaged and quantified using fluorescently tagged cargoes such as dextran and albumin linked to Alexa dyes (Fig. 2). For routine analysis, we use a 3 mL solution of 50 μg/mL 10 kDa dextran-Alexa^{488} (made with HBSS), which is added to dissected abdomens to cover the entire preparation in the dissecting dish.
2. This is then incubated at 25 °C for 0–30 min, depending on the experiment. Under these conditions the signal for Alexa-conjugated 10 kDa dextran does not increase significantly after about 20 min (*see* **Note 4**).
3. Endocytosis is stopped by placing the dishes onto ice, aspirating the dextran solution (*see* **Note 5**), and briefly rinsing dissections three times with ice-cold HBSS. The nephrocytes can then be fixed with cold 2% formaldehyde in HBSS for 10 min and then rinsed three times with HBSS (*see* **Note 6**).
4. Nephrocytes are counterstained with a cell-surface marker to confirm internalization of the endocytic cargo. The final HBSS

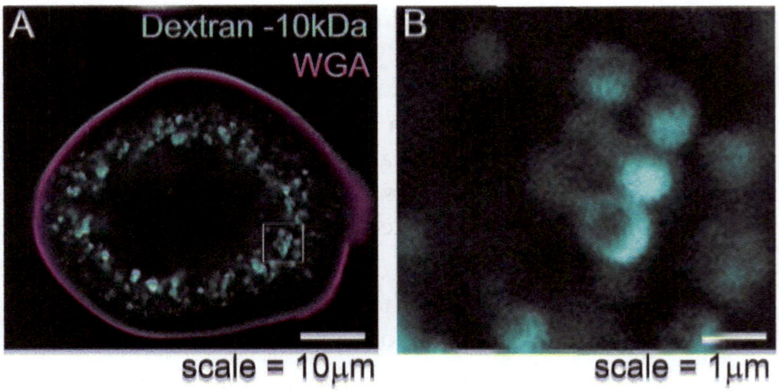

Fig. 2 Analysis of pericardial nephrocyte function using 10 kDa dextran. Pericardial nephrocytes were imaged by confocal microscopy after a 20-min incubation (25 °C) with 10 kDa fluorescently conjugated dextran. Cells were fixed with formaldehyde and then counterstained with wheat germ agglutinin (WGA). Dextran can be seen within vesicles with an approximate diameter of 1 μm

rinse is replaced with 3 mL of 5 μg/mL wheat germ agglutinin (WGA) conjugated to the Alexa[594] fluorochrome. A 30-min incubation of WGA at ambient temperature is sufficient to obtain excellent signal-to-noise ratio (*see* **Note 7**).

5. Fixed abdomens are then transferred to a glass chamber slide. These are prepared beforehand by adhering two glass coverslips (No. 1 size) to a standard microscopy slide so that the distance between the coverslips is approximately 1 cm. The coverslips are adhered to the slide using clear nail polish.
6. A thin layer of vacuum grease is smeared onto the glass slide in order to facilitate placement of the dissected abdomens. Applying abdomens to bare glass will cause problems later because coverslipping will displace them.
7. The fixed abdomen is cut from the thorax and the cuticle trimmed on either side of the heart tube using curved Vannas scissors.
8. The trimmed abdomen is then taken from the dish using forceps that hold the corner of the tissue. It is then placed onto the glass slide and gently flattened out (*see* **Note 8**).
9. A confocal microscope is used to obtain optical section through the midpoint of nephrocytes; the resulting micrographs can be used for image analysis using ImageJ software.

3.4 Analysis of Pericardial Nephrocyte Morphology and Enumeration After Counterstaining with WGA

1. Flies should be dissected and counterstained with WGA as described above.
2. Morphometric analysis is best done using a confocal microscope so that the *z*-plane midpoint of nephrocytes can be established.
3. Although pericardial nephrocytes show a range of folds and indentations, their overall morphology approximates an ellipse. For this reason we typically measure both the longest and shortest axes at the cell's midpoint. These numbers are combined to provide an estimate of nephrocyte size at the cell's midpoint (μm^2) or volume (μm^3).
4. We aim to quantify at least five nephrocytes from five to six flies per experimental cohort to provide a minimum of 25 measurements.
5. Enumeration of pericardial nephrocyte abundance can be done using wide-field fluorescence optics, usually with a 10× objective (assuming the use of a 10× eyepiece).
6. It is sometimes not possible to see all nephrocytes due to overlapping fat body or because the dissection has disrupted heart morphology; quantification is avoided when this problem is encountered.

7. In adult flies, pericardial nephrocyte abundance ranges between 20 and 30 nephrocytes per fly, with the mode approximating 26 per fly.

3.5 Staining for the Slit Diaphragm Proteins Duf and Sns

1. *Drosophila* are dissected and fixed as described and then incubated with 3 mL of polyclonal antisera to Duf or Sns (made in PBS with 0.1% Triton-X100 in order to permeabilize cells; *see* **Note 9**).
2. Antisera are batch specific; our current batch of anti-Duf antisera was raised in rabbit against a synthetic polypeptide corresponding to amino acids 32–46 Kirre/Duf (KSKKNKSSQSSHHGD); and anti-Sns was raised in goat against a synthetic polypeptide corresponding to amino acids 1180–1196 (DMPPPRYQKDGTLPVNY).
3. These antisera are used at 1:100 (Duf) and 1:10 (Sns) dilutions of 1.2 and 1.5 mg/mL stock affinity-purified solutions, respectively.
4. Antisera should be incubated with tissues overnight at 4 °C.
5. Antisera are then rinsed from the dissected tissue by three washes with PBS (each 5 min).
6. Secondary anti-rabbit or anti-goat antibodies conjugated to a fluorescent Alexa dye are then incubated for 1 h at 25 °C and rinsed off using three washes of PBS.
7. Nephrocytes and overall heart morphology are best visualized after being counterstained with wheat germ agglutinin and mounted on slides as described above.

3.6 Assessment of Food Intake and Modulation of Dietary Sugar

One of the issues with modulating diets is quantifying food ingestion. Numerous assays have been developed, one of the most useful being the capillary feeder (CAFE) assay [9]. However this relies on measurements of liquid food intake, rather than intake of the solid food that flies are routinely propagated on. We have developed a simple solid food intake assay (SOFI) that works to quantify food intake by flies on a daily basis (Fig. 3). It is limited to the use of groups of male flies because females will lay eggs on the food and singleton flies provide data that is too variable. Nonetheless it provides a reliable, quantitative measure of food ingestion for a group of flies over several days. It is simple to set up and easily monitored.

1. To a 7 mL plastic bijou tube 2 mL of 1% agar is added in order to maintain hydration of the flies.
2. Five holes are then punched into one half of the bijou tube's cap using a 25G needle.
3. A small bolus of molten *Drosophila* food is placed into the cap so that none is obstructing the air holes and all the food is

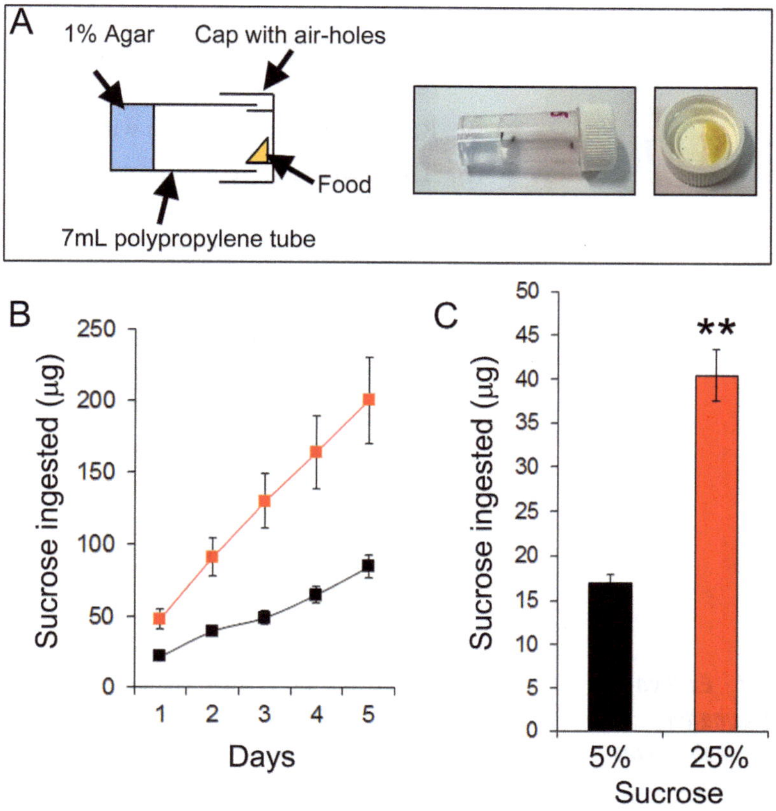

Fig. 3 Quantification of sucrose intake by male flies provided with solid food diets containing either 5 or 25% sucrose. (**a**) Male flies were maintained as groups of ten in a solid food ingestion assay (SOFI) tube for several days. (**b**) Ingestion of food was recorded for 5 days and the total amount of sucrose ingested per fly per day is shown (+/−SEM). (**c**) Flies provided with the higher sucrose diet ingest more sugar than flies on the low-sucrose diet. $**P < 0.001$. $n = 10$ SOFI assay vials

within the bevel demarking the thread of the cap's screw (*see* **Note 10**).

4. Typically, ten male flies are added to a tube (*see* **Notes 11** and **12**).
5. To control for evaporation from food, each experiment should have an equal number of tubes that do not contain flies but whose caps do contain food.
6. Vials should be placed horizontally so that the air holes in the cap are uppermost and food is closest to the horizontal plane.
7. Maintain flies and control vials at 25 °C on a 12-h:12-h light-dark cycle.

8. To quantify solid food ingestion the cap of a tube is removed and weighed on a microbalance. The first measurement is regarded as "day zero" (*see* **Note 13**).
9. Replace the weighed cap without trapping flies in the thread.
10. The caps are reweighed each day for several days. The amount of food eaten is calculated by establishing the difference in weight between each day and subtracting the amount that has also evaporated in the control tubes. This figure can then be divided by the number of flies in the vial to obtain the milligrams of food eaten per day per fly. The mean sucrose intake (±SEM) of ten SOFI assays is presented (Fig. 3).
11. Using this assay it is possible to ascertain that flies adjust their food intake according to the amount of sucrose in the diet (e.g., they reduce overall intake when the concentration rises from 5 to 25% sucrose). While this satiety feedback is tightly regulated, there appears to be a limit as to how much flies can compensate. We find that, despite reducing food intake, flies will over-ingest sucrose when at 25% in the diet (Fig. 3).

3.7 Ex Vivo Incubation of Nephrocytes

This method does not necessarily require specialist cell culture incubators or aseptic technique, although it does require antibiotics to reduce the risk of infection in cultures. Dissected abdominal preparations can be maintained for short periods of time (typically overnight but sometimes up to 48 h), which is sufficient to assess the impact of genotypes or pharmacological agents or both, on nephrocyte function, slit diaphragm homeostasis, and nephrocyte viability.

1. Schneider's medium should be aliquoted and frozen until required (usually as 13 mL aliquots in 15 mL centrifuge tubes; this is sufficient for three independent cultures using 4 mL per dish).
2. Antibiotics are added to the culture medium (100 units/mL of a 5000 units/mL stock of penicillin/streptomycin), so too is fetal calf serum (to a final concentration of 10%).
3. Flies should be dissected as described above. Different genotypes can be grouped within the same culture dish so that any pharmacological treatments are applied equally (*see* **Note 14**).
4. Rinse the dissected abdomens with HBSS.
5. Add 4 mL of culture medium to the dish(es), place lids on them, and transfer to a 150 mm petri dish (also containing wetted paper, if the incubator is not humidified). The use of a larger petri dish is simply for ease of carriage.
6. Make sure that the surface you are placing the culture dish on is level; if not medium will be unequally distributed in the culture dish.

7. Cultures can be maintained at 25 °C for 24–48 h; after 24 h the heart is still beating, nephrocytes are still endocytically active, and slit diaphragms (as evidenced by anti-Duf staining) are largely intact/expressed at the cell surface as regular linear arrays.
8. Nephrocytes can be stained, fixed, and imaged as described.

3.8 Monitoring Intracellular Calcium in Nephrocytes

Regulation of intracellular calcium is crucial to podocyte function in mammalian models and humans and there have been impressive inroads made to the imaging of podocyte calcium in vivo [10]. *Drosophila* nephrocytes are well suited as models of podocyte calcium handling and we have developed a reporter system (Fig. 4) based on nephrocyte-restricted expression of the latest generation of genetically encoded calcium indicators, *GCaMP6* [8].

1. Dissection is as described with one major difference: the buffer used contains no calcium or magnesium—this is added prior to stimulation of intracellular calcium.
2. A single fly should be dissected for each experiment because imaging can capture only one field of view from a single fly. However, this collects calcium data from 20+ pericardial nephrocytes.
3. A water dipping objective (×10) is required for live imaging of nephrocytes and a standard camera and corresponding software capable of a frame rate of >30 fps is adequate for data capture.
4. After dissection in calcium-free buffer, more calcium-free buffer is added to a final volume of 3 mL. The petri dish with the fly is then situated on the microscope stand and the objective placed into the buffer.

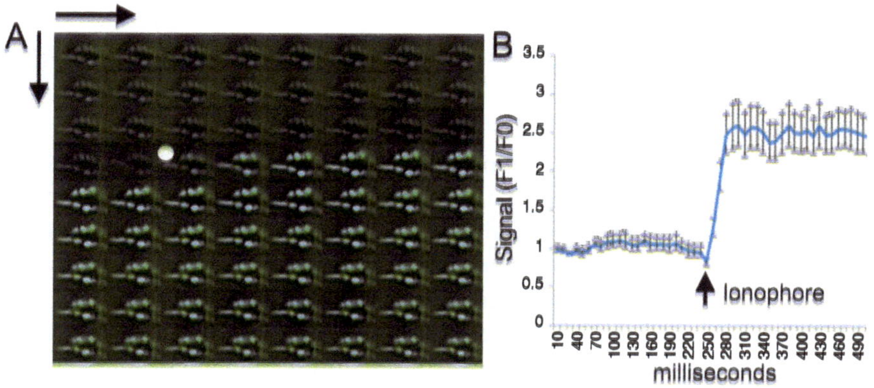

Fig. 4 Monitoring intracellular calcium in pericardial nephrocytes. (**a**) Raster plot of fluorescence signal in which nephrocytes expressing *GCaMP6* calcium reporter under the control of *dKlf15-Gal4* were dissected in calcium-free buffer and then stimulated with 20 mM $CaCl_2$ and calcium ionophore (10 μm A23187, white dot). Frames are temporally ordered from left to right, top to bottom; there are 25 frames per second—so each row is 1/3rd of a second. (**b**) A sustained rise in intracellular fluorescence is detected in response

5. Prior to the next step the camera should be set to record the pre-transient fluorescence. A typical delay of 10 s is used before the initiation of the transient.
6. To initiate a calcium transient 1 mL of buffer is added (this should contain 4× the final concentration of calcium required (e.g., 10 mM for 2.5 mM) in the experiment and 4× the amount of any agonist required).
7. At this point the heart will start to beat and, as a consequence, pericardial cells will also move. It is therefore important to try some test runs so that a field of view is captured which includes pericardial nephrocytes at both the heart's diastole and systole.
8. Dissections can be preincubated for several minutes with pharmacological agents prior to initiation of a transient.
9. Data is then analyzed using ImageJ "measure stack" plug-in [11]. Using the pre-transient fluorescence signal as a baseline (F0), a calculation for the relative signal increase (F1/F0) can be calculated (where F1 is the fluorescence being recorded during the transient). It is important to also subtract any background signal from both F1 and F0 readings before establishing the ratio of change. For an excellent, in-depth review of calcium imaging please refer to Bootman et al. [12].
10. Before the next fly is analyzed it is important to wipe the objective free of any calcium-containing buffer using a lens cloth dampened with distilled water.

4 Notes

1. Although anesthesia can be achieved with CO_2, this has a major effect on heart function and can limit analyses should quantification of cardiac function be needed. Typically, we use triethylamine as the agent of choice. Additionally, a regular heart beat is a good indicator that dissection did not damage the heart and adjacent nephrocytes.
2. Routine genotyping should be done on stocks but, unlike mice, most transgenes are maintained over chromosomal balancers carrying dominant markers; that is, one chromosome carries the transgene or modified gene of interest/mutation; the other chromosome's sequence is "scrambled" due to multiple translocations that reduce the risk of crossing over; this balancer also carries a dominant genetic marker so it can be identified in offspring—those flies not expressing the dominant marker carry the allele of interest. This means that segregation of transgenes/alleles of interest is easily followed from F_0 to F_1 progeny. For more information on using *Drosophila*

chromosomal balancers and routine *Drosophila* husbandry please refer to the book "Fly Pushing" by Ralph Greenspan [13].

3. Aspiration is the step that most likely disrupts the overall architecture of the heart and nephrocytes. Novices can avoid this step in order to retain architecture but remaining tissues may obscure some nephrocytes. This issue is a problem when counting nephrocytes but not necessarily so when assessing individual nephrocyte morphology or staining.
4. As the dextran is trafficked into more acidic compartment the fluorescence is quenched. Dyes that fluoresce in lower pH environment such as the pHrodo-conjugated dextrans can also be utilized to assess endocytosis.
5. This can be reused several times as long as results are not compared between assays. Typically we use the same staining solution several times over 1 week, if stored at 4 °C.
6. We find that the signal for fixable endocytic cargoes such as dextran wanes over longer periods of incubation (e.g., overnight), so nephrocytes are imaged on the day of the assay.
7. Wheat germ agglutinin binds N-acetylglucosamine and N-acetylneuraminic acid (sialic acid) residues on cell-surface proteins; it preferentially binds to pericardial nephrocytes but will also bind the surfaces of other cell types, making it a useful counterstain for immunofluorescent imaging. WGA is available conjugated to a wide range of fluorescent molecules with different excitation and emission spectra. The Thermo Fisher/ Molecular Probes website has an extensive list of resources regarding vital dyes and fluorescence molecules.
8. As the abdomen comes out of the liquid in the dissecting dish it will curl up and this can be fiddly but by gently pressing the tissue into the grease on the glass slide the tissue should come off the forceps and remain in place on the slide.
9. Triton-X100 is crucial because staining is dependent on the antibodies' access to the cytoplasmic regions of the proteins; hence cells must be permeabilized. Also, it is easy to forget adding triton to the solutions; its addition can be confirmed by gently shaking the solution; if bubbles develop—you have added the Triton.
10. This is easily achieved if the food is molten and pipette tips are pre-warmed to approximately 60 °C in a benchtop heat block.
11. Add flies that have been anesthetized with CO_2 and place them in the tube when it's horizontal; then flies can't get stuck on the agar, which can sometimes happen while they recover from anesthetic.

12. Males are used because females will lay eggs on the food and this affects the weighing.
13. Removing the cap can be troublesome as flies will want to escape; with a little practice and dexterity it is possible with the leading hand to remove the cap and place it on the balance while capping the tube with the thumb of the other hand; the leading hand is then free to right down the measurement.
14. For lab book and reference purposes it is useful to have a small sketch/diagram of the dish showing which fly is which genotype.

References

1. Zhuang S et al (2009) Sns and Kirre, the *Drosophila* orthologs of Nephrin and Neph1, direct adhesion, fusion and formation of a slit diaphragm-like structure in insect nephrocytes. Development 136(14):2335–2344
2. Weavers H et al (2009) The insect nephrocyte is a podocyte-like cell with a filtration slit diaphragm. Nature 457(7227):322–326
3. Hartley PS et al (2016) SPARC-dependent cardiomyopathy in *Drosophila*. Circ Cardiovasc Genet 9(2):119–129
4. Hermle T et al (2017) Modeling monogenic human nephrotic syndrome in the *Drosophila* garland cell nephrocyte. J Am Soc Nephrol 28 (5):1521–1533
5. Ivy JR et al (2015) Klf15 is critical for the development and differentiation of *Drosophila* Nephrocytes. PLoS One 10(8):e0134620
6. Brand AH, Perrimon N (1993) Targeted gene expression as a means of altering cell fates and generating dominant phenotypes. Development 118(2):401–415
7. Kimbrell DA et al (2002) The Dorothy enhancer has Tinman binding sites and drives hopscotch-induced tumor formation. Genesis 34(1-2):23–28
8. Chen TW et al (2013) Ultrasensitive fluorescent proteins for imaging neuronal activity. Nature 499(7458):295–300
9. Ja WW et al (2007) Prandiology of *Drosophila* and the CAFE assay. Proc Natl Acad Sci U S A 104(20):8253–8256
10. Reiser J et al (2005) TRPC6 is a glomerular slit diaphragm-associated channel required for normal renal function. Nat Genet 37 (7):739–744
11. Schneider CA, Rasband WS, Eliceiri KW (2012) NIH image to ImageJ: 25 years of image analysis. Nat Methods 9(7):671–675
12. Bootman MD et al (2013) Ca2+–sensitive fluorescent dyes and intracellular Ca2+ imaging. Cold Spring Harb Protoc 2013(2):83–99
13. Greenspan, R.J., Fly pushing: the theory and practice of *Drosophila* genetics. 2. 2004, New York: Cold Spring Harbor Laboratory Press

Chapter 3

A Technique for Studying Glomerular Filtration Integrity in the Zebrafish Pronephros

Maria Kolatsi-Joannou and Daniel Osborn

Abstract

With the advances in next-generation sequencing and rapid filtering of candidate variants in diseased patients, it has been increasingly important to develop translatable in vivo models to study genetic changes. This allows for functional validation of pathogenic mutations and establishes a system to understand the etiology of disease. Due to the ease of genetic manipulation and rapid *ex utero* development, the zebrafish has become a valuable resource to study important biological processes, including nephrogenesis. The development and function of the zebrafish pronephros are akin to that of mammals. As such, they offer a tractable model to study kidney disease, especially diabetic nephropathy. However, in order to study kidney dysfunction in zebrafish it is imperative that an appropriate readout is available. The appearance of macroproteins in patient's urine is indicative of defective kidney function. In this technical chapter, we describe the in vivo use of fluorescently tagged dextrans of different molecular weights to reveal the integrity of the zebrafish glomerular filtration barrier.

Key words Diabetes, Glomerular filtration, Zebrafish, Nephropathy, Proteinuria

1 Introduction

The zebrafish provides a comprehensive vertebrate model for studying human genetic disease. Due to conserved kidney-specific gene expression, function, and relative simplicity of nephron organization, the zebrafish embryo offers a versatile tool for studying nephrogenesis [1]. The zebrafish kidney develops initially as a simple pronephros consisting of two nephrons fused at the midline by their glomeruli, permitting the filtration of blood [2]. The pronephric tubules then run bilaterally along the body axis (absorbing or secreting solutes) and re-fuse at the cloaca, allowing waste to be excreted [3]. While mammalian kidneys progress through three stages of embryonic development (pronephros, mesonephros, and metanephros) each marked by increased complexity, the zebrafish embryonic kidney remains in the most immature form [3]. The zebrafish pronephros does eventually develop into a mesonephros

Luigi Gnudi and David A. Long (eds.), *Diabetic Nephropathy: Methods and Protocols*, Methods in Molecular Biology, vol. 2067, https://doi.org/10.1007/978-1-4939-9841-8_3, © Springer Science+Business Media, LLC, part of Springer Nature 2020

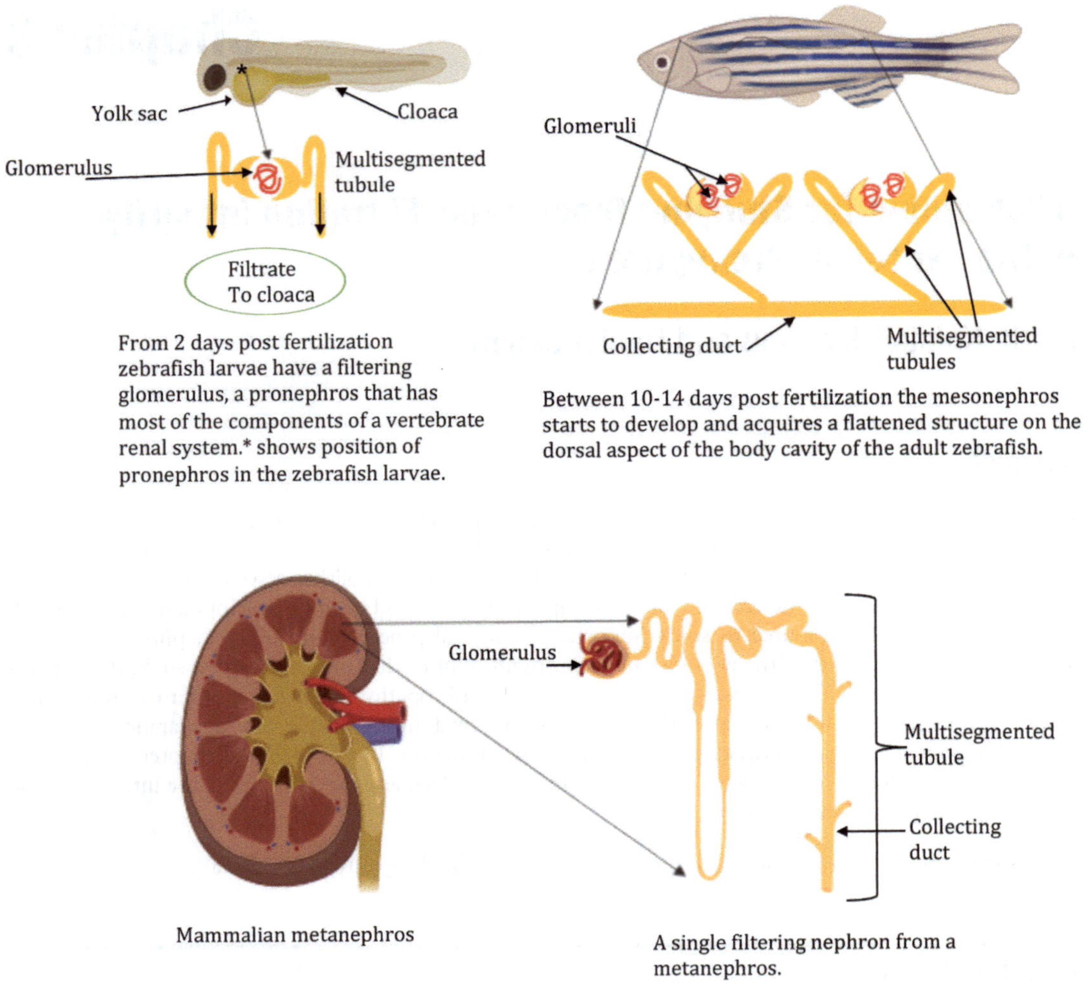

Fig. 1 Schematic diagram showing the zebrafish pronephros (larval stage), mesonephros (juvenile-adult stage), and mammalian metanephros

during juvenile stages of development, and by adulthood contains several hundred nephrons [4] (Fig. 1). Despite these differences, the genetic patterning of the zebrafish kidney and the function of different conserved components are remarkably similar with those of higher vertebrates [5]. Like in mammals, the zebrafish glomerulus consists of fenestrated endothelial cells, a glomerular basement membrane, and podocytes [6]. By 4 days postfertilization (dpf), these components can be visualized by transmission electron microscopy (TEM), suggesting the establishment of the filtration barrier [7].

These features make the zebrafish an attractive animal model for diabetes. Diabetes is the leading cause of end-stage renal failure in the Western world. One of the first indications of diabetic nephropathy in patients is the inability of the glomeruli to filter macro-proteins such as albumin, and as such the presence of albumin in the urine is normally an indication of a dysfunctional kidney (assessed with a simple dipstick) [8]. Disruption of slit diaphragm proteins (e.g., nephrin and podocin) along with foot process effacement, glomerular basement thickening, and endothelial cell disturbance relates to early signs of diabetic nephropathy [9]. Thus, the zebrafish includes all the required components of a normal-functioning mammalian glomerulus that can be manipulated to phenocopy a diabetic kidney.

Acute and chronic models of hyperglycemia can be induced in zebrafish by various methods. Acute hyperglycemia is achieved in adult zebrafish by giving a single intraperitoneal (IP) injection of D-(+) glucose [10]. This can also be attained in larval zebrafish by bathing them in high concentrations of D-(+) glucose [11–13]. Chronic hyperglycemia is accomplished by alternate immersion of adult zebrafish in D-(+) glucose and freshwater for up to 28 days [14–16]. Overfeeding adult fish results in a type II model of diabetes [17], while an IP injection of the diabetes causing compound streptozotocin in adult zebrafish brings on hyperglycemia and mimics type I diabetes [18]. However, if zebrafish are to be utilized to mimic diabetic nephropathy, it is essential that appropriate methods are in place to evaluate kidney function. Furthermore, the development of quick and easy protocols to study kidney function facilitates future chemical screens, which may be used to ameliorate diseased kidneys. Unfortunately, the common dipstick is not applicable to zebrafish embryonic blood volumes. Here we describe methods for studying glomerular filtration barrier integrity in zebrafish by measuring the vascular clearance of different molecular weight fluorescent dyes by the pronephros and imaging the outcome using whole-mount and paraffin sections.

2 Materials

2.1 Animal Husbandry

Wild-type zebrafish should be maintained on a recirculating water system, with parameters optimized for breeding: set at pH 7, conductivity 500 μs, temperature 28.5 °C, 10% daily water change, and a 14-h day/10-h night photoperiod. A biological, particulate, carbon, and ultraviolet filter should be used to process the recirculating water. Adult zebrafish should be kept at a capacity of five fish per liter and a 1:1 male-to-female ratio. In general, we keep 20 females and 20 males per 8 L tank; several tanks set up like this will supply a small laboratory with a daily supply of eggs. Fish should be fed at least three times daily, ideally with live brine shrimp. To set up breeding, trays of marbles (to prevent eggs from being consumed by the fish) or breeding tanks can be placed into the stock tanks the night before the eggs are required. The subsequent morning, allow 30 min after the lights switch on for the fish to spawn. Harvest eggs using an appropriately sized strainer and incubate eggs in system water containing methylene blue at 28.5 °C until 4 days postfertilization (dpf).

2.2 Dextran Clearance Assay

2.2.1 Equipment

1. Flaming/Brown Micropipette puller model P-1000 (Sutter Instruments).
2. Air compressor (Jun-Air).
3. Picospritzer III (Parker Instruments).
4. Compact 3-Axis control micromanipulator (Marzhauser).
5. Dissecting stereomicroscope with epi-fluorescence illumination.
6. Borosilicate standard wall capillaries.
7. Microloader tips.
8. S8 Stage Micrometer 1 mm/0.1 mm.
9. Dumont #5 forceps.
10. Microinjection molds.
11. Glass microscope slides.

2.2.2 Reagents

1. Rhodamine B 10 KDa labeled dextran, dissolved in autoclaved water to a final concentration of 50 mg/mL.
2. Fluorescein 500 KDa lysine fixable dextran dissolved in autoclaved water to a final concentration of 50 mg/mL.
3. Methylcellulose made to 3% by agitating 6 g of methylcellulose in 70 mL of 80 °C hot water in a glass beaker. Make sure that all particles are wet and evenly dispersed before adding 130 mL of ice-cold water; mix and cool at 4 °C for 30 min, aliquot, and store at −20 °C.
4. Methylene blue 0.1% in H_2O.
5. Paraformaldehyde (PFA), made to a 4% solution by dissolving 40 g PFA in 700 mL of H_2O stirring gently on a heating block at ~80 °C with 5 mL 5 M NaOH. Adjust to pH 7.4 using HCl. Add 100 mL 10× PBS and top up volume to 1 L with H_2O.
6. Ethyl 3-aminobenzoate methanesulfonate salt (Tricaine): Dissolve 440 mg Tricaine powder in 97.9 mL double-distilled water. Add 2.1 mL 1 M Tris and adjust pH to ~7. This can be stored in a freezer. To use Tricaine as an anesthetic, mix 4.2 mL Tricaine stock solution with 100 mL fish water.
7. N-phenylthiourea (PTU): Dissolve PTU to a final concentration of 0.003% by heating to 60 °C.
8. Agarose.

2.3 Fixation and Dehydration of Tissue

2.3.1 Reagents

1. 4% PFA.
2. Phosphate-buffered saline.
3. 70, 85, 95, 100% ethanol.

2.3.2 Equipment

1. Glass bijous with snap on lid.
2. Plastic Pasteur pipettes.

2.4 Paraffin Embedding

2.4.1 Reagents

1. Histo-Clear II.
2. Paraffin wax pellets.

2.4.2 Equipment

1. Metal base molds 15 × 15 × 5 mm.
2. Embedding cassettes.
3. Embedding center.
4. Magnifying glass on stand.
5. Glass Pasteur pipettes.
6. Incubator/small oven at 60 °C.
7. Metal forceps or needle.

2.5 Sectioning

1. Microtome.
2. Electrothermal paraffin section mounting bath.
3. Slide-drying hot plate.
4. Double-distilled water.
5. Superfrost Plus microscope slides.
6. Pencil.
7. Thin-pointed brush (art ones).
8. Razor blade.
9. Medium-tip forceps.
10. Disposable microtome blades.
11. Stereomicroscope (to view cut sections).

2.6 Observing Dextran-Injected Zebrafish Larvae

2.6.1 Reagents

1. Histo-Clear.
2. 100, 70% ethanol
3. Double-distilled water.
4. Antifade Mountant.
5. Nail varnish.

2.6.2 Equipment

1. Staining dishes and racks.
2. Glass coverslips.
3. Fluorescent microscope.

2.7 Hematoxylin Eosin staining

2.7.1 Reagents

1. Histo-Clear.
2. 100, 70% ethanol.
3. Tap water.
4. Harris hematoxylin.
5. Eosin.
6. Acid alcohol solution (70% ethanol, 1% hydrochloric acid).
7. Histomount (Histo-Clear-based mounting media).
8. Glass coverslips.

2.7.2 Equipment

Staining dishes and racks.

2.8 Immunofluorescence

2.8.1 Reagents

1. Histo-Clear.
2. 100, 70% ethanol
3. Double-distilled water.
4. Sodium citrate tribasic dihydrate.
5. 0.2 M HCl.
6. PBS, phosphate-buffered saline.
7. Fetal calf serum.
8. Bovine serum albumin.
9. Tween-20.
10. Rabbit polyclonal Podocin (NPHS2, Protein Tech).
11. Mouse mono clone 6F-H2 Wilms' Tumor 1 (WT-1, Merck Millipore).
12. Goat serum.
13. Donkey serum.
14. Alexafluor® 488 donkey anti-rabbit.
15. Alexafluor® 594 goat anti-mouse.
16. Hoechst dye.
17. Sudan black.
18. Antifade mountant.
19. Nail varnish.

2.8.2 Equipment

1. Microwavable container.
2. Pap pen.
3. Glass coverslips.
4. Slide-staining tray.

3 Methods

3.1 Dextran Clearance Assay

1. Pull the borosilicate needles to an appropriate length for microinjection using the micropipette puller; the P-1000 model has preset programs specifically for zebrafish microinjections and can be easily optimized to the user's preferences.
2. Set up the injection rig as indicated in Fig. 2.
3. Pour 2% molten agarose into a 90 mm petri dish and float one of the custom molds on the surface until the agarose has cooled and solidified. Remove the mold and fill the dish with fish system water containing Tricaine (4.2 mL stock in 100 mL fish water).
4. Mix 1 μL of 10 KDa rhodamine dextran and 1 μL 500 KDa fluorescein dextran with 8 μL of nuclease-free water. Mix, and briefly centrifuge. Load 6 μL of the dextran mix into a pulled needle using a microloader pipette tip, insert into the needle holder, and secure in place using the provided nut and seal.

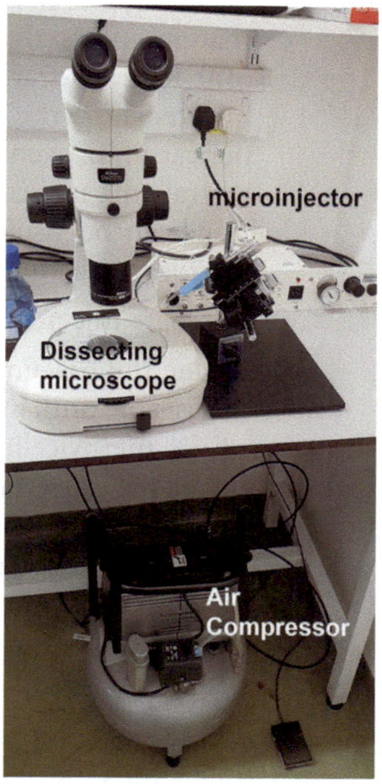

Fig. 2 A typical microinjection setup. An air compressor is attached to a regulator, which accurately controls the amount of liquid expelled from a glass needle. The needle holder is housed on top of a micromanipulator, allowing three-dimensional axial movements. A fluorescent stereomicroscope with digital imaging capabilities should be used to perform the microinjection and confirm fluorescent dextran-positive vessels

5. Break the tip of the needle (to allow an opening) under the microscope and expel the air from the needle (by selecting 1-min duration and using manual pulse) to permit the solution to enter the tip (once the mixture begins to exit the needle quickly change pulse duration back to microseconds).
6. Adjust the droplet size to a diameter of 100 μm using the micrometer reticule. This equates to a volume of 0.5 nL. You may need to adjust the thickness of the needle tip by breaking the tip further. The optimal needle length and thickness will give a 0.5 nL volume with a duration time of between 30 and 50 μs.
7. Place ten 4 days postfertilization embryos into the agarose plate containing the anesthetic. Monitor embryos until they become immobile with a regular heartbeat. Man oeuvre embryos into the agarose trough so that the yolk abuts the vertical agarose wall.
8. Inject 1 nL of dextran mix (two pumps on the foot pedal) into the flow of blood cells within the duct of Cuvier. Blood can be seen to split at the posterior cardinal vein where it fans out across the yolk reconvening at the sinus venosus of the heart. By injecting into this pool of cells, the dextran is immediately taken into the heart and around the vasculature. It is important that it enters the heart and not the pericardial space; the 500 KDa dextran will not enter the cardiovascular system if injected into the pericardium. The intersection between the pericardium, ventro-caudal pharyngeal arches, and dorso-rostral yolk makes a good needle entry point. Successful injections can be visualized immediately using the epi-fluorescent microscope setup (*see* **Note 1**).
9. Incubate injected embryos for 3 h at 28.5 °C.
10. Image the baseline fluorescence by anesthetizing the embryos in Tricaine until immobile. Place an individual embryo in a dish of 3% methylcellulose. Orientate embryos on their side and image the dorsal aorta and posterior cardinal vein (Fig. 3a, b) in both the red (fluorophore excitation: 570 nm, emission: 590 nm) and green (fluorophore excitation: 494 nm, emission: 521 nm) channels. Remove embryo from methylcellulose using a blunt instrument and place in freshwater in a 24-well plate. Label accordingly for future monitoring (*see* **Note 2**).
11. Repeat imaging procedure for the remaining embryos.
12. Incubate embryos at 28.5 °C until 24 h postinjection (hpi).
13. Repeat **steps 10** and **11**.
14. Glomerular filtration integrity can be quantified by measuring the fluorescent intensity from either the dorsal aorta (DA) or the posterior cardinal vein (PCV) using NIH's ImageJ software and the acquired images (*see* **Note 3**). Fluorescent intensity can

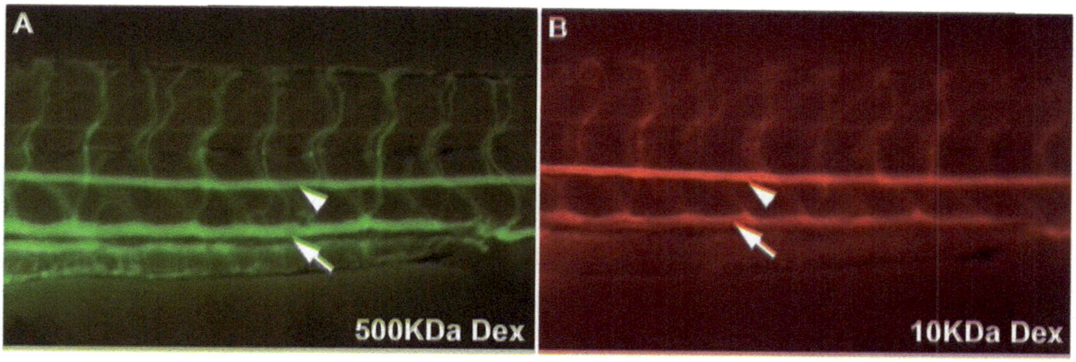

Fig. 3 Embryos correctly injected with fluorescently conjugated dextrans will localize to the vasculature. Image acquisition of (**a**) 500 KDa dextran (green) and (**b**) 10 KDa dextran (red) in the zebrafish trunk. The dorsal aorta (arrow head) and posterior cardinal vein (arrow) offer appropriate points to measure relative fluorescence intensity

then be compared between 3 and 24 h postinjection (hpi) for the two sizes of conjugated dextran. To perform a measurement for fluorescent intensity in ImageJ:

(a) Open the desired image and specify a region of interest (roi) using Edit/Selection/Specify from the software tabs. It is important to keep the size of the roi consistent between images.

(b) Position the roi over the DA or PCV; make sure that whichever one is chosen is used for every sample. In addition, select a landmark that can be used to position the roi at the same axial position, for example at the somite ten position.

(c) Set measurement parameter to include mean gray scale and area, using analyze/set measurements from the software tabs.

(d) Take the measurement by using the Analyze/measure tabs.

(e) Repeat **steps 1–4** for multiple embryos in both the red (10 KDa dextran) and green (500 KDa Dextran) channels at 3 hpi at 24 hpi time points.

(f) Compare the percentage remaining fluorescence intensity for each dextran, for each individual embryo, using the following equation: 100/3 hpi value × 24 hpi value. A dramatic loss in the 10 KDa dextran should be seen, while little to no loss in the fluorescence of the 500 KDa dextran should be observed.

3.2 Fixation and Dehydration of Tissue

1. Place zebrafish larvae (5 day postfertilization) into a glass bijous containing 4% PFA. Leave overnight at 4 °C.

2. Remove the PFA and dispose safely. Wash the zebrafish larvae 3X in PBS, 5 min each to remove traces of PFA.
3. Dehydrate the fixed zebrafish larvae through increasing concentrations of ethanol starting with 70%, 85%, 95%, and 100% for 45 min each.
4. Keeping the zebrafish in the glass bijou, remove 100% ethanol and replace with two changes of Histo-Clear, 45 min each.

3.3 Paraffin Embedding

1. Replace the Histo-Clear with 50:50 Histo-Clear/wax for 1 h at 60 °C (use a prewarmed glass pipette for wax changes so the wax does not solidify).
2. Replace with three changes of neat paraffin wax, 1 h each. Label embedding cassettes with the date and the genotype of the fish and a few experiment details.
3. Place a metal mold on the heated stage of the embedding center. Using a prewarmed glass pipette, transfer a little wax to the mold.
4. Very quickly using a prewarmed glass pipette gently suck up the zebrafish larvae and transfer to the metal mold.
5. Using prewarmed metal forceps or needle, flick the zebrafish until it stands on its head (magnifying glass can be used here) and slide the mold to the cold plate of the embedding center so as to solidify a thin layer of wax and the zebrafish is standing on its head. The zebrafish can be repositioned by returning the mold to the hot plate and melting the wax.
6. Once the correct orientation has been obtained move the mold onto the cold stage of the embedding center, place a labeled embedding cassette on top of the mold, and top up with molten wax using the prewarmed glass pipette.
7. When the wax has hardened, the mold can be removed and the wax blocks can be stored in a box at room temperature.

3.4 Sectioning

1. Fill the section mounting bath with fresh double-distilled water, and heat to 48 °C. The slide-drying hot plate should be on at 40 °C.
2. Using the razor blade, trim away excess wax trying to keep the edges parallel.
3. Put the paraffin blocks on ice for 30 min. The colder the block the smoother the sectioning and the better the ribboning.
4. Label the superfrost plus slides with the details that correspond to the blocks to be cut.
5. Insert a new blade into the microtome and keep the safeguard plate up when adjusting and inserting blocks.

6. Insert the cold wax block into the microtome block holder. Adjust the blade so it is just touching the block.
7. Set the section thickness on the microtome to 10 μm. This is to trim into the block until the zebrafish head comes into view.
8. Once the zebrafish head is in view, change the thickness to 5 μm and start sectioning at a steady speed to obtain a decent ribbon. Use forceps to hold the start of the ribbon.
9. Once there are 5–6 sections in a ribbon, with the thin-pointed brush gently lift off the ribbon on the blade, slowly transfer it to the mounting bath, and allow to float and stretch for a minute.
10. Use a labeled superfrost plus slide to pick up the sections by dipping the slide behind the floating sections until one end sticks to the top of the glass and lift the slide out of the water. Check the slide to see whether the tissues of interest are in view using a stereomicroscope. Since we are interested in the pronephros, it is easier to section from the head down as there are organs to use as landmarks as you cut closer to the single glomerulus that the zebrafish larvae have at this particular stage of development. Usually as you get to the esophagus start collecting the sections. The glomerulus is between the esophagus and the intestine, whereas the pronephric tubules run down on either side of the intestine to the cloaca.
11. Place the slide onto the drying hot plate for 20–30 min, then place them into racks, and allow to dry overnight at 37 °C to facilitate adherence onto the slide.

3.5 Observing Dextran-Injected Zebrafish Larvae

1. Put slides in a rack and place in oven at 65 °C. This reduces the time the slides spend in the Histo-Clear.
2. Rehydrate in two changes of 100% ethanol, 5 min each, and 70% ethanol 2 min, followed by a wash in double-distilled water.
3. Mount the sections in mounting media (30 μL per slide).
4. Gently apply the nail varnish around the edges of the coverslip to seal it down and stop the sections from dehydrating. The slides can be stored in a slide box in the dark at 4 °C.
5. Images taken using an AxioImager Z1 fluorescent microscope (Fig. 4a, b).

3.6 Hematoxylin Eosin staining

1. Put slides in a rack and place in the oven at 65 °C. This reduces the time the slides spend in the Histo-Clear.
2. Deparaffinize sections in two changes of Histo-Clear, 5 min each.
3. Rehydrate in two changes of 100% ethanol, 5 min each, and 70% ethanol 2 min.

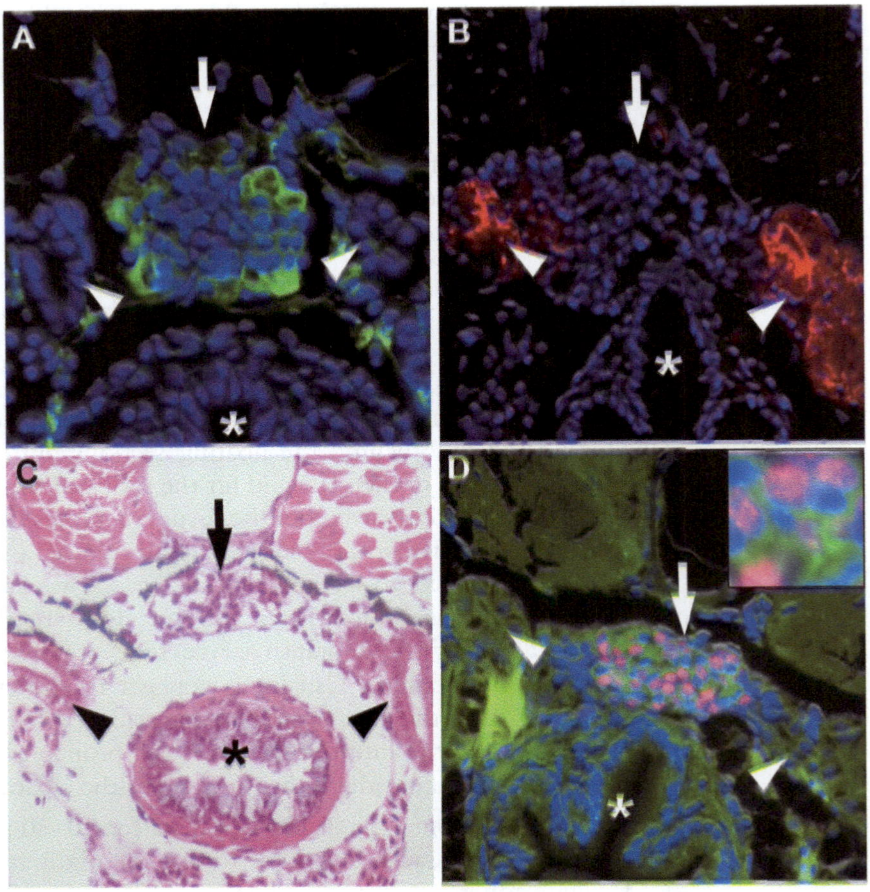

Fig. 4 Paraffin transverse sections though a 72 hpf zebrafish embryo. (**a**) 500 KDa Dextran (green) remains in the vasculature, shown in the blood vessels of the glomerulus (arrow), and is absent from the pronephric tubules (arrow heads). (**b**) 10 KDa Dextran (red) filters through the glomerulus and accumulates in the pronephric ducts. Nuclear staining is shown in blue. (**c**) Hematoxylin and eosin staining highlights general cell morphology. (**d**) Podocin (pink) and WT1 (green) localize to the nuclei (blue) of the glomerulus (arrow), emphasized in the inset panel

4. Wash in tap water briefly.
5. Stain in Harris hematoxylin solution for 5 min.
6. Wash in running tap water for 5 min.
7. Differentiate in 1% acid alcohol for 30 s.
8. Wash in running tap water for 5 min.
9. Counterstain in eosin solution for 30 s.
10. Dehydrate through 70% ethanol, and two changes of 100% ethanol, 5 min each.
11. Clear in two changes of Histo-Clear, 5 min each.
12. Mount in histomount.

13. Images taken using an Axioplan bright-field microscope (Zeiss) (Fig. 4c).

3.7 Immunofluorescence

1. Deparaffinize sections in two changes of Histo-Clear, 5 min each.
2. Rehydrate in two changes of 100% ethanol, 5 min each, and 70% ethanol 2 min followed by a wash in double-distilled water.
3. Make up the antigen retrieval treatment solution.
4. From 1 L of double-distilled water take out 22 mL and replace with 22 mL of 0.2 M HCl. Dissolve 2.94 g sodium citrate tribasic dihydrate in this solution. Pour this into a microwavable container that can hold a rack of slides with the lid not completely closed so as to let steam out. Heat the solution for 10 min on a high setting. Once the solution is boiling the rack of slides are ready to be carefully placed in the citrate buffer. Turn the microwave setting to medium heat for 15 min. Allow the slides to cool down in the buffer for 20–30 min (*see* **Note 4**).
5. Wash in two changes of double-distilled water, 5 min each.
6. Using the pap pen, draw around the section to be stained. The pap pen provides a hydrophobic barrier around the section allowing for less spread of antibody so as it concentrates on the tissue section.
7. Wash the slides in PBS-Tween-20 (0.1%) (PBS-T) for 5 min.
8. Apply block to the slides (50 mL fetal calf serum, 5 g bovine serum albumin dissolved in 1 L PBS-Tween-20 (0.1%)). (This can be made in advance and aliquoted and kept at −20 °C.) Incubate for an hour at room temperature in a humidified (damp tissue) slide-staining tray.
9. Dilute the primary antibodies, podocin (slit diaphragm), 1:75 in block plus 10% donkey serum, and WT-1 (podocytes), 1:50 plus 10% goat serum. Apply the antibodies onto the sections and incubate overnight at 4 °C in the humidified slide-staining tray.
10. Wash the primary antibodies off in three changes of PBS-T, 5 min each.
11. Dilute the secondary antibodies in block Alexafluor 488 donkey anti-rabbit for podocin and Alexafluor 594 goat anti-mouse for WT-1. Incubate for an hour at room temperature in the dark.
12. Wash the secondary antibodies off in three changes of PBS, 5 min each.
13. Add 30 μL Hoechst dye to 200 mL PBS and incubate for 5 min at room temperature in the dark. This stains the cell nuclei.
14. Wash the slides in several changes of PBS.

15. Incubate the slides in Sudan black (0.1% Sudan black, 70% ethanol) for 20 min. This reduces autofluorescence.
16. Wash the slides in several changes of double-distilled water.
17. Mount the sections in mounting media (30 μL per slide).
18. Gently apply the nail varnish around the edges of the coverslip to seal it down and stop the sections from dehydrating. The slides can be stored in a slide box in the dark at 4 °C.
19. Images were taken using an AxioImager Z1 fluorescent microscope (Fig. 4d).

4 Notes

1. If the needle is resisting to enter the tissue, gently tap several times on the head of the micromanipulator. This provides enough force that causes the needle to jolt forward enough to break the surface of the tissue and allow the needle to penetrate through.
2. It is important that all images are taken using the same parameters (i.e., magnification, pixel resolution, and exposure time).
3. The dextran clearance assay can be used to compare the effects of different pharmaceutical agents on kidney function or to model genetic perturbations.
4. Not every antibody works with microwaving in citrate buffer to unmask the antigen site. Enzymatic treatments can be used for example proteinase K (20 mg/mL in distilled water) and trypsin (0.5% in distilled water). Tissue sections are incubated in these at 37 °C for 10–15 min.

References

1. Outtandy P, Russell C, Kleta R, Bockenhauer D (2019) Zebrafish as a model for kidney function and disease. Pediatr Nephrol 34:751–762
2. Drummond I (2003) Making a zebrafish kidney: a tale of two tubes. Trends Cell Biol 13:357–365
3. Drummond IA, Majumdar A, Hentschel H, Elger M, Solnica-Krezel L, Schier AF, Neuhauss SC, Stemple DL, Zwartkruis F, Rangini Z, Driever W, Fishman MC (1998) Early development of the zebrafish pronephros and analysis of mutations affecting pronephric function. Development 125:4655–4667
4. Gerlach GF, Wingert RA (2013) Kidney organogenesis in the zebrafish: insights into vertebrate nephrogenesis and regeneration. Wiley Interdiscip Rev Dev Biol 2:559–585
5. Wingert RA, Davidson AJ (2008) The zebrafish pronephros: a model to study nephron segmentation. Kidney Int 73:1120–1127
6. Ichimura K, Bubenshchikova E, Powell R, Fukuyo Y, Nakamura T, Tran U, Oda S, Tanaka M, Wessely O, Kurihara H, Sakai T, Obara T (2012) A comparative analysis of glomerulus development in the pronephros of medaka and zebrafish. PLoS One 7:e45286
7. Fukuyo Y, Nakamura T, Bubenshchikova E, Powell R, Tsuji T, Janknecht R, Obara T (2014) Nephrin and Podocin functions are highly conserved between the zebrafish

pronephros and mammalian metanephros. Mol Med Rep 9:457–465

8. Christou-Savina S, Beales PL, Osborn DP (2015) Evaluation of zebrafish kidney function using a fluorescent clearance assay. J Vis Exp: e52540
9. Reidy K, Kang HM, Hostetter T, Susztak K (2014) Molecular mechanisms of diabetic kidney disease. J Clin Invest 124:2333–2340
10. Dorsemans AC, Lefebvre d'Hellencourt C, Ait-Arsa I, Jestin E, Meilhac O, Diotel N (2017) Acute and chronic models of hyperglycemia in zebrafish: a method to assess the impact of hyperglycemia on neurogenesis and the biodistribution of radiolabeled molecules. J Vis Exp:e55203
11. Powers JW, Mazilu JK, Lin S, McCabe ER (2010) The effects of hyperglycemia on adrenal cortex function and steroidogenesis in the zebrafish. Mol Genet Metab 101:421–422
12. Elo B, Villano CM, Govorko D, White LA (2007) Larval zebrafish as a model for glucose metabolism: expression of phosphoenolpyruvate carboxykinase as a marker for exposure to anti-diabetic compounds. J Mol Endocrinol 38:433–440
13. Jörgens K, Hillebrands JL, Hammes HP, Kroll J (2012) Zebrafish: a model for understanding diabetic complications. Exp Clin Endocrinol Diabetes 120:186–187
14. Gleeson M, Connaughton V, Arneson LS (2007) Induction of hyperglycaemia in zebrafish (Danio rerio) leads to morphological changes in the retina. Acta Diabetol 44:157–163
15. Alvarez Y, Chen K, Reynolds AL, Waghorne N, O'Connor JJ, Kennedy BN (2010) Predominant cone photoreceptor dysfunction in a hyperglycaemic model of non-proliferative diabetic retinopathy. Dis Model Mech 3:236–245
16. Carnovali M, Luzi L, Banfi G, Mariotti M (2016) Chronic hyperglycemia affects bone metabolism in adult zebrafish scale model. Endocrine 54:808–817
17. Zang L, Maddison LA, Chen W (2018) Zebrafish as a model for obesity and diabetes. Front Cell Dev Biol 6:91
18. Olsen AS, Sarras MP, Jr RVI (2010) Limb regeneration is impaired in an adult zebrafish model of diabetes mellitus. Wound Repair Regen 18:532–542

Chapter 4

Modeling Human Diabetic Kidney Disease by Combining Hyperglycemia and Hypertension in a Transgenic Rodent Model

Carolynn Cairns and Bryan Conway

Abstract

Traditional animal models mimic only the earliest stages of human diabetic nephropathy (DN), which limits their utility to dissect the pathogenesis of progressive disease or test novel therapeutics. In this chapter we describe in detail the experimental procedures required to conduct the *Cyp1a1mRen2* rodent model, in which hyperglycemia and renin-dependent hypertension synergize to promote moderate proteinuria, renal fibrosis, and induction of many of the transcriptomic changes observed in the kidney of patients with progressive DN.

Key words Animal model, Diabetes, Hypertension, Nephropathy, Renin

1 Introduction

Diabetic nephropathy (DN) is the most common cause of end-stage kidney disease. Traditional animal models, such as induction of type 1 diabetes with streptozotocin in the C57BL/6J mouse or the leptin-receptor-deficient *db/db* type 2 diabetic mouse, are limited as they do not exhibit many of the key biochemical, pathological, or transcriptomic changes observed in patients with progressive DN [1, 2]. Treatment of hypertension is at least as important as glycemic control in slowing the progression of nephropathy [3]. Indeed, hypertension may be a prerequisite for progressive nephropathy to occur: in patients with diabetes and unilateral renal artery stenosis, the kidney downstream of the normal renal artery may exhibit typical nephropathic changes, while the kidney downstream of the stenosis may remain unaffected despite identical levels of hyperglycemia, suggesting that the transmission of systemic hypertension to the kidney is an absolute requirement for the development of nephropathy [4, 5]. Most animal models of DN do not develop hypertension [1] and we

Luigi Gnudi and David A. Long (eds.), *Diabetic Nephropathy: Methods and Protocols*, Methods in Molecular Biology, vol. 2067, https://doi.org/10.1007/978-1-4939-9841-8_4,

hypothesized that the addition of hypertension to hyperglycemia may accelerate nephropathy and mimic changes of progressive DN. We have described how this hypothesis was tested using the *Cyp1a1mRen2* rat, in which the mouse renin cDNA is genomically integrated under an inducible promoter [6]. Induction of hyperglycemia and renin-dependent hypertension synergistically promotes heavy proteinuria, renal fibrosis, and many of the transcriptomic changes observed in the kidneys of patients with progressive DN [7]. Furthermore, tight control of glycemia and blood pressure reduced albuminuria and renal expression of genes implicated in the fibrotic response in this model; however there was no reduction in the established renal scarring [8]. In this chapter we describe in detail the methodology required to conduct this useful model of DN. The methods will be detailed in sections including induction, monitoring, and management of both diabetes and hypertension; measurement of proteinuria and renal function; and finally how to model regression of albuminuria through reversal of hyperglycemia and hypertension.

2 Materials

2.1 Cyp1mRen2 rat

The *Cyp1a1mRen2* rat on the Fisher background was generated by our collaborators as described previously [6] (*see* **Note 1**). Briefly, the mouse renin cDNA is genomically integrated under the *Cyp1a1mRen2* promoter, enabling renin gene expression to be activated in the liver by administration of Cyp450 inducers, such as indole-3-carbinol.

2.2 Induction of Hyperglycemia

1. 25 mg Streptozotocin (STZ, enough for four 250 g rats, with extra to spare): Place into an Eppendorf tube; cover with aluminum foil (to protect against light sensitivity). Store at −20 °C until needed.
2. 10 mM Sodium citrate (1.47 g of sodium citrate in 49.5 mL ddH_2O): Use a pH meter to adjust pH to 4.5 by slowly adding 1 mol/L citric acid solution (typically 0.5 mL is required).
3. Place into a conical flask the volume of sodium citrate buffer required for the number of rats to be injected (need 1 mL/kg body weight, so 250 μL for a typical 250 g rat). Add 20 mg STZ per 1 mL of sodium citrate buffer. Dissolve the STZ by mixing with a 23G needle and syringe for a couple of minutes and then sterile filter this solution through a 22 μM filter; use immediately (*very important see* **Note 2**).

2.3 Monitoring of Diabetes

1. Blood glucose monitor with test strips: Ideally, all blood glucose measurements should be taken using non-fasting morning samples (*see* **Note 3**).

2.4 Management of Diabetes

1. Isoflurane anesthetic.
2. Anesthetic rig with induction chamber and nose cone.
3. Betadine (10% povidone-iodine solution).
4. 16G disposable hypodermic needle.
5. Sterile forceps.
6. Trocar/stylet for implant insertion.
7. Insulin implants.

2.5 Induction of Hypertension

1. Weigh the required amount of indole-3-carbinol (I-3-C): For a 0.125% strength diet, 1.25 mg I-3-C is required per kg of diet and typically we made 5 kg (need 6.25 mg I-3-C) per session. Grind the crystalline I-3-C into a powder using a pestle and mortar (*see* **Note 4**).
2. Standard ground rat chow ground: Place 5 kg of RM1 diet into a container with a lid.
3. Sprinkle the I-3-C onto the ground RM1 diet, stirring constantly until it is completely mixed.
4. 50 mL Glass jars.
5. Each day remove the weight of diet required to fill the total number of glass containers necessary to feed all animals and place into a new receptacle. Slowly add water and continue to mix until it develops the consistency of a paste (*see* **Note 5**).
6. Decant the 0.125% I-3-C RM1 diet paste to fill each 50 mL glass jar which can then be placed in the rat cages.

2.6 Monitoring of Hypertension

1. A noninvasive tail-cuff blood pressure monitor, which consists of apparatus required to measure tail cuff including:
   (a) A controller with capability of monitoring up to two rats.
   (b) An occlusive cuff which can be inflated to greater than systolic blood pressure to impede blood flow to the tail.
   (c) A volume pressure recorder (VPR) cuff to measure distal blood flow.
   (d) A rodent restrainer.
   (e) An animal-warming platform.

2.7 Measurement of Proteinuria and Creatinine Clearance

1. To accurately measure food intake, water intake, and urine output a rat metabolic cage is required.
2. Lithium heparin tube.
3. 1 mL Insulin needle for venepuncture.
4. Creatininase-based enzymatic assay.
5. Rat albumin ELISA.

3 Methods

3.1 Induction of Diabetes

1. Rats should be fasted for 12 h prior to induction of diabetes with STZ. Inject 1 mL/kg of the 20 mg/mL into the tail vein of the rat (typically 250 μL for a 250 g rat, *see* **Notes 6** and 7).
2. Supply rats with 10% sucrose in drinking water for 48 h to avoid hypoglycemia post-injection, due to release of insulin from damaged β-cells.
3. Rats should be tested for sufficient levels of hyperglycemia 2 days after injection (*see* below). We defined hyperglycemia as blood glucose concentration >15 mmol/L. Exclude rats that do not achieve this level.

3.2 Monitoring of Hyperglycemia

1. Monitor blood glucose levels using blood glucose monitor with test strips. We typically monitored blood glucose weekly. Nick the tail vein with a 21G needle and milk the tail to provoke a small drop of blood, which can be drawn by capillary action into the test strip.

3.3 Management of Hyperglycemia

1. The first insulin implant is required once blood glucose concentration is >30 mmol/L, typically 1–2 weeks after induction of diabetes. Insertion of half an implant was usually sufficient to bring the blood glucose concentration down to the target range of 20–30 mmol/L (*see* Fig. 1).
2. Implants are inserted under light general anesthesia. Place the rat in induction chamber with oxygen flow at 1 L/min and 4% isoflurane until rat is unconscious, then transfer to nose cone, and reduce isoflurane concentration to 2%.
3. Shave a 2–3 cm square area of dorsal skin and clean the shaved area with Betadine antiseptic solution.
4. Pinch the skin between the thumb and index fingers and pierce the elevated skin with a 16G disposable hypodermic needle to create a track and withdraw (*see* **Note 8**).
5. Briefly immerse the trocar/stylet in a 2% Betadine solution, then push it through the skin orifice created by the hypodermic needle to a length of at least 2 cm, and remove the stylet.
6. Using forceps, immerse the implant briefly (5 s) in Betadine solution and insert it into the proximal end of the trocar.
7. Use the stylet to push the implant down the trocar until it exits subcutaneously from the distal end of the trocar.
8. Pinch the skin over the inserted implant, before withdrawing the trocar and stylet.
9. Apply a drop of the Betadine solution over the skin opening.

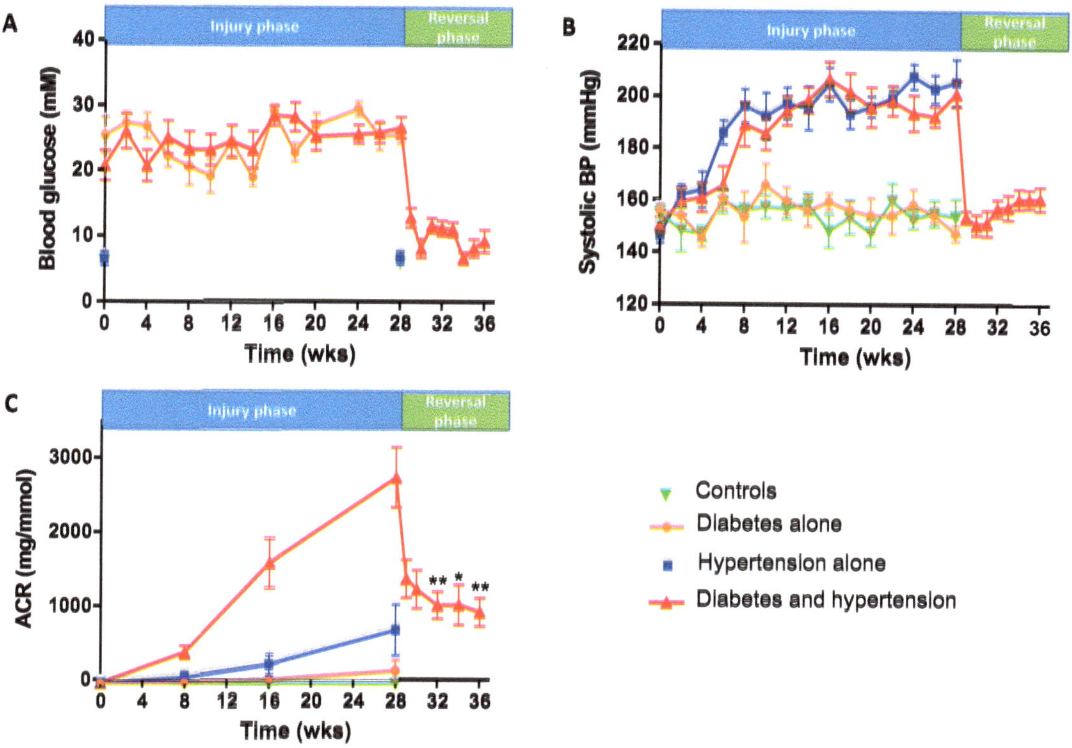

Fig. 1 Mean (**a**) blood glucose, (**b**) blood pressure, and (**c**) urinary albumin:creatinine ratio in rats with diabetes only, hypertension only, or the combination of diabetes and hypertension compared with control rats over the course of 28 weeks (injury phase). Diabetes and hypertension synergized to augment albuminuria. At the end of 28 weeks, optimization of blood glucose and blood pressure in the previously diabetic and hypertensive group promoted regression of albuminuria. Data are means (±SEM). $*p < 0.05$, $**p < 0.01$ vs. albuminuria in diabetic and hypertensive rats at 28 weeks

10. The skin defect will soon contract and requires no suturing or clips for closure.
11. If blood glucose concentration 1 week later remains >30 mmol/L, insert an additional one-half or one-quarter implant (*see* **Note 9**).
12. The timing of subsequent implant insertions was based on the weekly blood glucose readings and twice-weekly weights. A new implant was inserted if blood glucose is >30 mmol/L or if weight falls by >5% in order to prevent excessive weight loss and ketosis (*see very important* **Notes 10** and **11**).

3.4 Induction of Hypertension

1. 2 weeks after induction of hyperglycemia, add 0.125% I-3-C by weight to the diet to induce hypertension (*see* **Note 12**).
2. Each day place two 50 mL glass jars containing 0.125% I-3-C in chow in each cage per three diabetic animals (*see* **Notes 13** and **14**).
3. Monitor blood pressure weekly (*see* below).

4. 0.125% I-3-C was sufficient to slowly induce hypertension equilibrating after 4 weeks at a systolic blood pressure of approximately 180–200 mmHg (*see* Fig. 1 and **Note 15**).
5. The diabetic animals will typically require a dose reduction to 0.09–0.1% I-3-C after 3–4 weeks if blood pressure exceeds 200 mmHg (*see* **Note 16**).

3.5 Monitoring of Hypertension

1. Tail-cuff blood pressure should be monitored twice weekly in order to detect any increases in blood pressure above target (*see* **Note 17**).
2. Animals should remain conscious and be restrained in holders wrapped in a heat blanket to increase core body temperature (*see* **Note 18**). Two cuffs are placed over their tails: a proximal occlusive cuff which inflates to impede blood flow into the tail and a distal VPR which monitors the waveform of returning blood flow after release of occlusion. The blood pressure at the point of onset of blood flow after occlusion is taken as the systolic BP and the pressure at the point at which the increase in blood flow stops is taken as the diastolic blood pressure.
3. Animals should be trained in the apparatus for 10–15 min over 3 consecutive days to reduce the degree of stress, which would otherwise artificially elevate the blood pressure (*see* **Note 19**).
4. Prior to each recording, the animal should be allowed to acclimatize in the restrainer for 5–10 min before measuring the blood pressure (*see* **Note 20**).
5. The blood pressure should be taken on a minimum of three occasions or until consecutive readings are no longer falling and the mean of the lowest two readings should be calculated and recorded.
6. We aimed for a systolic blood pressure of 180–200 mmHg. If systolic BP exceeded >200 mmHg, the concentration of I-3-C was reduced by 25%, or if it was <180 mmHg, the dose was increased by 25% (*see* **Note 21**). We maintained the rats diabetic and hypertensive for a total of 8 months (*see* **Note 22**).

3.6 Measurement of Proteinuria and Creatinine Clearance

1. Set up the metabolic cage as per the manufacturer's instructions. Ensure that there is sufficient food and water available for the 24-h duration and that the receptacle for collecting urine is sufficiently large (*see* **Note 23**).
2. Place a single rat in the cage and house for 24 h in a warm environment.
3. After 24 h, measure the urine output and collect urine for analysis, including albumin (*see* **Note 24**) and creatinine (*see* **Note 25**).

4. To assess creatinine clearance a blood sample will also be required to measure serum creatinine. Place the animal in a heat box for 5 min to promote vasodilation of the tail vein, before placing in a restrainer and drawing blood by tail-vein venepuncture using an insulin syringe.
5. Calculate the creatinine clearance using the formula: 24-h urine vol (mL) × urine creatinine concentration (mmol/L)/plasma creatinine concentration (μmol/L) × 0.001 × 60 × 24, which simplifies to 24-h urinary volume (mL) × urine creatinine concentration (mmol/L)/(plasma creatinine concentration (μmol/L) × 1.44). Typical values are 2 mL/min for a 250 g rat (*see* **Note 26**).

3.7 Reversal of Hyperglycemia and Hypertension

One advantage of this model is that the severity of blood pressure can be readily regulated by adjusting the dietary I-3-C concentration and indeed the hypertension be completely reversed by removing the I-3-C from the diet. Together with employing increased dose or frequency of insulin implants, this can be used to model the pathophysiological effects of improved blood pressure and blood glucose control.

1. To normalize blood pressure, place the rat back on normal chow. Expression of the murine renin transgene will fall rapidly, such that blood pressure typically normalizes within 1 week (*see* Fig. 1).
2. Normalization of blood glucose concentration is more challenging. We slowly titrated up the dose of the insulin pellet, typically by inserting one-half pellet subcutaneously and rechecking blood glucose 48 h later. If blood glucose remained >10 mL/L we inserted a further one-quarter pellet and if it remained >15 mmol/L, we inserted a further one-half pellet (*see* **Note 27**).

4 Notes

1. We employed Fisher rats as they have been found to develop more severe hypertension in response to indole-3-carbinol than other strains such as Lewis [9].
2. The STZ-Na citrate buffer solution should be prepared immediately before injection as the drug degrades after 15–20 min in the Na-citrate buffer.
3. Non-fasting samples provide a better indication of the severity of hyperglycemia induced by feeding.
4. I-3-C is a skin, eye, and inhalational irritant; therefore wear safety glasses and protective disposable gloves and mix in a fume cupboard.

5. The paste should be made up fresh daily, although it is possible to make up 2 days of diet on a Saturday to cover the weekend.
6. To induce vasodilation of the tail vein to facilitate intravenous injection, we recommend warming the rats for 3–5 min in a heat box prior to injection.
7. Many investigators choose to anesthetize the rat using isoflurane prior to injection to facilitate the injection, although placing the rat in a restrainer is normally suffice.
8. The hole in the skin made by the 16G needle facilitates the insertion of the trocar/stylet.
9. We found that half an insulin implant was usually sufficient to keep blood glucose level in the target 20–30 mM range. We were reluctant to insert full implants as they typically caused blood glucose to fall below the target range. If blood glucose remained above target range, an additional half implant was inserted (occasionally we implanted one-quarter of an implant if the blood glucose was only marginally above target). Implants can readily be cut in half or quarters using a scalpel.
10. We found that the pellets typically were deplete of insulin after approximately 6 weeks and at this point blood glucose concentration increased and weight fell rapidly. We were reluctant to test blood glucose more than once weekly as this may have caused trauma to the tails; therefore, to detect insulin deficiency, we weighed the rats twice weekly and checked blood glucose in any rat with >5% weight loss between measurements. For models of diabetes alone, weekly weights and blood glucose recording would likely be suffice but we consider that this is too infrequent in the combined diabetes and hypertension model. In this model, when the rats become hyperglycemic, they also become hyperphagic and hence consume more indole-3-carbinol; therefore, they may become rapidly unwell due to a combination of hyperglycemia and malignant-phase hypertension.
11. The remnants of the insulin-depleted implant will be completely absorbed in a few weeks and removal is not necessary.
12. We induced hypertension after the onset of hyperglycemia to mimic the chronology of type 1 diabetes in humans.
13. We tended to keep 3–6 animals per cage for companionship. The animals did not thrive as well when caged singly.
14. Always place unused diet into waste bins; do not dispose of down the sink as blockage may occur to outflow pipes.
15. One of the advantages of the model is that the induction of the renin transgene and hence severity of blood pressure can be adjusted by titrating the concentration of I-3-C in the diet.

Lower concentrations will produce a milder blood pressure phenotype, while higher doses induce malignant-phase hypertension [10]. After pilot experiments, we opted for a dose of 0.125% as this induced moderate hypertension, but avoided malignant-phase hypertension, which confounded the interpretation of the results in the constitutive mouse renin-expressing (*mRen2*) rat [11, 12]. The slow induction of hypertension permitted arterial adaptation to occur so that even though the systolic blood pressure was high, no onion-skinning features, typical of malignant-phase hypertension, were observed.

16. Diabetic rats tend to eat up to 50% more than their normoglycemic counterparts (30 g/day compared to 20 g/day) when their blood glucose levels are maintained in the 20–30 mmol/L range. 0.125% I-3-C in the diet results in a blood pressure of 180–200 mmHg in nondiabetic rats; therefore in diabetic rats the concentration of I-3-C needs to be reduced by up to one-third (typically 0.09–0.1%) in order to obtain the same daily I-3-C dose. Limiting the mass of food available for the diabetic rats to match food intake to the nondiabetic counterparts was not feasible as this resulted in marked weight loss in the diabetic rats. We did not feel that daily gavage was feasible given the long timescale over which the study was run.

17. We employed tail-cuff plethysmography; the length of the study exceeds the battery life of a standard radiotelemetry device.

18. Tail plethysmography requires sufficient blood flow in the tail to obtain a reliable signal, therefore increasing core body temperature assists by inducing vasodilation and increased blood flow.

19. It may be helpful to incorporate a dark nose cone at the end of the tube to limit the animal's view and alleviate stress.

20. Typically we operated with two restrainers and while measuring blood pressure on one rat we allowed another rat to become acclimatized in an adjacent restrainer.

21. If the systolic blood pressure is >200 mmHg on two consecutive occasions ensure that the blood glucose concentration is <30 mmol/L as severe hyperglycemia is associated with hyperphagia; if blood glucose concentration is >30 mmol/L then an insulin implant should be inserted and blood pressure rechecked 2–3 days later as this is preferable to reducing the dose of I-3-C.

22. At the end of 8 months of diabetes and hypertension, the rats are profoundly albuminuric (*see* Fig. 1); they exhibit glomerulosclerosis and tubulointerstitial fibrosis (*see* Fig. 2) and many

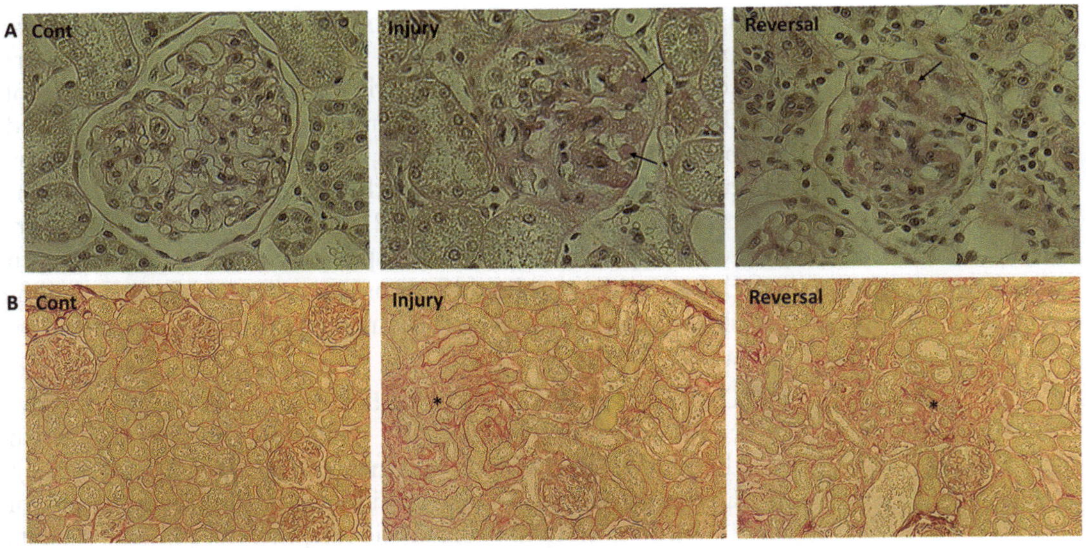

Fig. 2 Representative (**a**) periodic acid Schiff (PAS) and (**b**) picrosirius red images from control rat kidney, kidney from rats after 28 weeks of diabetes and hypertension (injury) and rats in which the diabetes and hypertension were subsequently reversed for 8 weeks (reversal). The PAS staining demonstrates that compared with control rats, there was an increase in mesangial matrix in the injury phase, which persists through reversal. Many glomeruli exhibit fibrin caps (arrow). In addition, the picrosirius red staining indicates patchy tubulointerstitial fibrosis (asterisk) after 28 weeks of diabetes and hypertension, which persists despite normalization of blood glucose and blood pressure for a further 8 weeks

of the transcriptomic changes observed in the kidney in patients with diabetic kidney disease [7].

23. Our diabetic and hypertensive rats were very polyuric, with the largest 24-h urine volume recorded at 160 mL. Hence, a larger receptacle than usual is required and even this may need to be emptied within the 24-h period.

24. To measure albumin, we used an immunoturbidimetric assay, which we adapted for a Cobas Fara centrifugal analyzer. An albumin ELISA is also a reasonable option. By 28 weeks, the diabetic and hypertensive rats become heavily albuminuric; therefore, despite the increased urinary volume, the urinary albumin concentration in the rats was 100-fold higher than for controls and the urine from the diabetic and hypertensive rats may need to be diluted to remain within the range of the assay.

25. Assays that employ the Jaffe reaction to measure plasma creatinine will overestimate the true creatinine concentration due to non-creatinine chromogens in the serum. Therefore we recommend using a creatininase-based assay to measure creatinine [13].

26. Creatinine clearance is straightforward to perform; however, it is a relatively inaccurate measure of renal function in rats. More

accurate alternatives include measurement of GFR by inulin clearance, performed either under terminal anesthesia [9] or by generating FITC-inulin decay curves by blood sampling at multiple time points immediately after injection of FITC-inulin [14]. Alternatively, GFR can be determined by the use of an optical device which transcutaneously measures the elimination kinetics of FITC-sinistrin [15].

27. We were concerned that the rats may be susceptible to hypoglycemia due to overtreatment with insulin. However, at no time did the blood glucose concentration in any rat fall <3 mmol/L. Perhaps this was because the glucagon response remained intact. Despite this, we would recommend titrating up the dose of insulin pellet, monitoring blood glucose readings thrice weekly during the period of tight glycemic control, and having 10% sucrose water available for any animal whose blood glucose concentration is <3 mmol/L.

Acknowledgments

Dr. Conway was supported by a MRC Clinician Scientist Award, a Scottish Senior Clinical Fellowship, a British Heart Foundation Transition Fellowship Award, and grants from Kidney Research UK and the Edinburgh and Lothians Health Foundation Renal Fund.

References

1. Brosius FC 3rd, Alpers CE, Bottinger EP et al (2009) Mouse models of diabetic nephropathy. J Am Soc Nephrol 20:2503–2512
2. Betz B, Conway BR (2016) An update on the use of animal models in diabetic nephropathy research. Curr Diab Rep 16:18
3. Mogensen CE (1998) Combined high blood pressure and glucose in type 2 diabetes: double jeopardy. British trial shows clear effects of treatment, especially blood pressure reduction. BMJ 317:693–694
4. Berkman J, Rifkin H (1973) Unilateral nodular diabetic glomerulosclerosis (Kimmelstiel-Wilson): report of a case. Metabolism 22:715–722
5. Beroniade VC, Lefebvre R, Falardeau P (1987) Unilateral nodular diabetic glomerulosclerosis: recurrence of an experiment of nature. Am J Nephrol 7:55–59
6. Kantachuvesiri S, Fleming S, Peters J et al (2001) Controlled hypertension, a transgenic toggle switch reveals differential mechanisms underlying vascular disease. J Biol Chem 276:36727–36733
7. Conway BR, Rennie J, Bailey MA et al (2012) Hyperglycemia and renin-dependent hypertension synergize to model diabetic nephropathy. J Am Soc Nephrol 23:405–411
8. Conway BR, Betz B, Sheldrake TA et al (2014) Tight blood glycaemic and blood pressure control in experimental diabetic nephropathy reduces extracellular matrix production without regression of fibrosis. Nephrology 19:802–813
9. Liu X, Bellamy CO, Bailey MA et al (2009) Angiotensin-converting enzyme is a modifier of hypertensive end organ damage. J Biol Chem 284:15564–15572
10. Kantachuvesiri S, Haley CS, Fleming S et al (1999) Genetic mapping of modifier loci affecting malignant hypertension in TGRmRen2 rats. Kidney Int 56:414–420
11. Kelly DJ, Wilkinson-Berka JL, Allen TJ et al (1998) A new model of diabetic nephropathy with progressive renal impairment in the

transgenic (mRen-2)27 rat (TGR). Kidney Int 54:343–352

12. Hartner A, Cordasic N, Klanke B et al (2007) Renal injury in streptozotocin-diabetic Ren2-transgenic rats is mainly dependent on hypertension, not on diabetes. Am J Physiol Ren Physiol 292:F820–F827
13. Keppler A, Gretz N, Schmidt R et al (2007) Plasma creatinine determination in mice and rats: an enzymatic method compares favorably with a high-performance liquid chromatography assay. Kidney Int 71:74–78
14. Qi Z, Whitt I, Mehta A et al (2004) Serial determination of glomerular filtration rate in conscious mice using FITC-inulin clearance. Am J Physiol Ren Physiol 286:F590–F596
15. Herrera Perez Z, Weinfurter S, Gretz N (2016) Transcutaneous assessment of renal function in conscious rodents. J Vis Exp 109:e53767

Chapter 5

Isolating and Culturing Mouse Podocyte Cells to Study Diabetic Nephropathy

Elisavet Vasilopoulou

Abstract

Diabetic nephropathy is associated with injury and loss of podocytes, specialized epithelial cells that are critical for glomerular filtration. This chapter describes a method of isolating and culturing podocyte cells from mouse adult kidneys. In this way, podocytes with genetic modifications can be obtained from transgenic animals and they can be used to study the effects of the diabetic environment in vitro.

Key words Diabetes, Diabetic nephropathy, Glomerulus, Kidney, Podocyte

1 Introduction

Animal models are essential for the study of diabetic nephropathy (DN) and have been utilized extensively to understand the mechanisms that lead to DN and develop new therapeutic targets [1]. However, the study of individual cells in vitro is also instrumental in dissecting relevant mechanisms and pathways in a cell-specific manner. One of the earliest signs of DN is albuminuria, which arises due to defects of the glomerular filtration barrier consisting of podocyte cells, glomerular basement membrane, and endothelial cells. Podocyte injury is one of the early hallmarks of DN. In the context of DN, podocyte injury involves perturbation of the podocyte cytoskeleton leading to foot process effacement and podocyte loss [2] and changes to podocyte secretion of vascular growth factors (vascular endothelial growth factor A, angiopoietins) [3] and pro-inflammatory cytokines (monocyte chemoattractant protein-1) [4, 5].

To enable the study of podocytes in vitro, immortalized cell lines of human [6] and mouse [7] podocytes have been established. This chapter describes the procedure of isolating and culturing primary podocytes from mouse adult kidneys. The procedure involves isolating glomeruli by perfusing mice with magnetic Dynabeads that are trapped in the glomerular capillaries, followed by

Luigi Gnudi and David A. Long (eds.), *Diabetic Nephropathy: Methods and Protocols*, Methods in Molecular Biology, vol. 2067, https://doi.org/10.1007/978-1-4939-9841-8_5, © Springer Science+Business Media, LLC, part of Springer Nature 2020

glomerular purification by magnetic separation. Once in culture, the first cells to grow out of the glomeruli are podocyte cells, which can be separated from the glomeruli by filtration according to size. Podocytes obtained in this way display a differentiated phenotype and can be cultured at different conditions to mimic the diabetic environment in vitro and study podocyte morphology and function [8–10].

2 Materials

2.1 Perfusion

1. Dynabeads (M-450 Epoxy magnetic beads, 4.5 μm bead size).
2. DynaMag-2 magnet.
3. Phosphate-buffered saline (PBS).
4. 0.1% (w/v) Bovine serum albumin (BSA) in PBS.
5. 0.1% BSA (w/v) in 0.2 M Tris pH 8.5.
6. Sterile distilled water.
7. Anesthesia system for isoflurane administration.
8. Dissection equipment.
9. Venflon catheter.
10. 20 mL Syringes.

2.2 Tissue Digestion

1. 10 mg/mL Collagenase A in Hanks balanced salt solution (HBSS); aliquots can be frozen at −20 °C.
2. DNase I.
3. Digestion solution: 1 mg/mL Collagenase A, 200 units/mL DNase I in PBS.
4. Shaking water bath.
5. 100 μm Cell strainer.
6. 50 mL Falcon tubes.
7. 5 mL Syringes.

2.3 Cell Culture

1. Matrigel matrix.
2. Culture media: DMEM/F12 with 10% fetal bovine serum (FBS), 1% penicillin-streptomycin, 1% L-glutamine, and 1% insulin-transferrin-selenium.
3. P100 cell culture dishes.
4. Trypsin-EDTA (0.25%).
5. 30 μm Cell strainer.
6. Normal glucose media: RPMI (powder reconstituted in 1 L sterile dH_2O, no glucose) containing 0.2% (w/v) $NaHCO_3$, 25 mM Hepes, 3.3 mM NaOH, 10% FBS, 1% penicillin-

streptomycin, 1% L-glutamine, 1% insulin-transferrin-selenium, 5 mM D-glucose, 20 mM mannitol.

7. High-glucose media: RPMI (powder reconstituted in 1 L sterile dH_2O, no glucose) containing 0.2% (w/v) $NaHCO_3$, 25 mM Hepes, 3.3 mM NaOH, 10% FBS, 1% penicillin-streptomycin, 1% L-glutamine, 1% insulin-transferrin-selenium, 25 mM D-glucose.
8. Antibodies: Anti-nephrin, anti-nestin, anti-WT1.
9. Phalloidin.

3 Methods

3.1 Perfusion

The perfusion solution has to be prepared fresh on the day before the perfusion. Amounts are per mouse unless specified otherwise.

1. Resuspend Dynabeads by vortexing for 2 min.
2. Immediately pipette 250 μL into an Eppendorf tube.
3. Place in a DynaMag-2 magnet, remove the supernatant, and wash twice with 0.1% (w/v) BSA in PBS.
4. Resuspend in 250 μL 0.1% BSA (w/v) in 0.2 M Tris pH 8.5 and incubate overnight with rotating at room temperature.
5. The next day, centrifuge for 10 min at 2000 × *g*, remove supernatant, place on the DynaMag-2 magnet, and wash three times with PBS. Resuspend in 250 μL distilled water and add to 40 mL PBS in a Falcon tube.
6. Take perfusion solution up in two 20 mL syringes with a Venflon catheter (22G) attached and cut the catheter to a length of 5 mm.
7. Anesthetize the mouse and use toe-pinch response method to determine the depth of anesthesia. Animal must be unresponsive before continuing.
8. Secure in the supine position on a dissecting board.
9. Make an incision at the lower abdomen through the skin and abdominal wall with sharp scissors, and extend to the left and right sides of the rib cage and clamp open.
10. Cut through the connective tissue at the bottom of the diaphragm to allow access to the thoracic cavity and expose the heart, which should still be beating.
11. While holding the heart steady with forceps, incise the right atrium and make a small incision at the apex of the left ventricle.
12. Cannulate the left ventricle of the heart using the syringe with the perfusion solution prepared as above and perfuse with

40 mL of the Dynabeads solution. A successful perfusion is evident by a lightened color of the liver (*see* **Note 1**).

13. Remove the kidneys and keep in PBS on ice.

3.2 Glomerular Isolation

Work under a class II biological safety cabinet and use sterile solutions.

1. Decapsulate the kidneys and mince into small (1 mm^3) pieces on a petri dish using a scalpel.
2. Digest each pair of kidneys in 1 mL of digestion solution for 30 min at 37 °C water bath with gentle agitation.
3. Press digest through a 100 μm cell strainer on a 50 mL Falcon tube using the plunger of a 5 mL syringe as a pestle.
4. Wash three times with PBS.
5. Centrifuge the cell suspension at 2000 × *g* for 5 min.
6. Discard the supernatant and resuspend the pellet in 1 mL PBS.
7. Transfer to an Eppendorf and place in the DynaMag-2 magnet. The glomeruli containing Dynabeads will be collected at the side of the Eppendorf facing the magnet.
8. Remove the supernatant and wash three times with PBS.
9. Remove from magnet and resuspend glomeruli in 1 mL culture media.

3.3 Culture and Podocyte Isolation

Work under a class II biological safety cabinet and use sterile solutions.

Prepare a Matrigel-coated P100 tissue culture dish in advance.

1. Thaw Matrigel on ice and keep on ice at all times (*see* **Note 2**).
2. Dissolve Matrigel in cold media (without serum and supplements) at 1/100 and add 6 mL of this solution to the P100 dish to coat with Matrigel.
3. Incubate at 37 °C for at least 1 h.
4. Remove Matrigel solution and add 6 mL of cell culture media to the P100 dish.
5. Add the glomeruli and incubate at 37 °C in a 5% CO_2 humidified atmosphere (*see* **Note 3**).
6. Do not disturb the dishes to allow the glomeruli to attach to the bottom of the dish.
7. The glomeruli collected in this way are decapsulated (Fig. 1a). Once they attach, the first cells to grow out of the glomeruli are podocytes. This starts approximately 3 days after plating (Fig. 1b).

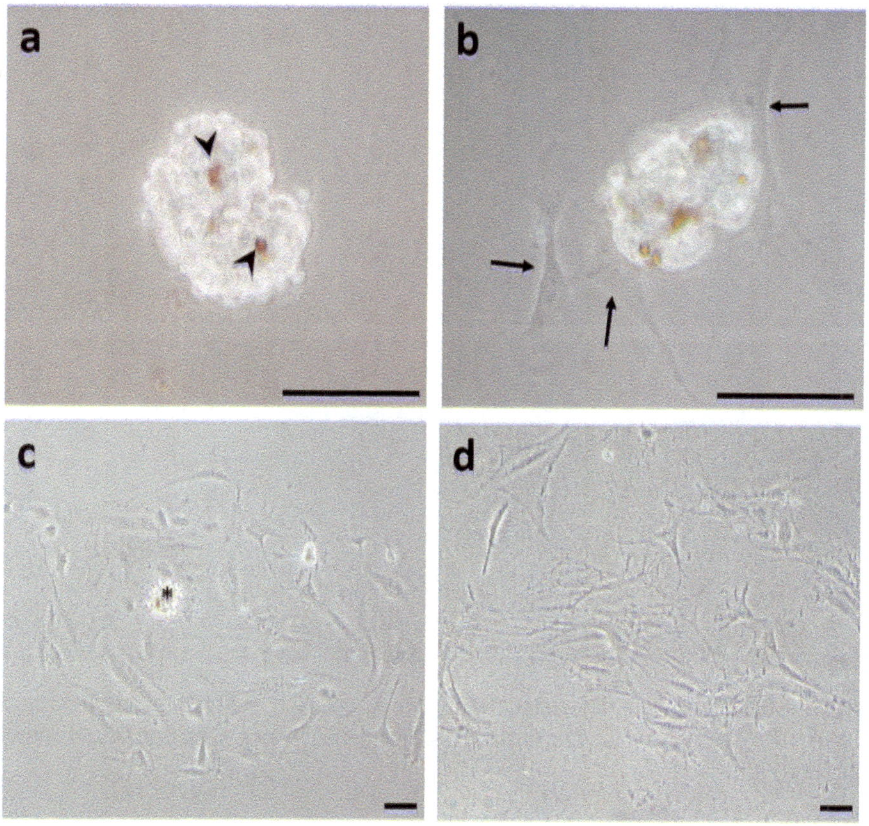

Fig. 1 Glomerular podocyte outgrowth. (**a**) A glomerulus in culture immediately post-isolation, magnetic beads trapped in the glomerulus are indicated by arrowheads. (**b**) Podocytes growing out of a glomerulus at day 3 post-isolation are indicated by arrows. (**c**) Podocytes growing out of a glomerulus (indicated by $*$) on day 7 post-isolation. (**d**) Podocytes in culture following separation from glomeruli by filtration. Scale bar = 50 μm

8. Seven days after plating, most of the podocytes will have grown out of the glomeruli and can be separated from them by filtration (Fig. 1c).
9. To collect the podocyte cells, remove the culture media and rinse with PBS.
10. Add 2 mL 0.25% trypsin-EDTA to detach cells and glomeruli.
11. Add 8 mL culture media to deactivate the trypsin and filter through a 30 μm cell strainer on a 50 mL Falcon tube. The glomeruli should stay on the top of the filter whereas the podocytes will pass though the filter and get collected in the filtrate.
12. Centrifuge the filtrate at 200 × *g* for 5 min.
13. Discard the supernatant and resuspend the pellet (podocytes) in 10 mL culture media.
14. Plate into a new P100 dish coated with Matrigel (Fig. 1d).

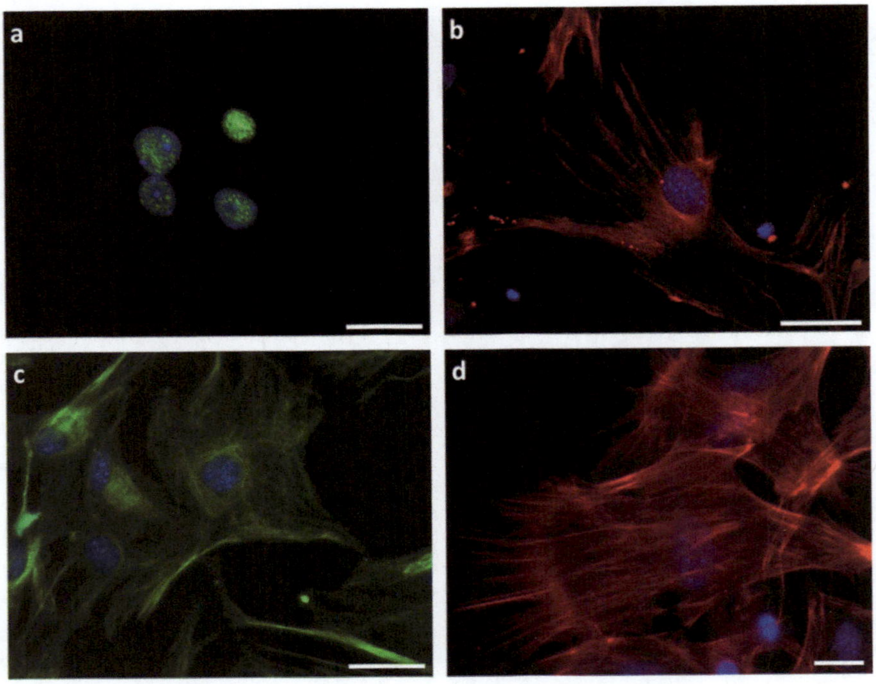

Fig. 2 Podocyte characterization. Representative pictures showing cultured podocytes stained for the podocyte markers WT1 (**a**), nephrin (**b**), and nestin (**c**). Actin filaments were visualized by staining for phalloidin (**d**). Scale bar = 20 μm

15. The podocytes obtained in this way express WT1, and mature podocyte markers nephrin and nestin, and have prominent actin fibers (stained with phalloidin) (Fig. 2). To assess the effects of the diabetic environment, the podocytes can be cultured with media containing normal (5 mM) or high (25 mM) glucose.
16. Isolated podocytes can be cryopreserved in liquid nitrogen in culture media containing 5% DMSO.

4 Notes

1. A successful perfusion is essential for efficient glomerular isolation. Ensure that the Venflon catheter is short enough (5 mm) to avoid puncturing the cardiac septum. Following a successful perfusion, the kidneys will have a pale color.
2. When handling Matrigel, work quickly as it readily turns into a gel at room temperature.
3. The preparation of glomeruli can be assessed immediately after plating under the microscope to ensure that there is no contamination from other kidney structures.

Acknowledgment

This work was supported by a Kidney Research UK Post-Doctoral Fellowship (PDF8/2015) to EV.

References

1. Alpers CE, Hudkins KL (2011) Mouse models of diabetic nephropathy. Curr Opin Nephrol Hypertens 20:278–284
2. Gnudi L (2012) Cellular and molecular mechanisms of diabetic glomerulopathy. Nephrol Dial Transplant 27:2642–2649
3. Gnudi L, Benedetti S, Woolf AS, Long DA (2015) Vascular growth factors play critical roles in kidney glomeruli. Clin Sci (Lond) 129:1225–1236
4. Lim AK, Tesch GH (2012) Inflammation in diabetic nephropathy. Mediat Inflamm 2012:146154
5. Tesch GH (2008) MCP-1/CCL2: a new diagnostic marker and therapeutic target for progressive renal injury in diabetic nephropathy. Am J Physiol 294:F697–F701
6. Saleem MA, O'Hare MJ, Reiser J, Coward RJ, Inward CD, Farren T, Xing CY, Ni L, Mathieson PW, Mundel P (2002) A conditionally immortalized human podocyte cell line demonstrating nephrin and podocin expression. J Am Soc Nephrol 13:630–638
7. Mundel P, Reiser J, Zuniga Mejia Borja A, Pavenstadt H, Davidson GR, Kriz W, Zeller R (1997) Rearrangements of the cytoskeleton and cell contacts induce process formation during differentiation of conditionally immortalized mouse podocyte cell lines. Exp Cell Res 236:248–258
8. Lay AC, Hurcombe JA, Betin VMS, Barrington F, Rollason R, Ni L, Gillam L, Pearson GME, Østergaard MV, Hamidi H, Lennon R, Welsh GI, Coward RJM (2017) Prolonged exposure of mouse and human podocytes to insulin induces insulin resistance through lysosomal and proteasomal degradation of the insulin receptor. Diabetologia 60 (11):2299–2311. https://doi.org/10.1007/s00125-017-4394-0
9. Kim Y, Lim JH, Kim MY, Kim EN, Yoon HE, Shin SJ, Choi BS, Kim Y-S, Chang YS, Park CW (2018) The adiponectin receptor agonist adiporon ameliorates diabetic nephropathy in a model of type 2 diabetes. J Am Soc Nephrol 29 (4):1108–1127
10. Qi W, Keenan HA, Li Q, Ishikado A, Kannt A, Sadowski T, Yorek MA, Wu I-H, Lockhart S, Coppey LJ, Pfenninger A, Liew CW, Qiang G, Burkart AM, Hastings S, Pober D, Cahill C, Niewczas MA, Israelsen WJ, Tinsley L, Stillman IE, Amenta PS, Feener EP, Vander Heiden MG, Stanton RC, King GL (2017) Pyruvate kinase M2 activation may protect against the progression of diabetic glomerular pathology and mitochondrial dysfunction. Nat Med 23(6):753–762

Part III

Techniques to Image the Diabetic Kidney

Chapter 6

Histological Examination of the Diabetic Kidney

Camillo Carrara, Mauro Abbate, Sara Conti, Daniela Rottoli, Paola Rizzo, and Gianfranco Marchetti

Abstract

The increasing prevalence of diabetes worldwide has led to a concomitant rise in diabetic kidney disease (DKD) as a major cause of end-stage renal disease. Glomerular lesions constitute the most striking and consistent features identified in biopsies from patients with DKD, although tubulointerstitial injury has an important and often under-recognized role in the progression to overt nephropathy. In advanced stages of the disease, podocyte detachment is a pivotal event in the loss of glomerular filtration barrier integrity and may explain, at least in part, the inability of current therapies to halt renal function decline. This chapter details the systematic method that can be used to study renal tissue samples from diabetic patients, and the specific role of different imaging techniques, such as light microscopy, immunofluorescence microscopy, and transmission and scanning electron microscopy in detecting histologic lesions specific to DKD.

Key words Diabetic kidney disease, Renal biopsy, Glomerulus, Podocyte, Light microscopy, Immunofluorescence microscopy, Transmission electron microscopy, Scanning electron microscopy

1 Introduction

Diabetic kidney disease (DKD) develops in 30–40% of patients with diabetes and is a leading cause of chronic kidney disease worldwide [1, 2]. Improved health care and living standards have increased the elderly population, which is at considerable risk for type 2 diabetes and carries a high burden of comorbid conditions that may affect the kidneys [3]. Patients with DKD most typically show glomerular hyperfiltration, progressive albuminuria, and declining glomerular filtration rate (GFR) which eventually results in end-stage renal disease [4]. However, in a subset of cases, GFR loss has been shown to occur independently of albuminuria or even in its absence [5]. In this cohort, risk factors other than albuminuria/proteinuria, related more specifically to diabetes, might contribute to GFR deterioration, including female sex (possibly related to estrogens), obesity, hypertriglyceridemia, hypertension, and insulin resistance.

Luigi Gnudi and David A. Long (eds.), *Diabetic Nephropathy: Methods and Protocols*, Methods in Molecular Biology, vol. 2067, https://doi.org/10.1007/978-1-4939-9841-8_6,

The constellation of renal structural lesions occurring in diabetes is unique and predominantly affects the glomeruli, with thickening of the glomerular basement membrane (GBM), and mesangial expansion, although the renal tubules, interstitium, and arterioles also undergo substantial changes within a few years of diabetes onset (Fig. 1a–e) [6]. Histological lesions in type 1 and type 2 diabetic patients share many similarities, but renal structure changes in type 2 diabetes are more heterogeneous and less predictably associated with clinical presentation [7]. In the earliest stage of DKD, light microscopy (LM) may show only glomerular hypertrophy without any other apparent sign of injury. The first morphological change, as detected by transmission electron microscopy (TEM) in glomeruli, consists of thickened GBM, which is apparent within 1.5–2 years of diabetes diagnosis, followed by other glomerular and tubular lesions, including loss of endothelial fenestrations, mesangial matrix expansion (Fig. 2), and severe tubular basement membrane thickening [8]. Diffuse mesangial matrix expansion is the hallmark lesion of diabetic glomerulopathy, is progressive, and, in about 25% of patients with advanced DKD, takes the form of mesangial nodules, so-called Kimmelstiel-Wilson nodules [9]. Furthermore, three-dimensional scanning electron microscopy (SEM) surface observation can be used to demonstrate the progressive damage to the podocyte's cytoarchitecture, another crucial contributor to progressive proteinuria and glomerular filtration barrier deterioration in DKD (Fig. 3) [10]. SEM is not intended to be used as a clinical pathology diagnostic tool, but as an effective research tool that may be instrumental in evaluating the extent of glomerular damage in patients with DKD and could provide pathologists with more dynamic information and insightful details than those given by TEM.

Renal biopsy is required for a definitive diagnosis of DKD and the use of ancillary techniques such as immunofluorescence (IF) microscopy and TEM is often decisive in ruling out other medical conditions affecting the kidney. Notably, in a large cohort of diabetic patients, over 60% of biopsies revealed nondiabetic renal disease, alone or alongside concomitant DKD [11]. The high prevalence of nondiabetic renal disease in diabetic patients is not surprising considering that patients often undergo diagnostic renal biopsy when the clinical course is not typical for DKD [6, 12]. In addition to clinical needs, access to kidney tissue is important for research purposes, in an effort to characterize the underlying mechanisms of DKD, identify new therapies to target these mechanisms, and discover new biomarkers that will more accurately reflect whether a patient with DKD is likely to progress or not [13]. An important and unsolved question is whether DKD is reversible. In one detailed report, typical lesions of advanced DKD (GBM thickening, mesangial expansion, and tubular lesions) recovered partially 10 years after pancreas transplantation, together with an

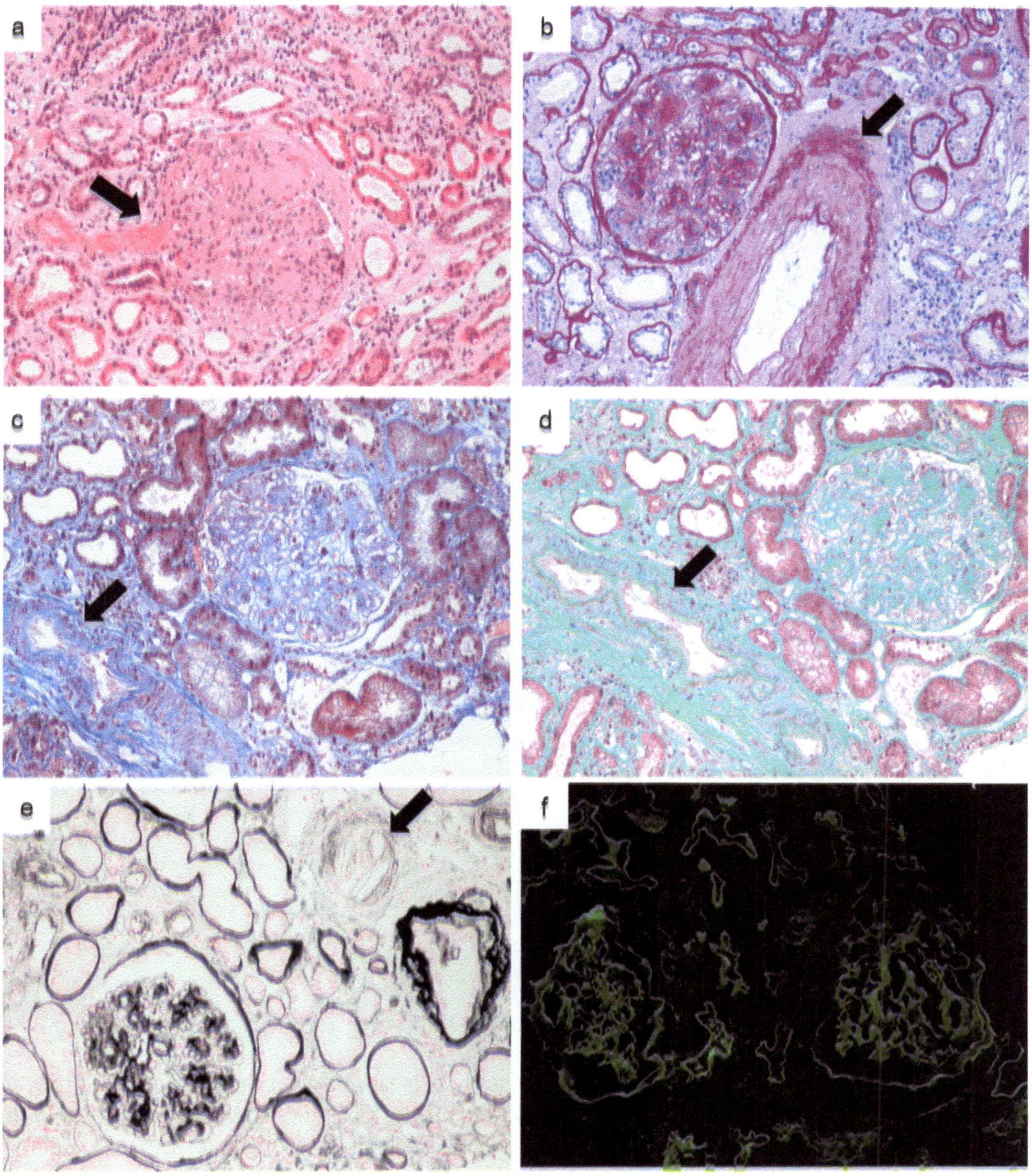

Fig. 1 Low-power view of renal cortical parenchyma by light microscopy in patients with advanced DKD. (**a**) An enlarged glomerulus shows nodular expansion of the mesangium and severe hyalinosis of the afferent arteriole. The surrounding parenchyma reveals diffuse interstitial fibrosis and tubular atrophy with a scattered, predominantly mononuclear, inflammatory infiltrate (hematoxylin and eosin stain; original magnification, ×100). In addition to the typical glomerular changes, severe atherosclerosis of the interlobular arteries (*arrows*) is a hallmark of advanced DKD (**b**, periodic acid-Schiff stain, original magnification, ×100; **c**, Masson's trichrome stain, original magnification, ×100; **d**, Gomori trichrome stain, original magnification, ×100). (**e**) An interlobular artery is occluded by an organizing atheroembolus (*arrow*), consisting of cholesterol clefts (silver methenamine stain, original magnification, ×100). (**f**) Immunofluorescence studies in patients with advanced DKD show dull linear staining of glomerular and tubular basement membranes for IgG (original magnification, ×100)

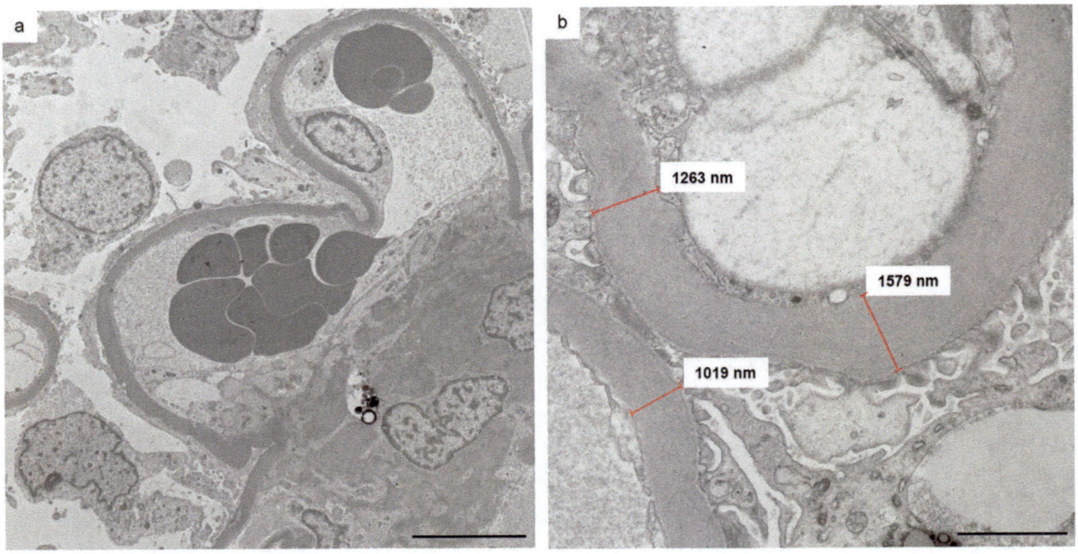

Fig. 2 (**a**) Transmission electron microscopy of a glomerular area in a patient with DKD shows thickening of the glomerular basement membrane and podocyte damage with effaced foot processes. Scale bar, 1000 nm. (**b**) Transmission electron micrograph at higher magnification in another case mainly showing a severely thickened glomerular basement membrane. Scale bar, 2000 nm

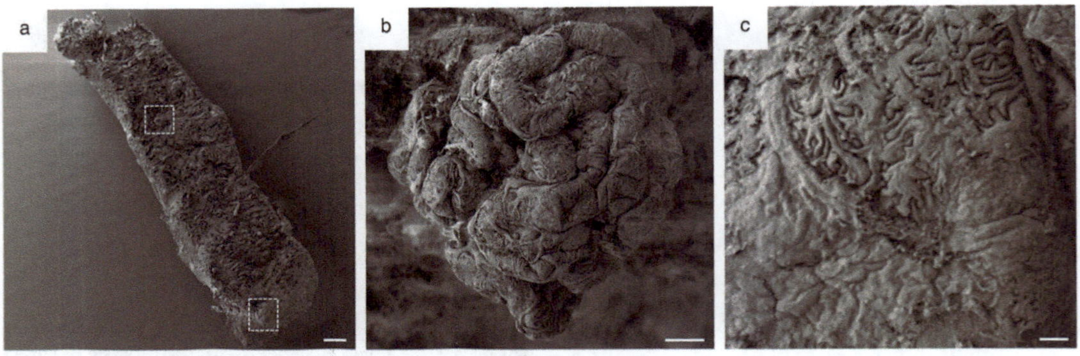

Fig. 3 (**a**) Low-power view of scanning electron microscopy of renal cortical parenchyma core in a case of early DKD showing superficial glomeruli (insets). Scale bar, 200 μm. High-power view of renal glomerulus (**b**, scale bar, 20 μm), showing an initial effacement of the interdigitating foot processes (**c**, scale bar, 1 μm)

improvement in clinical and laboratory parameters [14]. In addition, in an experimental mouse model of DKD, the leptin-deficient BTBR *ob/ob* mouse, Pichaiwong et al. showed that leptin replacement resulted in near-complete reversal of both structural and functional measures of injury [15]. Immunohistochemical labeling with the podocyte markers Wilms tumor 1 and p57 identified parietal epithelial cells as a possible source of regenerating podocytes. These findings indicate phenotypic plasticity in podocyte and parietal epithelial cell populations, suggesting that podocytes may regenerate from parietal epithelial cells/progenitors in DKD, although this hypothesis is still being debated [16].

This chapter aims to describe a method that can be applied to renal biopsies from diabetic patients, focusing on the procedures of tissue fixation, processing and production of good sections for LM, IF, and TEM, and preparations for SEM, but also exploring their combined application in DKD. In this respect, it should be pointed out that automation is rapidly changing histology practice, trying to make manual techniques obsolete. Recent advances in technology have led to the development of constant-throughput processors and microwave energy systems [17]. Some of the main advantages of these processors include improved tissue turnaround time in an age of increased workload, no additional staffing, and a reduction of toxic vapors in the laboratory. Although we agree that addressing all these issues is crucial, in this chapter we opted to focus on traditional full manual procedures, which, if performed by specially trained technicians, can provide renal tissue sections of the highest quality, and additional information with significant investigative potential.

2 Materials

2.1 Tissue Processing and Staining for Light Microscopy

1. Dubosq-Brasil: Combine 12 mL aqueous picric acid (saturated 8.96% alcoholic), 108 mL absolute ethanol, 60 mL concentrated formalin, and 15 mL acetic acid.
2. Absolute ethanol (ETOH): Use distilled water (dH_2O) to make dilutions of 90% and 70% ETOH.
3. Xylene.
4. Paraffin (melting point 53 °C).
5. Histology oven for laboratory use (working temperature from +20 °C to +100 °C through electronic thermostat with microprocessor).
6. Slide warmer for paraffin tissue section mounting.
7. Stainless steel mold.
8. Embedding ring made of high-impact polystyrene that fits well in the microtome chuck adapter.
9. Glass slide racks.
10. Glass Coplin jars (standard 10-slide Coplin jars hold approximately 50 mL of solution).
11. Glass histology cap containers (50 mL).
12. Glass measuring beaker (300 mL) used for paraffin storage.
13. Manual rotary microtome.
14. Microtome blades.
15. dH_2O.

16. Mayer's hematoxylin.
17. 1% Eosin Y aqueous solution.
18. 0.5% Periodic acid: 1 g Periodic acid in 200 mL dH_2O.
19. Schiff's reagent Hotchkiss McManus.
20. 5% Sodium thiosulfate: 5 g Sodium thiosulfate pentahydrate in 100 mL dH_2O.
21. Weigert's hematoxylin: Combine equal volume of Weigert's iron hematoxylin solution A and Weigert's iron hematoxylin solution B.
22. Ponceau Masson fuchsin.
23. Phosphomolybdic acid.
24. Aniline blue.
25. Gomori solution: Mix 1 g eosin Y, 0.2 g light green, 0.5 g phosphotungstic acid, 100 mL dH_2O, and 0.5 mL acetic acid.
26. Light green solution: Mix 1 g light green, 100 mL dH_2O, and 1 mL acetic acid.
27. Stock solution: Mix 3 g hexamethylenetetramine, 0.25 g silver nitrate, 220 mL dH_2O, and 1 g sodium tetraborate.
28. Golden chloride: 1 g Golden chloride in 500 mL dH_2O.
29. Nuclear fast red solution.
30. Xylene-based mounting medium.
31. Glass coverslips, 24 × 50 mm.

2.2 Tissue Processing for Immunofluorescence Microscopy

1. Liquid nitrogen Dewar with high thermal efficiency, equipped with suitable metallic canisters.
2. Phosphate-buffered saline (PBS) 10× at pH 7.4: Mix one part concentrated buffer to nine parts deionized water (1:10 dilution).
3. Optimal cutting temperature (OCT) compound.
4. Acetone.
5. An incubation chamber with a lid in which glass microscope slides can be laid flat and slightly raised off the bottom of the chamber. Place a dampened paper towel on the bottom of the chamber to maintain humidity and prevent the tissue sections from drying out.
6. Microscope slides, pre-coated.
7. Staining jars/slide holders.
8. Cryostat microtome (−25/−30 °C).
9. Cryotome blades.
10. Fluorochrome-conjugated primary antibodies to detect immunoglobulins (IgG, IgM, and IgA), complement components (C3 and C1q), fibrin, kappa and lambda light chains.

11. Glass Coplin jars (standard 10-slide Coplin jars hold approximately 50 mL of solution).
12. Aqueous mounting medium Fluoromount™.
13. Glass coverslips, 24 × 32 mm.

2.3 Tissue Processing for Transmission Electron Microscopy

1. Ultrapure distilled water (ddH_2O).
2. 0.1 M Cacodylate buffer, pH 7.4.
3. Primary fixative: 2.5% Glutaraldehyde in 0.1 M cacodylate buffer, pH 7.4.
4. Secondary fixative: 1% Osmium tetroxide (OsO4) in 0.1 M cacodylate buffer, pH 7.4.
5. Graded ETOH (10%, 50%, 70%, 90%, and 100%), prepared by mixing known contents of ddH_2O and ETOH.
6. Propylene oxide.
7. Epoxy resin.
8. Embedding molds.
9. Knifemaker.
10. Glass knife strips.
11. Ultramicrotome.
12. Diamond knife.
13. Toluidine blue.
14. Single-edge carbon steel.
15. Copper grids (100 mesh, square, or hexagonal mesh) washed with ETOH and dried prior to use.
16. Tweezers, #5 Dumont.
17. Uranyl acetate replacement (UAR).
18. Lead citrate.

2.4 Tissue Processing for Scanning Electron Microscopy

1. ddH_2O.
2. 0.1 M Cacodylate buffer, pH 7.4.
3. Primary fixative: 2.5% Glutaraldehyde in 0.1 M cacodylate buffer, pH 7.4.
4. Secondary fixative: 1% Osmium tetroxide (OsO_4) in 0.1 M cacodylate buffer, pH 7.4.
5. Graded ETOH (10%, 50%, 70%, 90%, and 100%), prepared by mixing known contents of ddH_2O and ETOH.
6. Fine-tipped forceps.
7. Dissecting tools (microscissors and razor blade): Dish for dissection.
8. Container for processing (sealable glass vials).
9. Carbon-conductive mounting tabs.

3 Methods

Once a renal biopsy is collected, the tissue is placed in a small petri dish containing enough cold saline to cover the tissue, and examined under a magnifying glass, in order to evaluate sample adequacy. Needle biopsy cores are then sent to the pathology laboratory for division and processing by placing in physiologic saline-moistened gauze. Once the tissue is available to the laboratory, it is important to identify, with a dissecting microscope or with a magnifying glass, the cortex to select a sample with glomeruli for LM, IF, and electron microscopy. The tissue is placed on a glass slide with normal saline and examined without a coverslip, producing a wet mount. The cortex appears irregular and the glomeruli are usually visible as small, reddish round structures with capillaries. If glomeruli are present, the tissue is divided using a clean scalpel so that at least a few glomeruli are fixed for study by electron microscopy and a few are frozen for IF; the remaining tissue is fixed for LM. The motion for cutting must be a slicing, not a crushing or tearing, movement. In theory, a single glomerulus each could be adequate for electron microscopy and IF studies. Therefore, where possible, the bulk of the specimen should be submitted for LM. Portions of tissue for TEM should not exceed 1 mm in thickness, ideally $1 \times 1 \times 1$ mm. Conversely, since SEM is a surface analysis imaging technique, the dimension of the sample may not be a limiting issue.

3.1 Tissue Processing and Staining for Light Microscopy

Place the fresh tissue specimen in a cap container filled with Dubosq-Brasil solution for 3 h.

1. Fixation is the most important step in the preparation of the tissue sample for LM. The main objective of fixation is to maintain clear and consistent morphological features of renal parenchyma. If tissue is inadequately fixed, the subsequent dehydration solutions may have detrimental effects on the process, possibly altering the staining characteristics of the tissue. The choice of a fixative is a compromise balancing beneficial and detrimental effects. Dubosq-Brasil fixative is particularly recommended for core needle biopsies, because of its good penetrating properties. Furthermore, it produces excellent cytoplasmic preservation, although the tissue is harmed by prolonged fixation (in general, avoid more than 4 h of fixation time). In addition, both ethanol and picric acid, which are important components of this solution, enhance the preservation of glycogen either by trapping it within protein or through precipitation (*see* **Notes 1** and **2**).
2. To properly embed the tissue in paraffin, it must first be dehydrated. This is done by passing the biopsy sample through a series of baths of increasing concentrations of ethanol,

culminating with 100% ethanol. For this purpose, we use histology cap containers. It is important to keep the containers closed during the procedure because ethanol is a volatile compound.

(a) Place the specimen in a cap container filled with 70% ethanol for 1 h.

(b) Transfer the specimen in a cap container filled with 90% ethanol for 50 min.

(c) Transfer the specimen in a cap container filled with 100% ethanol for 1 h.

3. Place the specimen in a cap container filled with xylene for 1 h. This agent acts as an intermediary between the dehydration and infiltration solutions. Indeed, following dehydration, the alcohol must be cleared from the tissue, making the tissue components receptive to the infiltrating medium. Remember that overexposure to xylene during processing will cause overhardening (*see* **Note 1**).

   Steps 1–3 must be carried out in a fume cupboard.

4. Remove the specimen from the clearing agent and lay it down flat on a paper towel for just a few seconds to remove the excess xylene. The tissue can now be infiltrated with a suitable histological wax.

5. Pour a small amount of molten paraffin into a suitably sized metallic mold. Paraffin is dispensed from a beaker stored at 56–58 °C in the histology oven. Keep the mold in the oven before use, and it should still be warm when paraffin is poured in it.

6. Lay the biopsy sample down flat at the bottom of the mold, completely submerged in paraffin, with the help of fine dissecting surgical forceps. The specimen is very carefully orientated in the mold because its placement will determine the "plane of section," an important consideration in both diagnostic and research histology. Try to minimize the compression and distortion of the biopsy core (*see* **Note 2**).

7. Place the mold in the histology oven at 58 °C for 1 h in order to obtain complete paraffin infiltration. Molten paraffin wax infiltrates the sample and replaces the xylene. Paraffin is a mixture of long-chain hydrocarbons produced in the cracking of mineral oil and can be purchased with melting points at different temperatures, the most common for histological use being about 56–58 °C. Hot paraffin wax is the major cause of shrinkage during paraffin processing. The temperature of the molten wax should be kept the lowest possible, consistent with complete infiltration during the available time.

8. An embedding ring is placed on top of the mold, topped up with more wax, and the whole thing is placed on a cold plate to

solidify (you can leave it in a refrigerator for 40 min at 4 °C to speed up the process).

9. When this solidification process is complete, the block with its attached ring can be removed from the mold and is ready for sectioning (be sure that the whole block has solidified completely before separating it from the mold). It should be noted that, if tissue processing is carried out properly, the wax blocks containing the tissue specimens are stable and are an important source of archival material.

10. Use a sharp microtome blade to manually carve the sides of the paraffin block. That will make it possible to reduce the surface area of the biopsy sections and it will facilitate the microtome cutting procedure.

11. Secure the embedding ring, which holds the tissue sample, in the microtome chuck adapter and orientate it so the blade will cut straight across the block.

12. Trim the block to expose the tissue surface to a level where a representative section can be cut. Trimming is normally done at a thickness of about 10 μm.

13. Serial sections that are 3 μm thick are cut, taking into account that three sections should be placed on each slide (we usually prepare three slides for hematoxylin–eosin stain, three for periodic acid-Schiff reaction, three for Masson's trichrome stain, three for Gomori trichrome, and three for silver methenamine stain). The long ribbon containing at least 45 sections should be collected, using a wet paintbrush, as soon as the knife reaches the level of the tissue (Fig. 4a). Optimal sections can be obtained only if the biopsy specimen is properly embedded and lies flat in the block; otherwise some artifacts can be introduced in the sectioning (tearing, holes, folding, and wrinkles). Thinness is a prerequisite of good renal biopsy sections.

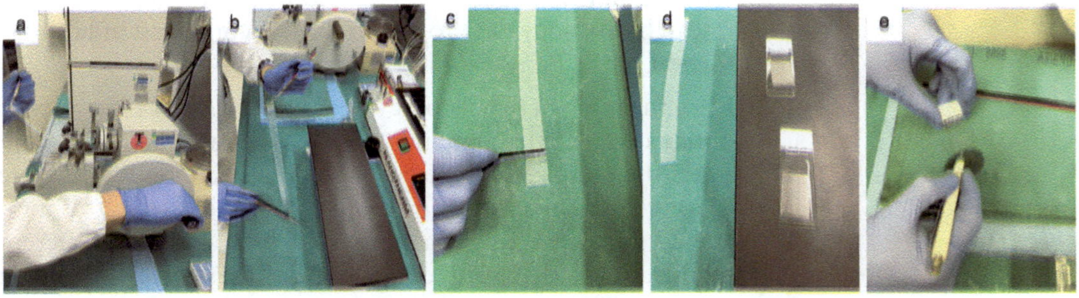

Fig. 4 This panel shows the technique of sectioning for light microscopy. (**a**) Block sectioning using a manual rotary microtome generates a long ribbon containing multiple sections; (**b**) the ribbon is transferred on the worktable with the help of two paintbrushes; (**c**) the ribbon is divided into three section pieces; (**d**) after having applied 1 mL of distilled water to the microscope slides, sections can be placed on water surface with the appropriate orientation; (**e**) extra water is removed from the slides being careful not to lose the sections

Standard histologic sections, which generally run 6–8 μm in thickness, are totally unsuitable. Sectioning tissues is a real art and takes much skill and practice.

14. With the help of two paintbrushes, pick up the long ribbon and lay it flat on a dry and clean piece of fabric. During transfer, the paintbrushes hold the ribbon at the extremities. Great care must be taken to avoid folds or tearing (*see* **Note 3**) (Fig. 4b).
15. Using a scalpel or a microtome blade, divide the ribbon in three-section pieces (Fig. 4c).
16. Using a plastic Pasteur pipette, apply approximately 1 mL of distilled water on the microscope slide and, with the paintbrush, gently drop off the three-section piece in the middle of the slide (each slide should be numbered consecutively before use) (Fig. 4d).
17. Incline the slide and pour off the extra water, being careful not to remove the section (you can hold the section using a thumb dressing forceps or another round-tip metallic tool). Transfer each slide onto the slide warmer at 40 °C for about 2 h. The section pieces should dry without forming wrinkles (Fig. 4e).
18. Tissue sections are then ready to be processed for histological stains. For LM, the elucidation of glomerular structure and lesions requires a variety of histochemical stains. We routinely employ five stains: hematoxylin and eosin, periodic acid-Schiff, Masson's trichrome, Gomori trichrome, and silver methenamine. Usually, we allocate three microscope slides for each stain (a total of 15 slides).
19. Place the slides in a jar filled with xylene three times for 5 min each, to completely dissolve the paraffin. Rehydrate gradually through a series of jars containing graded alcohols (100% ethanol twice for 10 min each, then 95% ethanol twice for 10 min each) and finally wash the slides by leaving the jar under a gentle jet of tap water. This procedure is preliminary to all the histochemical stains, and allows water-soluble dyes to penetrate the sections. All the dyes are filtered before use to enhance the colors and to avoid that any precipitated dye may appear as an artifact.
20. After tissue hydration (**step 19**), the slides are immersed in different soluble dyes according to the type of histological staining to be done:
    (a) Hematoxylin and eosin stain: The hematoxylin stains the nuclei light blue, and eosin Y imparts pink color to the eosinophilic structures, including the cell cytoplasm (Fig. 1a).

        Procedure: Place the slides in a jar filled with Mayer's hematoxylin for 5 min. Wash the slides with tap water for about 2 min, and then perform a quick wash in distilled water before putting the slides into eosin Y. This step is always necessary before going into any dye, in order not to pollute it with the impurities of the tap water. After incubation with eosin Y, wash the slides with running and then distilled water, and complete the procedure by dehydrating the sections and mounting the coverslips (*see* **steps 21–23**).

(b) Periodic acid-Schiff (PAS): It is used to detect polysaccharides such as glycogen, and mucosubstances such as glycoproteins, glycolipids, and mucins. In the kidney, the PAS stain highlights in magenta the basement membranes, the hyaline substance, and the area of sclerosis, while nuclei are counterstained in blue with hematoxylin (Fig. 1b).

(c) Procedure: Immerse the slides in 0.5% periodic acid for 10 min. Wash the slides with tap water for 2 min and quickly with distilled water, and move the slides in the Schiff reagent solution for 15 min, after which a 15-min wash is performed with 5% sodium thiosulfate. Perform a further wash with running and then distilled water, and move the slides in Mayer's hematoxylin solution for 5 min. After an additional wash, complete the procedure by dehydrating the sections and mounting the coverslips (*see* **steps 21–23**).

(d) Masson's trichrome: Three-color staining protocol which highlights collagen in blue, while cytoplasm and nuclei are stained in pink and black, respectively (Fig. 1c).

Procedure: Place the slides in a jar filled with Weigert's hematoxylin for 10 min. After washing the slides with tap water for 2 min and quickly with distilled water, place the slides in Ponceau Masson fuchsin solution for 4 min, and then in phosphomolybdic acid for 13 min. Perform a further wash with running and then distilled water, and leave the slides in a jar containing aniline blue at 37 °C in an oven for 10 min. After an additional wash, immerse the slides in acetic acid for 3 min and complete the procedure as described in **steps 21–23**.

(e) Gomori trichrome: It is a variant of Masson's trichrome, in which collagen is highlighted in green, cytoplasm is stained in red/brown, and nuclei are black (Fig. 1d). Procedure: Place the slides in a jar filled with Weigert's hematoxylin for 5 min. Wash the slides with tap water for 2 min and quickly with distilled water, and move the slides in the Gomori solution for 30 min, after which a further wash is performed. When slides are immersed in distilled water, take one slide at a time, and quickly dip it into a jar filled with light green solution (for approximately 2 s) and immediately spray absolute ethanol on each slide by using a wash bottle. Then, complete the procedure by dehydrating the sections and mounting the coverslips (*see* **steps 21–23**).

(f) Silver methenamine: It is an excellent stain for the demonstration of glomerular and tubular basement membranes, which are highlighted with an intensive silver color (Fig. 1e).

Procedure: Place the slides in 0.5% periodic acid for 30 min, and then wash the slides with tap water for 2 min and quickly with distilled water. Move the slides in a jar filled with stock solution kept at 50 °C in an oven. After 3 h check the sections under a microscope, and eventually repeat the check every 15 min, until the glomerular capillaries have taken on an intense gray/black color. Perform a rapid wash in distilled water, and rapidly place the sections in a jar filled with golden chloride for 1 min, after which a further rapid wash is performed with distilled water. Rinse the slides in 5% sodium thiosulfate for 1 min and then in distilled water, and then move in nuclear fast red solution for 5 min. After an additional wash, complete the procedure by dehydrating the sections and mounting the coverslips (*see* **steps 21–23**).

21. Once the steps in the soluble dyes have been performed, dehydrate the sections by dipping them into two jars filled with absolute ethanol, and one with xylene (approximately 5 s for each passage). The dehydration is complete when no streak of water is visible on the slide. This step is crucial to preserve the morphology of the tissue, and to enable an effective mounting of the coverslip.
22. Lay a glass coverslip on a paper towel, and using a plastic pipette place two drops of xylene-based mounting medium on it. Lower the slide over the coverslip, starting from one side of the slide, and going slowly down to prevent the formation of air bubbles. Turn the slide and apply a slight pressure to favor mounting medium distribution and coverslip adhesion.
23. Let the slides dry at room temperature on a flat surface.

3.2 Tissue Processing for Immunofluorescence Microscopy

The principle of IF is based on the specific binding of labeled antibody to antigen in tissue. Direct IF microscopy on renal tissue detects and localizes immunoglobulins (primarily IgG, IgM, IgA, kappa, and lambda light chains), complement components (primarily C3, C1q, and C4), and fibrin-related antigens by first reacting tissue sections with FITC-labeled antisera, followed by observation of specific fluorescent staining. IF is best performed on unfixed sections that can be transported to the laboratory in a physiologic saline-moistened gauze inside a petri dish. In DKD, IF can be a decisive tool for ruling out any other medical conditions affecting the kidney, which can be associated with or superimposed on diabetes. Usually there are no immune complexes by IF in glomeruli from diabetic patients. Cases of overt DKD may show the characteristic linear homogeneous staining of IgG along glomerular and tubular basement membranes (Fig. 1f). This staining is not thought to be indicative of immune injury, but may represent "stickiness" of the enlarged GBM to antisera used for IF [9].

1. Snap freeze fresh renal tissue (alone or pre-immerged in optimal cutting temperature compound—OCT) by submerging it directly in liquid nitrogen. During the freezing procedure, you can protect the needle core in a small aluminum foil inserted in the suitable canister and folded into the shape of a "boat." The sample will quickly snap freeze, producing a typical noise ("frying-like"). When the noise disappears, you can extract the canister and its content from the nitrogen Dewar (*see* **Note 4**).
2. Using pre-cooled forceps, remove the specimen from the aluminum foil and lay it down flat at the bottom of the cryostat, where the temperature is kept at −25 °C (*see* **Note 5**). In the meantime, mount a disposable blade and place all necessary items in the cryostat: usually 3–4 kimwipes and a couple of paintbrushes. Never touch the specimen with warm tools (*see* **Note 6**).
3. For crude frozen tissue, apply a small base of OCT compound to a specimen chuck inside the cryostat and place the frozen tissue sample in the center of the chuck, keeping track of tissue orientation (Fig. 5a, b). Adjust the orientation with pre-cooled forceps if necessary. Avoid bubbles in the OCT (*see* **Note 7**).

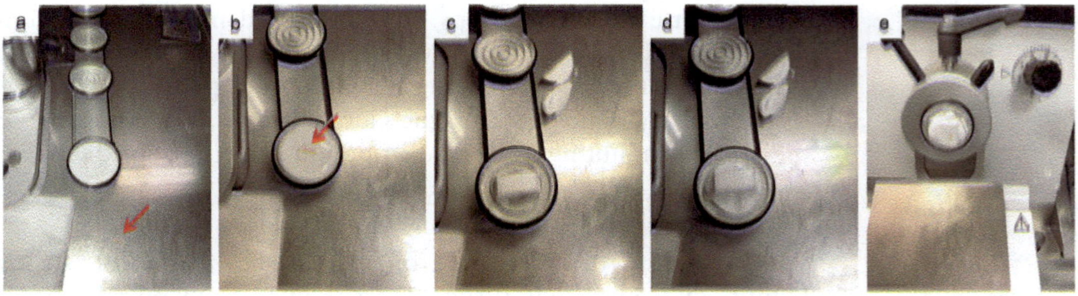

Fig. 5 This panel shows the frozen embedding method for immunofluorescence. (**a**) A small base of OCT compound is applied to a specimen chuck inside the cryostat (red arrow indicates the snap-frozen specimen); (**b**) the specimen is placed in the center of the chuck (red arrow); (**c**) a rectangular block is carved in solidified OCT; (**d**) a new base of OCT compound is applied to the specimen chuck and the block is placed in the center of the chuck; (**e**) the block is mounted in the cryostat holder, ready for sectioning

4. Quickly cover the sample with additional OCT compound before it starts to solidify and, then, wait for complete gel solidification.
5. Using a disposable blade, hand carve a rectangular block of OCT that perfectly encases the tissue core sample (Fig. 5c). Try to circumscribe the sample and avoid cracking of the block. Finally, remove the block from the specimen chuck.
6. Apply a small base of OCT compound to a second specimen chuck inside the cryostat and place the OCT block containing the tissue sample in the center of the chuck (Fig. 5d). Wait for complete gel solidification. This procedure will create an ideal support for block sectioning. Make sure that the cryostat sectioning arm is moved sufficiently back from the blade, so that the block can be mounted without touching the blade. Mount the chuck with the block in the holder, with the desired orientation (Fig. 5e).
7. Rotating the cryostat wheel, the specimen advances toward the cutting blade. Slowly raise the sectioning arm until it is almost touching the blade. Proceed further, advancing the arm as though sectioning, until the blade begins to cut into the OCT block. Wipe away unwanted or damaged sections with a paintbrush or kimwipes, always moving from the back of the blade to the front. Serial sections of 2 μm of thickness are cut. Sections may be collected singly or in a short string of two, holding a pre-warmed slide just above the sections on the blade. Check sections under a light microscope and keep notes about section location and quality on specific numbered slides for later reference. When glomeruli have been located, a total of 8–10 sections are cut. Three to five slides with two sections each will be obtained for staining and storage. Remember to pre-warm the slides and label them with the name of the antigen used. Always clean the blade with brush or kimwipes after collecting sections and allow temperature to rebalance.
8. Lay the slides down flat to dry. Slides should be allowed to dry for approximately 1 h or may be stored in a slide box at −80 C°.
9. Place the slides in a Coplin jar with acetone for 10 min (*see* **Note 8**).
10. Lay the slides flat for 2 min to dry.
11. Rinse in PBS for 10 min, then extract the slides, and wipe excess PBS from slides, thereby avoiding the tissue of drying.
12. Lay the slides flat, tissue side up, in the incubation chamber. Take fluorochrome-conjugated primary antibodies from the −20 ° C refrigerator (appropriately diluted antibodies are kept in separate and easily recognizable test tubes; for the

dilutions, combine instructions from antibody data sheet with end-user optimization experiments). Using a glass Pasteur pipette, apply 4–5 drops of antibody so that it will distribute itself evenly over the tissue sections.

13. Place the lid on the chamber and incubate the sections in the dark at room temperature for 30 min. After 15 min check that the antibody is completely covering the tissue sections and, if necessary, add a drop of antibody to the glass slides.
14. Pour the primary antibody solution off the sections and place the slides in a Coplin jar filled with PBS for 15 min. Repeat once more to wash all unbound primary antibody from the sections. Extract the slides and wipe excess PBS avoiding the tissue to dry.
15. Lay the slides flat on a paper towel. Apply 3–4 drops of Fluoromount on the tissue section and gently lower a glass coverslip, using slow movements to prevent air bubbles from forming and being trapped on the section. Allow Fluoromount to dry for 5 min at room temperature and, then, lay the slides flat on a tray in the refrigerator in the dark at +4 °C (*see* **Note 9**).

3.3 Tissue Processing for Transmission Electron Microscopy

1. Place the portion of the biopsy (tissue pieces 1 × 1 × 1 mm) for TEM in a glass vial for fixation in freshly prepared 2.5% glutaraldehyde in 0.1 M cacodylate buffer, pH 7.4 (*see* **Note 10**). Take care to transfer quickly the fresh tissue with no or minimum delay of fixation. Never let the tissue dry. Wooden sticks may help avoiding other harmful contacts with the fragments. Fill the vial with 1 mL of fixative and check that all fragments are fully submerged by solution. Seal the cap container. Fixation for TEM is complete after 4 h in a refrigerator at 4 °C (*see* **Note 11**).
2. Wash 2× for 10 min with cacodylate buffer. Each solution can be removed and replaced with a plastic transfer pipette very carefully and gradually to avoid the loss or drying of small samples. Theoretically, processing is started overnight. If necessary, the tissue for TEM can be stored in buffer at 4 °C, for instance before it is mailed to an external laboratory.
3. Replace the buffer solution with 1% osmium tetroxide in cacodylate buffer for 1 h postfixation. Seal the vial cap. At the end, the tissue has turned completely black (*see* **Note 12**).
4. Dehydrate the tissue with graded ETOH: 10% ETOH × 5 min, 50% × 10 min, 70% × 10 min, 90% × 15 min, and finally 100% × 15 min (*see* **Note 13**).
5. Replace 100% ETOH with propylene oxide for 15 min. Use a plastic pipette carefully because the liquid has a tendency to leak out. The sample must undergo the treatment with propylene oxide that acts as an intermediate liquid miscible with

ETOH and with the solvent of the non-water-soluble epoxy resin. It acts with the anhydride component of the hardener of the including medium, becoming an integral part of the cross-linked polymer.

6. Replace the propylene oxide with 50% resin and 50% propylene oxide mixture (v/v, 1 mL per sample) and leave the tissue immersed for 4 h. This mixture is freshly prepared in advance at room temperature in a glass tube, by mixing both components with a plastic pipette until a clear solution is obtained. The epoxy resin must be prepared at least 24 h before use (*see* **Note 14**). It is important to check that the polymerization of newly prepared resin in the oven will produce adequate blocks. We periodically pre-assess the quality of the epoxy resin, by testing the polymerization of each new stock in the absence of tissue.
7. Replace the intermediate solution with epoxy resin 12 h (overnight), for infiltration of the tissue. Epoxy resin must be pre-warmed at room temperature a few hours before.
8. Transfer each fragment gently to the tip of the embedding mold using a smoothened needle or wooden sticks. Finally, fill completely each mold with resin, using the needle in order to remove any possible bubble. We place a small paper label with numbered code written in pencil in each mold to identify each tissue fragment.
9. Place the molds in oven at 60 °C for 72 h to obtain polymerized blocks (Fig. 6a). This critical step requires tight control of working temperature (58–60 °C).
10. In the ultramicrotome, remove excess resin from the face of the block using a single-edge carbon steel. Cut a few sections with

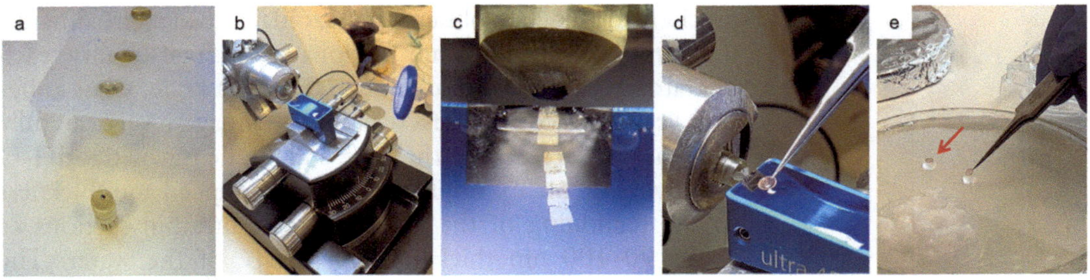

Fig. 6 This panel shows the technique of sectioning and staining for transmission electron microscopy. (**a**) The tip of a block, taken from the embedding mold and containing the osmicated tissue (black), can be trimmed for selection of an area of interest; (**b**) the block (top left) and the knife are secured on the ultramicrotome and carefully aligned with each other, prior to filling the knife tray with ultrapure water; (**c**) thin sections are cut by the best area of the knife edge to form a floating ribbon of sections in the presence of the correct meniscus; (**d**) collection of the sections on a grid; (**e**) staining on the top of drops (arrow) in a petri dish, in the presence of NaOH pellets (bottom left) if lead citrate is used

a glass knife and discard them until the tissue is reached. Trim the block further to obtain a truncated pyramid with a trapezoidal base. Glass knives to cut these semithin, also called "thick" sections (1 μm), can be made from a glass strip by a knifemaker. Select always a knife with good edge under a stereomicroscope and apply a water-resistant adhesive tape to the knife in order to build a tray or "boat" to be sealed with dental wax. Alternatively, a special diamond knife can be used (semithin sections cut at 0.5 μm thickness) as illustrated in Fig. 6b. Before cutting, carefully orient the block with respect to the knife and fill the tray with ddH_2O that will completely cover the knife edge (Fig. 6b). The technique for cutting thick or final ultrathin sections is mostly identical, although the ability to cut final sections suitable for TEM will require practice with the ultramicrotome, under initial supervision by an expert technologist (*see* also **step 14**). As the knife edge cuts through the resin, it causes the sections to become compressed. This may be alleviated by exposing the sections to vapors of organic solvents such as chloroform. The sections will appear to become smooth and large (Fig. 6c).

11. Collect the semithin sections by a pipette and transfer them to a drop of water on a microscope slide. One can use a glass pipette with a smoothened tip (briefly being heated over a flame).
12. Heat the slide on a heating plate and add a drop of 1% toluidine blue (in 5% borax, filtered) to stain on the plate for 10 s.
13. Wash gently the sections with ddH_2O using a plastic pipette. Dry again the slide on the hot plate. Examine the sections under a light microscope to identify areas of interest. We usually proceed by one or more sessions of approximately 30 cuts, 25–35 μm, in attempts to find glomeruli.
14. Once the area of interest is found, remove the knife and trim precisely the block to obtain a trapezoidal face of approximately 0.5 mm^2. To cut ultrathin sections of optimal quality, each operator uses a personal, dedicated diamond knife. Glass knifes with very good edge are less reliable. Orient again very carefully the block with respect to the knife and fill the tray with ddH_2O as above (Fig. 6b, c). Adjusting the cutting speed and thickness to the sectioning of the fragment, cut ultrathin sections of about 90–100 nm thick on the surface of the water. The thickness of the sections is determined by their refractive color. Good sections will appear silver (60 nm) to gold color (100 nm).
15. The ultrathin sections may form a ribbon on the water surface (Fig. 6c). An eyelash mounted on a stick is used for clustering the sections into small groups to be collected on the glossy side of copper grids by tweezers (Fig. 6d). Place gently the grid on a filter paper to dry in a covered plastic dish.

16. Place the required number of drops of UAR (diluted 4× in ddH_2O) on parafilm in a dish, one drop per grid. Using tweezers, place each grid face-down, with the sections in direct contact with the surface of the drop (Fig. 6e). Stain for 15 min. We use 10 cm petri dishes covered with aluminum foil. Optimal contrast of the EM image can be obtained by staining the sections with heavy metals. We use UAR stain which is specific for nucleic acids, and lead citrate which binds nucleic acids, membranes, and glycogen. UAR is used as an alternative to uranyl acetate stain due to environmental problem of radioactivity [18]. We filter the solution with a 0.22 μm filter applied to a syrinx.
17. Rinse each grid in ddH_2O by gently dipping and stirring. Use tissue culture dishes or a series of three small beakers; blot dry by pressing the surface of the grid on a piece of filter paper.
18. Place the grids on drops of lead citrate onto new parafilm in the petri dish with NaOH pellets which prevents formation of precipitates (Fig. 6e) (*see* **Note 15**). Stain for 10 min. Grids are best protected in numbered grid boxes before examination under the electron microscope. Avoid leaving them not protected, in free contact with air or too long in a plastic dish.
19. Rinse again the grids in ddH_2O and dry each grid as above.

3.4 Tissue Processing for Scanning Electron Microscopy

Fixation and initial steps of dehydration procedures for TEM and SEM are identical (Subheading 3.3, *see* **steps 1–4**).

1. Place the holder specimen of critical point dryer in a plastic container filled with 100% ETOH. Very quickly, place the tissue in the critical point drying holder slot. This is a crucial step and it is important that tissue be handled with care to avoid damaging or drying it. Insert specimen holder into the critical point drying instrument, fill the chamber with 100% ETOH, and cool to approximately 9–10 °C, as indicated in the manufacturers' recommendations (Fig. 7a). When the chamber is at the right temperature, add liquid carbon dioxide from a CO_2 cylinder to replace all ETOH with liquid CO_2. At this point, the chamber is slowly heated to the critical point under pressure. Once CO_2 is in the gas phase, it is slowly drained from the chamber (*see* **Note 16**).
2. Samples were mounted very carefully on aluminum SEM specimen stubs (12.5 mm diameter), taking care not to damage the biopsy with the fine-tipped forceps (*see* **Note 17**). Carbon-conductive mounting tabs, double-sided adhesive disks, can be pressed onto a specimen stub and leave a conductive carbon adhesive when the backing material is removed. This adhesive maintains the sample's mechanical stability (Fig. 7b).

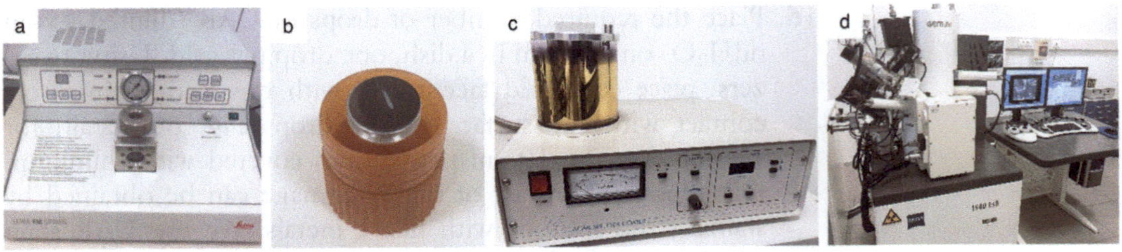

Fig. 7 This panel shows the technique of sample processing for scanning electron microscopy. (**a**) Dehydration with a critical point dryer; (**b**) the sample is mounted very carefully on an aluminum scanning electron microscope specimen stub; (**c**) the specimen is coated with a deposition of a thin layer of gold using a sputter coater; (**d**) the biopsy, ready for examination, is inserted into the sample chamber of the scanning electron microscope

3. Dehydrated samples need to be electrically conductive. To this end, the specimen is coated with a deposition of a thin layer of conductive metal, such as gold. The layer of gold increases the amount of secondary electrons that can be detected from the surface of the sample and it needs to have a fine grain and to be distributed evenly across the specimen surface with a sputter coater (Fig. 7c).
4. After metallization, place the stub in a SEM storage box. It is recommended that, until they are ready for examination, specimens be allowed to dry overnight in a desiccator.
5. Insert the stub into the sample chamber of the SEM (Fig. 7d). When the specimen is finally ready for examination, the operator must adjust several parameters that can greatly affect the quality of the images and consequently the quality of the analysis. Among these factors, the most important include voltage, depth of field, microscope aperture, focus and astigmatism, noise, and background. It is good practice to adjust electron beam alignment, focusing, and proper stigmation at magnifications higher than those used for imaging (*see* **Note 18**).

4 Notes

We suggest that a specially trained technologist be present during the needle biopsy procedure and sample procurement to see that the tissue is handled properly and utilized to the greatest advantage.

1. Many of the fixatives and solvents in histochemistry are highly toxic (refer to material safety data sheets for correct and safe handling). Throughout the procedure wear gloves, goggles, and lab coat. Work under hood or well-ventilated area. Avoid contact and inhalation. Dubosq-Brasil fluid contains picric acid that is highly explosive when dry. It is therefore best handled as a commercially prepared saturated aqueous solution.

Formaldehyde is a severe eye and skin irritant, sensitizer by skin and respiratory contact, and toxic by ingestion and inhalation. Target organ effects are on respiratory system and it is proven to be a carcinogen. Label with "Formaldehyde warning" sticker. Acetic acid is corrosive, and its target organ effects are on respiratory system. Xylene, although not proven to be a carcinogen, may cause headaches as a side effect to inhalation of the vapor and is flammable and toxic through skin exposure.

2. The specimen must be processed carefully, avoiding compressing or fragmenting it. In addition, because renal biopsy specimens are very small, prolonged exposure to the dehydrating and clearing agents should be avoided.
3. After paraffin block sectioning, during the transfer of the ribbon from the microtome to the worktable, avoid any exposure to airflow. The ribbon is very fragile and thin; it can easily rip off, break, or fold.
4. Liquid nitrogen is one of the cryogenic liquids commonly used in research labs. The major hazards of liquid nitrogen are associated with the properties of extreme cold and evaporation. Use only approved containers that can withstand the extremely low temperatures. Dewars should not be filled to more than 80% of capacity, since expansion of gases during warming may cause excessive pressure buildup. While wearing eye/face protection and thermal resistant gloves, open the tank valve and carefully fill the Dewar flask with liquid nitrogen to approximately one-half. Close the valve, remove the dispensing hose, and cover the Dewar flask.
5. Tissue submitted for IF should not be fixed with cross-linking fixatives. Never use forceps that have been previously soaked in Dubosq-Brasil fluid while handling the IF specimen.
6. Throughout the procedures of processing and sectioning, keep the temperature inside the cryostat at −25 °C. Kimwipes and paintbrushes should be cooled in the cryostat before use.
7. The IF method described in this chapter can be easily modified embedding the specimen in an apposite plastic mold filled with OCT compound prior to freezing it in liquid nitrogen. Results between the two methods are comparable as long as one keeps in mind the importance of a proper specimen orientation during OCT embedding, which directly affects the quality of the sections.
8. Acetone is a colorless volatile liquid. Remember that it is highly flammable and can irritate eyes, nose, and throat. It is not known to cause cancer.
9. Quality control material for IF is not available commercially. Biopsy material is a very valuable resource and quality control should be performed just upon receipt of new lots of antibody

reagents [19]. A previously stained kidney biopsy specimen that is positive for the target antigen of the new antibody reagent will be pulled for testing reactivity of the new lot in comparison with the old lot of antibody reagents. A skilled and experienced observer can evaluate the intensity and localization of immunoreactants while recognizing the normal background and internal positive controls for each antigen tested. Each biopsy is evaluated on a case-by-case basis and examined for internal staining patterns. Internal controls exist for many of the antigens in routine use. For example, IgA is generally present in tubular casts, IgG in protein droplets, and C3 in blood vessels. Each biopsy will have a tissue section stained with a drop of PBS to act as the negative staining control.

10. The preparation of biological specimens for electron microscopy poses biological, chemical, and mechanical risks to the user. Understanding the requirements for proper protection is imperative in order to minimize exposure when handling infectious agents, hazardous tools, and chemicals, and operating high-voltage instrumentation. General protection measures include using appropriate fume hood; wearing adequate equipment including lab coats, gloves, and eye protection; and correct maintenance of the electron microscope. The reader is referred to data sheets and specific recommendations provided by manufacturers. Work in a hood for any electron microscopy procedure whenever possible, particularly involving materials for fixation, infiltration, embedding, and staining. Precise measures apply for waste disposal.
11. Glutaraldehyde penetrates the tissue slowly so a thickness of 1 mm serves to allow more rapid fixation. It does not fix lipids; therefore the postfixation in osmium is carried out to preserve the membranes. Prepare the fixative solution fresh and use it ice cold. Cacodylate buffer, 0.1 M, pH 7.4 is also prepared freshly. A 0.2 M stock solution of sodium cacodylate trihydrate ($C_2H_6AsNaO_2 \cdot 3H_2O$) can be made in a hood and stored at 4–8 °C in an amber glass bottle. Given the carcinogenic and mutagenic activity of glutaric aldehyde and the toxicity of osmium tetroxide, care must be taken in the use of these substances avoiding contact with the skin and inhalation of vapors through the supply of extractor hoods.
12. Osmium tetroxide solutions are commercially available. Less preferably, due to possible hazard, one can prepare the fixative starting from OsO4 crystals. The ampoule (1 g osmium) is inserted in an amber glass bottle which must be absolutely clean. Close tightly and shake the bottle to crush the ampoule. Add 50 mL ddH_2O. Prepare at least 1 day before use to ensure that the crystals dissolve completely. Store the solution at 4–8 °C. Prepare the working fixative just before use, mixing

equal parts of stock osmium tetroxide and 0.2 M cacodylate buffer resulting in 1% osmium tetroxide in 0.1 M cacodylate buffer. Residual osmium tetroxide after fixation can be fully neutralized by twice the volume of oil (corn oil is preferred because of its high percentage of unsaturated bonds).

13. The dehydration of the tissue is one of the most critical steps in the electron microscopy sample processing. The dehydration steps must be carried out as rapidly as possible to avoid the coarctation of lipid-containing tissue components.

14. Preparation of epoxy resin: In a glass cylinder pour 10 mL Durcupan ACM, add 36 mL of epoxy embedding medium DDSA, and mix gently by hand for 10 min. In another cylinder pour 12 mL of Epon 812, add 400 μL of Epon accelerator DMP30, and mix as before. Join the two solutions thus obtained in a 50 mL tube, coated with aluminum foil, and place on rotator/mixer for 10 min. Divide the resin in two plastic 25 mL syringes (discard the needles, seal with parafilm, and wrap with aluminum foil). The syringes can be stored in a refrigerator and used for up to 30 days. Bring the syringe to room temperature before each use and back to the fridge thereafter. It is essential to mix the various components of epoxy resin accurately, so as to obtain a single homogeneous phase, free of air bubbles, able to harden evenly. Epoxy resin has adequate viscosity, and is fairly stable under the intense electron beam. Resins when polymerized are virtually not destructible, as are the tissues once embedded in them. The purpose of the embedding medium is to provide a stable, hard matrix throughout a tissue to be cut into very thin sections. Epoxy resin can be irritating to skin and eyes and is known to be carcinogenic.

15. Preparation of lead citrate: Weigh 0.0225 g of lead citrate and dissolve in 1 mL of 1 N NaOH. Add 9 mL of sterile H_2O. Place in a 10 mL tin and centrifuge for 15 min at 3300 rcf. Store at room temperature in the dark. At the time of use place in a syringe equipped with a 0.22 μm filter. Be careful not to shake the tube. Do not collect the dye from the surface, which is rich in CO_2, the main cause of formation of precipitates.

    Notes 10–12 of TEM section apply also for SEM.

16. The dehydration of the sample is the most essential step in the SEM sample processing. For this reason, all dehydration steps, especially heating and venting with critical point drying, require patience and must be carried out very slowly and in a reproducible way to minimize the effects of surface tension forces that can cause specimen distortions and artifacts.

17. The exact localization of all superficial glomeruli present on the biopsy core surface is conducted under a stereomicroscope.

This is a very important step that enables the sample to be mounted in the correct position on the stub in order to view the few glomeruli that are usually present on its surface.

18. Although there are general guidelines for how to set up SEM for the observation of biological samples, in practice, optimal settings may vary greatly depending on the sample itself and on the application. Best microscope's settings vary for each sample that is observed.

References

1. Afkarian M, Zelnick LR, Hall YN, Heagerty PJ, Tuttle K, Weiss NS, de Boer IH (2016) Clinical manifestations of kidney disease among us adults with diabetes, 1988-2014. JAMA 316 (6):602–610. https://doi.org/10.1001/jama.2016.10924
2. WHO: Global status report on noncommunicable diseases 2014. http://www.who.int/nmh/publications/ncd-status-report-2014/en/
3. Chen L, Magliano DJ, Zimmet PZ (2011) The worldwide epidemiology of type 2 diabetes mellitus—present and future perspectives. Nat Rev Endocrinol 8(4):228–236. https://doi.org/10.1038/nrendo.2011.183
4. Ritz E, Zeng XX, Rychlik I (2011) Clinical manifestation and natural history of diabetic nephropathy. Contrib Nephrol 170:19–27. https://doi.org/10.1159/000324939
5. Porrini E, Ruggenenti P, Mogensen CE, Barlovic DP, Praga M, Cruzado JM, Hojs R, Abbate M, de Vries AP (2015) Non-proteinuric pathways in loss of renal function in patients with type 2 diabetes. Lancet Diabetes Endocrinol 3(5):382–391. https://doi.org/10.1016/S2213-8587(15)00094-7
6. Fioretto P, Mauer M (2007) Histopathology of diabetic nephropathy. Semin Nephrol 27 (2):195–207. https://doi.org/10.1016/j.semnephrol.2007.01.012
7. Fioretto P, Caramori ML, Mauer M (2008) The kidney in diabetes: dynamic pathways of injury and repair. The Camillo Golgi Lecture 2007. Diabetologia 51(8):1347–1355. https://doi.org/10.1007/s00125-008-1051-7
8. Alicic RZ, Rooney MT, Tuttle KR (2017) Diabetic kidney disease: challenges, progress, and possibilities. Clin J Am Soc Nephrol 12 (12):2032–2045. https://doi.org/10.2215/CJN.11491116
9. Najafian B, Alpers CE, Fogo AB (2011) Pathology of human diabetic nephropathy. In: Ronco C (ed) Contributions to nephrology, vol 170. Karger, Basel, pp 36–47. https://doi.org/10.1159/000324942
10. Conti S, Perico N, Novelli R, Carrara C, Benigni A, Remuzzi G (2018) Early and late scanning electron microscopy findings in diabetic kidney disease. Sci Rep 8(1):4909. https://doi.org/10.1038/s41598-018-23244-2
11. Sharma SG, Bomback AS, Radhakrishnan J, Herlitz LC, Stokes MB, Markowitz GS, D'Agati VD (2013) The modern spectrum of renal biopsy findings in patients with diabetes. Clin J Am Soc Nephrol 8(10):1718–1724. https://doi.org/10.2215/CJN.02510213
12. Gambara V, Mecca G, Remuzzi G, Bertani T (1993) Heterogeneous nature of renal lesions in type II diabetes. J Am Soc Nephrol 3:1458–1466
13. Gluck C, Ko YA, Susztak K (2017) Precision medicine approaches to diabetic kidney disease: tissue as an issue. Curr Diab Rep 17(5):30. https://doi.org/10.1007/s11892-017-0854-7
14. Fioretto P, Steffes MW, Sutherland DE, Goetz FC, Mauer M (1998) Reversal of lesions of diabetic nephropathy after pancreas transplantation. N Engl J Med 339(2):69–75
15. Pichaiwong W, Hudkins KL, Wietecha T, Nguyen TQ, Tachaudomdach C, Li W, Askari B, Kobayashi T, O'Brien KD, Pippin JW, Shankland SJ, Alpers CE (2013) Reversibility of structural and functional damage in a model of advanced diabetic nephropathy. J Am Soc Nephrol 24(7):1088–1102
16. Andeen NK, Nguyen TQ, Steegh F, Hudkins KL, Najafian B, Alpers CE (2015) The phenotypes of podocytes and parietal epithelial cells may overlap in diabetic nephropathy. Kidney Int 88(5):1099–1107. https://doi.org/10.1038/ki.2015.273
17. Suvarna K, Layton C, Bancroft J (2012) Bancroft's theory and practice of histological techniques, 7th edn. Churchill Livingstone Elsevier, London

18. Nakakoshi M, Nishioka H, Katayama E (2011) New versatile staining reagents for biological transmission electron microscopy that substitute for uranyl acetate. J Electron Microsc 60 (6):401–407. https://doi.org/10.1093/jmicro/dfr084

19. Jennette JC (1998) Crescentic glomerulonephritis. In: Jennette JC, Olson JL, Schwarz M, Silva FG (eds) Heptinstall's pathology of the kidney, 5th edn. Lippincott-Raven, New York

Chapter 7

Sample Preparation and Stereological Methods for the Study of Glomerular Ultrastructure Using Electron Microscopy

Kathryn E. White

Abstract

In this chapter we describe conventional methods used for preparing renal tissue for transmission electron microscopy. We also describe a relatively new technique, serial block face scanning electron microscopy. Protocols are given for processing, sectioning, and imaging of tissue along with methods for obtaining quantitative data from the results.

Key words Glomerulus, Mesangium, Podocyte, Stereology, Electron microscopy

1 Introduction

The classic lesions of diabetic glomerulopathy—mesangial expansion and thickening of the glomerular basement membrane—were described decades ago [1–5]. However they have continued to be of interest in multiple studies exploring development and treatment of diabetes [6–9]. Although the lesions can be identified by light microscopy, early changes can only be detected and accurately quantified using electron microscopy (EM). Transmission EM (TEM) can also allow detailed examination of the filtration surface of the glomerulus comprising the basement membrane, endothelial cells, and podocytes. Most studies have concentrated on the glomerulus but it is also recognized that the tubulointerstitium has a role in the development of diabetic nephropathy [10].

The first—and arguably the most important—stage in processing tissue for EM is fixation. Inadequate fixation of tissue leads to suboptimal results with images difficult to interpret due to the presence of artifacts. The primary fixative used is generally glutaraldehyde, which penetrates the tissue and cross-links proteins to "fix" the structures in as lifelike a state as possible.

Luigi Gnudi and David A. Long (eds.), *Diabetic Nephropathy: Methods and Protocols*, Methods in Molecular Biology, vol. 2067, https://doi.org/10.1007/978-1-4939-9841-8_7,

Fixation of renal tissue can be either by perfusion or by immersion. Perfusion fixation gives the best results but obviously cannot be carried out on human tissue. For animal studies it can be advantageous to remove one kidney to use, e.g., RNA analysis before perfuse-fixing the other kidney in situ. However this limits what can be done with other organs so immersion fixation is often the method of choice.

Glutaraldehyde is a relatively large molecule and penetrates tissue much slower than other aldehydes such as formaldehyde used in tissue fixation for light microscopy. Therefore with immersion fixation, the tissue pieces for EM must be very small (needle biopsy or approximately 1 mm^3) or the fixative will not reach the cells before they start to degrade. In addition, the subsequent processing involves dehydration of the tissue and, if fixation is not complete, excessive extraction of cellular components will occur.

The other component of the fixative is a buffer and there have been a variety of different buffers used in human renal biopsy studies—modified Tyrode [9], Millong [11], and cacodylate [12]—but all have a similar osmolality and pH. Phosphate buffers can sometimes produce deposits in tissue and therefore in our laboratory sodium cacodylate is often the buffer of choice. It has been used in a number of animal studies, again with a similar osmolality and pH. It should be noted that the proximal tubule is particularly sensitive to osmolality and a fixative-buffer combination that is adequate for the glomerulus may not be suitable for the tubules [13].

For transmission EM, primary fixation is followed by secondary fixation using osmium tetroxide. Osmium tetroxide is a strong oxidizing agent and binds lipids, including those in the cell membrane. As well as enhancing preservation of membranes, the osmium, being a heavy metal, adds contrast to the biological tissue when viewed under the TEM.

After primary and secondary fixation is complete, the tissue is dehydrated through a graded series of either acetone or ethanol. The removal of water and replacement with acetone or ethanol has to be a gradual process to reduce "shock" to the cells. Once in 100% solvent, the solvent is gradually replaced by epoxy resin. After 100% epoxy resin has penetrated the tissue, the tissue pieces are embedded in fresh resin and polymerized at 60 °C to form a hard block. This block is then sectioned on an ultramicrotome; ultrathin sections are picked up on copper grids, stained with uranyl acetate and lead citrate to increase the contrast, and viewed under the TEM.

With TEM, one generally examines a single section through the structure of interest, whether it be a glomerulus, podocyte, or mitochondrion. Therefore, unless serial sectioning is performed, the resulting 2D images are only "snapshots" of the whole structure. Serial sectioning for TEM is extremely time consuming and difficult and even the most experienced technician will lose some sections. However, new technologies have been developed that allow multiple images to be collected through a structure with much less effort and a great deal of more accuracy. These technologies are serial block face scanning electron microscopy (SBFSEM), focus ion beam scanning electron microscopy (FIBSEM), and automated tape collection ultramicrotome (ATUMtome). In each case a z-stack of images is collected using a scanning EM and structures of interest can then be segmented for 3D reconstruction.

This chapter includes protocols for one of these techniques: SBFSEM. For SBFSEM the tissue needs to be of high contrast as the technique works by collecting backscattered electrons from the surface of the resin block. After primary fixation, tissue undergoes a "heavy metal protocol" in which the tissue is impregnated with a number of different heavy metals, including osmium, before being dehydrated and embedded in resin as above. It is of even greater importance that the tissue pieces are small; otherwise the heavy metals will not penetrate into the center of the sample. For SBFSEM, a mini ultramicrotome is incorporated inside a SEM so that the sectioning and imaging take place in situ. Sections are taken from the block but they are discarded and it is the surface of the block that is imaged. The section, image, section, and image routine is repeated for a specified z distance, resulting in a stack of high-resolution images. The magnification, resolution, and distance z can all be optimized depending on whether the structure is a whole glomerulus or a single cell within the glomerulus for example.

2 Materials

2.1 Buffers

Phosphate buffers have been considered most suitable for renal tissue, with many modified versions used. Recipes for one modified buffer (Tyrode) and more commonly used buffers (cacodylate and Sorensen's) are given here. Buffer should be stored in the fridge and discarded if it becomes cloudy. They are all made up as 0.2 M stock solutions and used at a final working dilution of 0.1 M, pH 7.4.

2.1.1 Modified Tyrode Buffer

The following powders are dissolved in 500 mL deionized water (final volume):

Water-free glucose	1.0 g
KCl	0.2 g
NaH_2PO_4	0.05 g
$NaHCO_3$	1.0 g
NaCl	3.5 g
$CaCl_2$ (50% solution)	0.79 mL
$MgCl_2$ (50% solution)	0.2 mL

2.1.2 Sorensen's Phosphate Buffer (0.2 M)

Solution A: Monobasic $NaH_2PO_4.H_2O$ 27.6 g in 1000 mL deionized water; stir until dissolved.

Solution B: Dibasic $Na_2HPO_4.2H_2O$ 28.4 g in 1000 mL with deionized water; stir until dissolved.

Add 9.5 mL of solution A to 40.5 mL of solution B to give 50 mL 0.2 M phosphate buffer; adjust pH to 7.4.

2.1.3 Sodium Cacodylate Buffer (0.2 M)

Solution A: Sodium cacodylate 21.4 g in 500 mL deionized water.

Solution B: 1.7 mL HCl in 100 mL deionized water (0.2 N HCL).

Add 5 mL solution B to 100 mL solution A to obtain pH 7.4.

Filter using Nalgene filter and vacuum pump. (*Caution*: It is poisonous and carcinogenic; use in fume hood, and wear lab coat and gloves.)

2.2 Fixatives

2.2.1 2% Glutaraldehyde

1. 8 mL EM-grade glutaraldehyde (25%) (*caution*: irritant, use in fume hood, wear lab coat and gloves).
2. 50 mL 0.2 M Buffer cacodylate or Sorenson's.
3. 42 mL Deionized water.

2.2.2 1% Osmium Tetroxide

Osmium tetroxide is purchased as sealed ampoules of either 1 g crystal or 2% or 4% solution. It is highly toxic and should only be used in the fume hood and disposed of properly (*see* **Note 1**). The ampoules containing osmium already in solution are recommended over the solid osmium.

Transfer the solution from the ampoule to a clean 25 mL glass jar and dilute 1:1 with deionized water (*see* **Note 2**).

2.3 Heavy Metal Solutions for SBFSEM

2.3.1 Potassium Ferrocyanide in Osmium Tetroxide

Add

1. 0.3 g Potassium ferrocyanide to 5 mL 4% aqueous osmium tetroxide.
2. 5 mL Deionized water.

2.3.2 Thiocarbohydrazide (TCH) Solution

Add

1. 0.1 g TCH to 10 mL deionized water (enough for 4–6 samples) (*see* **Note 3**).

Place in sealed 25 mL glass jar in 60 °C oven for 1 h. Agitate occasionally to aid in dissolving of powder. Filter solution through 0.22 μm syringe filter and use when cooled.

2.3.3 Aspartic Acid Stock

Dissolve 0.998 g of L-aspartic acid in 250 mL of deionized water. Adjust to pH 5.5 by adding approximately 3.5 mL 1 M KOH to 125 mL of aspartic acid solution (*see* **Note 4**).

2.3.4 Lead Aspartate Solution (Stock Powder Weighed Out into Small Vials Ready for Use)

Add 0.12 g of lead nitrate to 20 mL of aspartic acid stock solution. Place in 60 °C oven for 30 min. No precipitate should form if the pH is correct.

2.3.5 Uranyl Acetate

Weigh 2 g uranyl acetate into a volumetric flask and fill to 100 mL with deionized water. Dilute 1:1 with deionized water to make a 1% working solution.

2.4 Acetone Solutions for Dehydration

25%, 50%, 75% acetone in deionized water.

100% acetone (stored in glass bottles in desiccator).

2.5 Resin

There are several different resins available from a number of manufacturers. They are comprised of three or four components that need to be mixed in the correct quantities—epoxy resin, hardeners, and accelerators. Some come in kit form so they require no measuring or weighing out of chemicals; the different components are simply added to each other. The resins also come in soft, medium, or hard, referring to their hardness once polymerized. For standard TEM, medium resin is recommended; for SBFSEM hard resin, such as 812, is required for best results (*caution*: irritant, use in fume hood, wear lab coat and gloves).

We recommend using the resin kits. Add all components to the largest bottle and mix well by shaking for several minutes. Transfer the resin to a polypropylene dropping bottle for dispensing (*see* **Note 5**). A resin series is required for impregnation—25%, 50%, 75%, and 100% in acetone.

2.6 Toluidine Blue for Light Microscopy

Dissolve 2.5 g borax (disodium tetraborate) in 500 mL distilled water. Add 5 g toluidine blue, and filter before use.

3 Methods

3.1 Processing

All processing is carried out in small clean flat-bottomed glass pots. At each stage the solution is decanted off and replaced with the next solution (*see* **Note 6**). Unless otherwise stated, pots are placed on a rotator at room temperature. Processing must be carried out in a fume hood.

3.1.1 Standard TEM Processing

1. Fix small pieces of renal cortex (1 × 1 × 1 mm) in 2% glutaraldehyde in 0.1 M cacodylate buffer overnight in refrigerator (*see* **Note 7**).
2. Rinse in three changes of 0.1 M cacodylate buffer, 15 min each, before secondary fixation in 1% osmium tetroxide for 1 h.

3. Rinse in two changes of deionized water, 15 min each, before starting the dehydration in acetone (25%, 50%, 75%, 30 min each; 100% two changes, 1 h each).
4. Using an epoxy medium resin kit, mixed to the manufacturer's specification, impregnate with 25% resin in acetone, and then 50%, 75%, and 100%, all for 1 h. Samples can be left overnight on the rotator at this stage.
5. Next day, do three changes of 100% resin over several hours before embedding the tissue in 100% resin in coffin molds or Beem capsules and place in 60 °C oven for 24–36 h to polymerize (*see* **Note 8**). Include a small label with sample number in the mold.

3.1.2 Serial Block Face Scanning Electron Microscopy Processing

1. Fix small pieces of renal cortex (1 × 1 × 1 mm) in 2% glutaraldehyde in 0.1 M cacodylate buffer overnight in refrigerator.
2. Rinse in three changes of buffer, 15 min each, before secondary fixation in 3% potassium ferrocyanide and in 2% osmium tetroxide for 1 h. Preparation of TCH solution should be started at this point.
3. Rinse in five changes of deionized water, 3 min each.
4. Place in filtered TCH for 20 min (this is the most critical step in terms of timing as the solution will precipitate out if left too long).
5. Rinse in five changes of deionized water, 3 min each.
6. Place in 2% osmium tetroxide in deionized water for 30 min.
7. Rinse in five changes of deionized water, 3 min each.
8. Place in 1% uranyl acetate at 4 °C (in refrigerator) overnight.
9. Rinse in five changes of deionized water, 3 min each (preparation of lead aspartate solution should be started at this point).
10. Place in lead aspartate solution for 30 min at 60 °C.
11. Rinse in five changes of deionized water, 3 min each.
12. Tissue can now be dehydrated through a graded series of acetone as for standard TEM (25%, 50%, 75%, 30 min each; 100% two changes, 1 h each).
13. Using an epoxy hard resin kit (*see* **Note 9**), mixed to the manufacturer's specification, impregnate with increasing resin concentration (25%, 50%, 75%, 100%) in acetone, each step for 1 h. Samples can be left overnight on the rotator at this stage.
14. Next day, do three changes of 100% resin over several hours before embedding the tissue in 100% resin in coffin molds or Beem capsules and place in 60 °C oven for 24–36 h to polymerize. Include a small label with sample number in the mold.

3.2 Sectioning

3.2.1 TEM Sectioning

Once the blocks have been polymerized they can be removed from the plastic molds and trimmed using a glass knife or razor blade to remove excess resin from the block face. Blocks for SBFSEM are also examined by TEM. Before cutting ultrathin sections for TEM it is advisable to cut "semi-thin" sections of 0.5–1 μm for light microscopy in order to ensure that there are glomeruli in the sectioned face. The block face is trimmed to a trapezoid shape, which reduces compression of the section and also aids in orientation. The semi-thin sections are cut with a diamond (or glass) knife; the sections float onto the attached water bath and can be picked up using a single-bristle brush (*see* **Note 10**) and refloated into a droplet of water on a glass slide. The sections are dried on a hot plate and stained with a drop of toluidine blue for 30 s while still on the hotplate. After rinsing in water the sections can be examined under the light microscope; if glomeruli are present then ultrathin sections can be taken; if there are no glomeruli the block can be trimmed further to reveal more tissue.

Once glomeruli are present in the block face, ultrathin sections of 70 nm are cut using a diamond knife and picked up onto copper washer grids (*see* **Note 11**). Sections from tissue that has been processed using the heavy metal process require no further staining and can be examined immediately on the TEM. Sections from tissue that has been processed using the standard protocol require staining with heavy metals to increase contrast. Grid staining is best carried out using an automatic staining machine; the stains used are 1% uranyl acetate and 3% lead citrate (*see* **Note 12**).

3.2.2 Pin Preparation for SBFSEM

Once glomeruli have been found in the block, the piece of resin containing the tissue is sawn off the rest of the block and glued onto a 3view pin. Silver glue is painted around the sample, which is then sputter-coated with 5 nm of gold to reduce charging in the SEM.

3.3 TEM Imaging

The number of images and magnification required is dependent on the objective. For qualitative data, images will be taken of any areas representative of the structure of interest, e.g., areas of GBM thickening and abnormalities in podocytes (Fig. 1). For quantitative data however, imaging must be unbiased, i.e., nothing must be selectively chosen. In order to estimate mesangial expansion, the whole glomerular profile is imaged at a relatively low magnification. For GBM thickening or podocyte foot process width however, a higher magnification is required to visualize the structures and it would be unrealistic to try and image the whole profile. Instead a systematic random sampling approach is taken to get an unbiased representation covering approximately 25% of the whole profile (it is possible to cover a greater area in mice). Starting at the top left of the glomerulus, an image is taken and the stage is moved a fixed number of microns in the x-direction and imaged again. This is repeated until the right-hand side of the glomerulus is reached

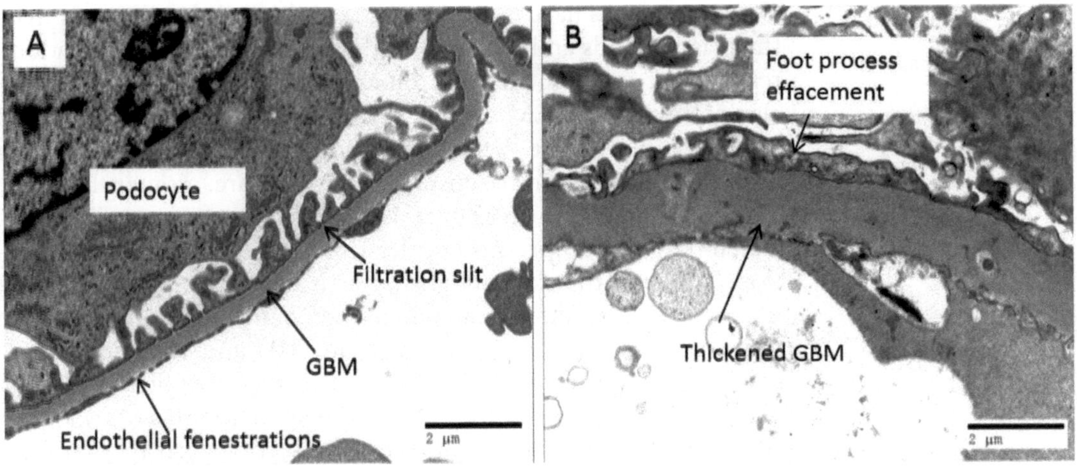

Fig. 1 Transmission EM images of (**a**) control and (**b**) type 1 diabetic patient showing the glomerular filtration barrier. In (**b**) the GBM is thickened and there is widening of the podocyte foot processes with loss of filtration slits

and the stage is moved a fixed number of microns in the y-direction and imaged and then movement returns back in the x-direction. Many electron microscopes have automated programs for this type of sampling; however it is very straightforward to do manually.

3.4 Quantification

There are a number of parameters that have been used to quantify the severity of diabetic glomerulopathy—mesangial volume fraction, GBM width, podocyte number, and podocyte foot process width (FPW) being the most often reported. There are several image analysis programs that can be used for quantification, e.g., ImageJ and Image Pro Plus.

Mesangial volume fraction gives an estimate of the extent of mesangial expansion in the glomerulus and is the ratio of the structure of interest (mesangium) to its reference volume (glomerulus). It is estimated using a grid of points randomly placed on a 2D section. The reference space is defined by the minimal string polygon outlining the glomerular tuft. The number of points hitting the reference space and on the structure of interest is counted. For efficiency, a coarse and fine grid with a ratio of 1:8 can be used—the coarse grid used to count points on the glomerular tuft and the fine grid used to count points on the mesangium (Fig. 2).

By the principle of Delesse (1847) [14], the area of a structure per unit area of the reference space (A_a) is directly related to the volume fraction of that same structure to the reference volume (V_v), i.e., $V_v \approx A_a$.

Therefore $V_v = \text{Pmes}/(\text{Pglom}*8)$ where Pmes is the number of points on mesangium and Pglom is the number of points on the glomerular tuft.

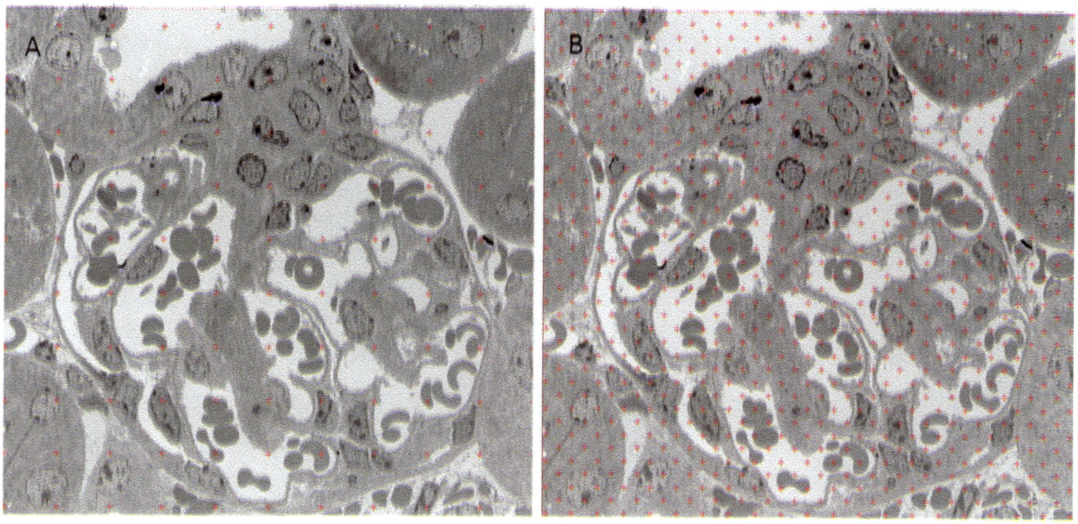

Fig. 2 Transmission EM images of a glomerular profile. The glomerular tuft is delineated with a minimal string polygon to define the reference space. (**a**) A grid of coarse points is superimposed on the image and the number of points landing on the glomerular tuft is counted. (**b**) A grid of fine points is superimposed on the image and the number of points landing on the mesangium is counted. The ratio of coarse to fine points is 1:8. Mesangial volume fraction is calculated as Pmes/(Pglom∗8)

Glomerular basement membrane width can be measured directly on the 2D images using the line tool. In order to select, without bias, the portion of GBM that will be measured, a grid of lines is superimposed on the image. The GBM is measured wherever a grid line intersects with the endothelium, perpendicular to the endothelium (Fig. **3**).

Podocyte number: The gold standard for estimating podocyte number is the dissector/fractionator method on serial sections and light microscopy [15, 16]. A more precise method would be to use SBFSEM to image a whole glomerulus, allowing the absolute number of podocytes to be counted. However it is time consuming and unlikely to be feasible on large numbers of glomeruli. An alternative using transmission EM is to estimate podocyte number density (N_v) and multiply this by glomerular volume to give podocyte number:

$$N = N_V \times V \tag{1}$$

When counting particles it is necessary to give each of them an equal chance of being sampled. Particles in 3D space that are cut by a 2D section will be seen as profiles. Each section will hit a particle in proportion to its size and more specifically its height normal to the section. This will therefore bias against smaller particles in a population (*see* **Note 13**).

The method of Weibel and Gomez [17] has attempted to overcome some of these problems using the equation

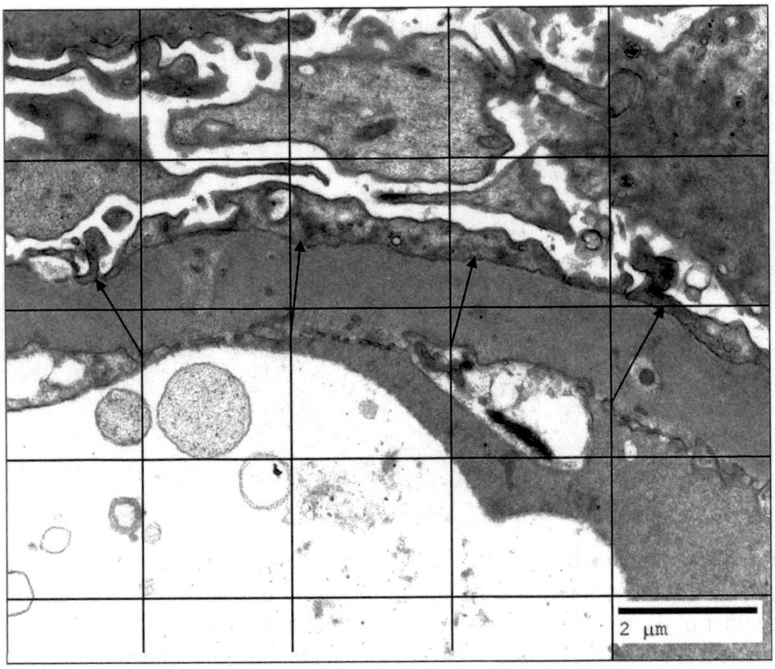

Fig. 3 Transmission EM image of the glomerular basement membrane. A grid of lines is superimposed on the image for the estimation of GBM width. The GBM is measured wherever a grid line intersects with the endothelium, perpendicular to the endothelium

$$N_V = K/\beta\sqrt{N_A^3/V_v} \quad (2)$$

where N_A is the profile density of the particles, V_v is the volume fraction of the particles, K is a size distribution coefficient, and β is a shape constant. For most biological applications the size distribution coefficient, K, varies between 1 and 1.05 and can therefore be neglected [12].

Measurements are performed on a single section through the glomerulus. A grid of coarse and fine points (ratio 1:X) is superimposed onto the glomerular profile. The numbers of podocyte nuclear profiles (n) (assuming one nucleus per cell) and coarse points (P_{tuft}) hitting the glomerular tuft are counted in order to estimate podocyte nuclear profile density (N_A):

$$N_A = \Sigma n/[\Sigma P_{tuft} \times \text{area per point}] \quad (3)$$

The number of fine points (P_{cell}) hitting podocyte nuclear profiles is counted to calculate the volume fraction of podocyte nuclei in glomerular tuft (V_V):

$$V_V = \Sigma P_{cell}/(\Sigma P_{tuft} \times X) \quad (4)$$

where X is the ratio of coarse to fine points

The number density of cells can then be calculated from Eq. 2, with a shape constant chosen depending upon whether the cells are considered to be spherical, an ellipse, or an ellipsoid. The shape constant used for podocyte nuclei for an ellipsoid is 1.55.

Foot process width can be measured directly on the images but a more efficient way is to measure the length of the GBM and divide it by the number of filtration slits (this assumes that the width of the slit itself is negligible). The mean of the FPW is calculated as

$$\text{FPW} = \Sigma\,\text{GBM length}/\Sigma\,\text{filtration slits}$$

where Σ filtration slits is the total number of filtration slits counted in each image and Σ GBM length is the total GBM length measured in each image.

3.5 SBFSEM Imaging and 3D Reconstruction

Although a great deal of information can be learnt from both qualitative and quantitative TEM analysis, it is inevitable that some assumptions have to be made when working with 2D images. With SBFSEM there is now the opportunity to obtain a z-stack of images and so reconstruct glomerular structures in 3D, revealing morphological arrangements that had not previously been apparent [18, 19]. There are a number of computer packages available to perform the initial segmentation of the structure of interest and subsequent 3D reconstruction (Fig. 4). Some of these (Fiji, Microscopy Image Browser) are free and others (Amira, Image Premier 3D) require licenses. These programs are not always intuitive; therefore workshops and online tutorials are recommended.

4 Notes

1. Osmium tetroxide waste is discarded into a glass bottle containing corn oil, which neutralizes the osmium. The ampoule and all containers coming into contact with osmium should be rinsed in corn oil before disposal.
2. The osmium can be diluted with buffer rather than water. However, we find that this increases the chance of buffer deposit. In addition, once in osmium, osmolality is no longer an issue as osmium renders membranes impermeable.
3. We recommend weighing out stock powders of all the heavy metal components into small vials ready for use.
4. Lead aspartate cannot be stored for long at pH 5.5. If there is a need to store, store prior to adding the KOH. The solution can form a precipitate if the pH is wrong.
5. Mixing the resin by shaking will result in bubbles in the resin, which will interfere with the embedding. Therefore always

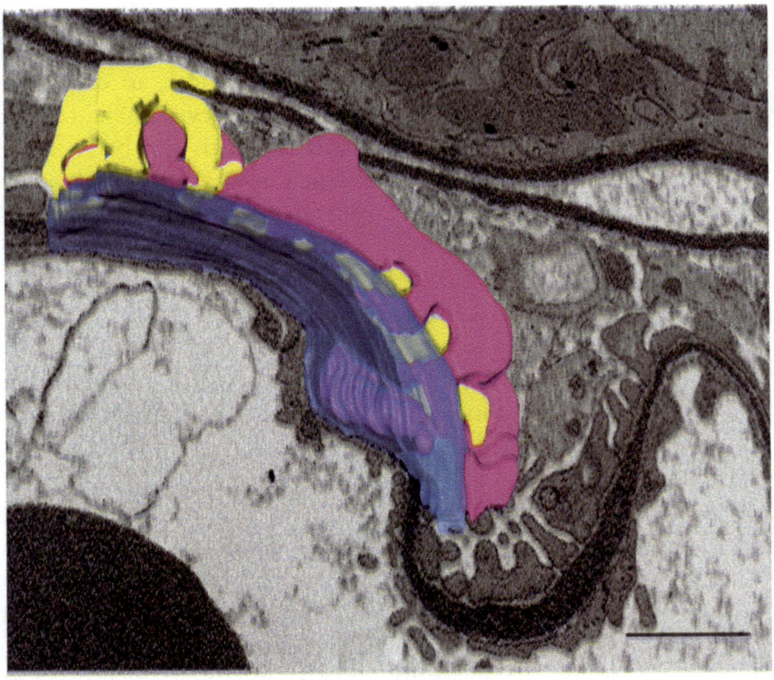

Fig. 4 SBFSEM image and 3D model of part of the glomerular filtration barrier from a diabetic mouse. The podocyte foot processes from two cells (yellow and pink) interdigitate with each other. A foot process from one podocyte (pink) is seen protruding through the GBM (blue). Scale bar 1 μm

allow enough time between mixing the resin components and embedding the samples for the bubbles to disappear.

6. Do not use plastic pots as plastic reacts with osmium and acetone. Ensure that there is enough volume of liquid to fully immerse the tissue pieces and allow adequate moving when on the rotator.
7. It is important that the pieces are small as glutaraldehyde is slow acting. Several pieces from one sample can be processed in the same pot. Tissue can be stored in the fixative for several days. If it is to be stored for longer periods (several weeks) replace fixative with a weaker solution of 1% glutaraldehyde in buffer.
8. Leftover resin can either be polymerized and disposed of or frozen for later use. If frozen, it is recommend to be used only for the acetone-resin infiltration steps and not for the 100% resin steps as it tends to be less viscous after freezing.
9. Hard resin is needed for SBFSEM as it is more resistant to the electron beam. If these blocks are also sectioned for TEM, care must be taken as the resin is more likely to "tear" if cut too quickly resulting in holes in the section. After rough trimming,

it is recommended that several thin, slow sections are taken from the block face to ensure a smooth surface.

10. The single-bristle brush is made by attaching a single bristle cut from a small paintbrush or (more traditionally) an eyelash onto a cocktail stick. We recommend using rapid correction fluid to attach the bristle to the stick.
11. There are a number of different grids available for picking up TEM sections. We recommend washer grids as opposed to mesh grids as none of the section will be obscured by the grid bars that make up a mesh grid. The washer grid has a thin support film of pioloform.
12. Grids can be stained by hand by placing them upside down onto a droplet of stain. Care should be taken with the lead citrate stain as deposits will form if carbon dioxide is present. Hand-staining should be carried out in a closed environment, e.g., petri dish, and a few pellets of sodium hydroxide added to absorb CO_2.
13. It is quite common to see podocyte number reported as the number of podocyte nuclei on a single section through a glomerulus. This is neither podocyte number nor podocyte density and is effectively meaningless. Further details on valid methods for estimation of podocyte number can be found in Ref. [20].

References

1. Basgen JM et al (1988) Measuring the volume density of the glomerular mesangium. Nephron 50(3):182–186
2. Gundersen HJ, Jensen TB, Osterby R (1978) Distribution of membrane thickness determined by lineal analysis. J Microsc 113 (1):27–43
3. Gundersen HJ, Osterby R (1977) Glomerular size and structure in diabetes mellitus. II. Late abnormalities. Diabetologia 13(1):43–48
4. Osterby R (1973) A quantitative electron microscopic study of mesangial regions in glomeruli from patients with short term juvenile diabetes mellitus. Lab Investig 29(1):99–110
5. Osterby R (1972) Morphometric studies of the peripheral glomerular basement membrane in early juvenile diabetes. I. Development of initial basement membrane thickening. Diabetologia 8(2):84–92
6. White KE, Bilous RW (2000) Type 2 diabetic patients with nephropathy show structural-functional relationships that are similar to type 1 disease. J Am Soc Nephrol 11(9):1667–1673
7. White KE et al (2002) Podocyte number in normotensive type 1 diabetic patients with albuminuria. Diabetes 51(10):3083–3089
8. Mauer M et al (2015) Glomerular structural-functional relationship models of diabetic nephropathy are robust in type 1 diabetic patients. Nephrol Dial Transplant 30 (6):918–923
9. (2001) Effect of 3 years of antihypertensive therapy on renal structure in type 1 diabetic patients with albuminuria: the European Study for the Prevention of Renal Disease in Type 1 Diabetes (ESPRIT). Diabetes 50 (4):843–850
10. Gilbert RE, Cooper ME (1999) The tubulointerstitium in progressive diabetic kidney disease: more than an aftermath of glomerular injury? Kidney Int 56(5):1627–1637
11. Steffes MW et al (2001) Glomerular cell number in normal subjects and in type 1 diabetic patients. Kidney Int 59(6):2104–2113
12. Lemley KV et al (2000) Evolution of incipient nephropathy in type 2 diabetes mellitus. Kidney Int 58(3):1228–1237

13. Maunsbach AB (1966) The influence of different fixatives and fixation methods on the ultrastructure of rat kidney proximal tubule cells. II. Effects of varying osmolality, ionic strength, buffer system and fixative concentration of glutaraldehyde solutions. J Ultrastruct Res 15 (3):283–309
14. Weibel ER, Bolender RP (1973) Stereological techniques for electron microscopy. In: Hayat MA (ed) Principles and techniques for electron microscopy. Van Nostrand Reinhold, New York, pp 273–296
15. Nyengaard JR (1999) Stereologic methods and their application in kidney research. J Am Soc Nephrol 10(5):1100–1123
16. White KE, Bilous RW (2004) Estimation of podocyte number: a comparison of methods. Kidney Int 66(2):663–667
17. Weibel ER, Gomez DM (1962) A principle for counting tissue structures on random sections. J Appl Physiol 17:343–348
18. Ichimura K et al (2015) Three-dimensional architecture of podocytes revealed by block-face scanning electron microscopy. Sci Rep 5:8993
19. Randles MJ et al (2016) Three-dimensional electron microscopy reveals the evolution of glomerular barrier injury. Sci Rep 6:35068
20. Lemley KV et al (2013) Estimation of glomerular podocyte number: a selection of valid methods. J Am Soc Nephrol 24(8):1193–1202

Chapter 8

Tissue Clearing and Deep Imaging of the Kidney Using Confocal and Two-Photon Microscopy

Daniyal J. Jafree, David A. Long, Peter J. Scambler, and Dale Moulding

Abstract

Microscopic and macroscopic evaluation of biological tissues in three dimensions is becoming increasingly popular. This trend is coincident with the emergence of numerous tissue clearing strategies, and advancements in confocal and two-photon microscopy, enabling the study of intact organs and systems down to cellular and sub-cellular resolution. In this chapter, we describe a wholemount immunofluorescence technique for labeling structures in renal tissue. This technique combined with solvent-based tissue clearing and confocal imaging, with or without two-photon excitation, provides greater structural information than traditional sectioning and staining alone. Given the addition of paraffin embedding to our method, this hybrid protocol offers a powerful approach to combine confocal or two-photon findings with histological and further immunofluorescent analysis within the same tissue.

Key words Confocal, Imaging, Kidney, Three-dimensional, Tissue clearing, Two-photon

1 Introduction

With the advent of novel wholemount immunofluorescence strategies, and improvements in microscope objectives and their working distances, three-dimensional imaging and analysis are becoming increasingly popular. Previously, obtaining three-dimensional images of organs would require sectioning, imaging, and alignment of serial sections to manually generate a z-stack, which is time consuming, laborious, and technically challenging. Now, intact imaging of entire organs or small organisms has been made possible by the wealth of tissue clearing strategies that are now readily available, and the advancements in confocal and light sheet imaging, enabling interrogation of intact biological structures down to cellular and even sub-cellular resolution. The principle of tissue clearing, also known as refractive index (RI) matching, and fluorescence imaging has been recently reviewed extensively [1, 2], even in the context of the kidney [3]. As light enters tissue, it scatters due to interaction with electrons and subsequent release of spherical

Luigi Gnudi and David A. Long (eds.), *Diabetic Nephropathy: Methods and Protocols*, Methods in Molecular Biology, vol. 2067,
https://doi.org/10.1007/978-1-4939-9841-8_8,

waves, with a concomitant slowing of the propagation of light through the tissue. The latter is the basis for the RI of the tissue. The aim of clearing tissues is to achieve minimal lateral scattering and enable all wavelengths of light to pass through the tissue [1]. These principles of RI matching have been integrated into preexisting wholemount immunofluorescence protocols, and most of these new protocols can be broken down into four steps [4]. Firstly, tissue may need to be pre-treated by, for example, decolorizing, bleaching, or other methods to quench autofluorescence. The second step enables penetration of subsequent reagents in the protocol and is critical for the immunolabeling and clearing of large volumes of tissue. This is achieved by permeabilizing agents, including detergents such as Triton X-100, or solvents such as dimethyl sulfoxide (DMSO). At this stage, some protocols also make use of hydrogel embedding to preserve tissue morphology and minimize protein loss. Thirdly, tissues can be immunolabeled, either passively by diffusion or aided by manipulation of pressure or electric fields within the reaction vessel. The final stage is clearing, after which volume imaging of the tissue is possible.

There are numerous tissue clearing techniques now available, each with their own advantages and disadvantages. Broadly, tissue clearing strategies can be grouped into four categories: solvent-based, simple immersion, hyperhydration, and hydrogel embedding. Some protocols combine different approaches from each category. Importantly, many of these protocols have been conceived, adapted, and optimized in neural tissue, which appears to be the most popular application for tissue clearing. Neural tissue has high lipid content; therefore delipidation is a priority for successful transparency. We have tried several of these protocols for clearing renal tissue with unsatisfactory results, including ScaleA2 [5], ScaleS [6], and ClearT2 [7]. It is unclear whether this is due to different properties of renal tissue, differences in reagents, insufficient incubation times, or subtle variations in experimental method. Regardless, the strategy that has yielded the most success, and one we have recently begun to implement regularly in our laboratory, is an older solvent-based approach, using a hybrid solution of benzyl alcohol and benzyl benzoate (termed BABB). Implemented in 2007 for the clearing and imaging of whole-mouse brains, mouse embryos, or fruit flies [8], BABB has largely gone out of fashion for neural tissue clearing due to its toxicity, incompatibility with water immersion objectives, and quenching of fluorescent proteins. BABB, however, remains a quick and effective method for clearing renal tissue, having recently been used for applications such as counting podocytes in mouse glomeruli [9] or comparing the developmental features of mouse and human embryonic kidneys [10].

In this chapter we describe a wholemount immunofluorescence labeling protocol that was designed and refined for solvent-based clearing using dibenzyl ether [11, 12]. This protocol, the latest iteration of which is termed immunolabeling-enabled three-dimensional imaging of solvent-cleared organs (iDISCO+) [13], is a powerful and quick tool for the immunolabeling renal tissue. We have combined the iDISCO pipeline with BABB-based clearing, given its low cost, ability to rapidly clear renal tissue, and high surface tension, making it useful when mounting samples between slides in preparation for confocal imaging. After acquisition of three-dimensional images, an image analysis pipeline can be developed using the range of commercial and open-access image analysis software now available [13–16], or custom approaches can be applied for renal images, such as TreeSurveyor for quantifying ureteric bud branching or automated segmentation and counting of glomeruli [17, 18]. Inspired by previous work using multidimensional approaches to study renal branching morphogenesis [19, 20], we have supplemented this protocol with a strategy to process and embed the immunolabeled and cleared renal tissue in paraffin. By combining this with traditional histology and immunohistochemistry techniques, one can assess three-dimensional structures of interest within the kidney using confocal imaging while also obtaining information about renal histology for disease phenotyping and can supplement observations in confocal imaging with further immunolabeling of serial sections. Thus using our protocol, a wealth of data can be gathered from a single kidney (Fig. 1).

2 Materials

Prepare all reagents in autoclaved glass containers or microcentrifuge tubes. All newly prepared reagents should be mixed thoroughly until fully dissolved. For reagents, individual storage time and safety considerations are provided in Table 1 (*see* **Note 1**).

2.1 iDISCO+ Wholemount Immunofluorescence

Many of the reagents here are 1× phosphate-buffered saline (PBS) based. We add 0.02% sodium azide to our stock 1× PBS solution prior to using it in subsequent reagents to prevent microbial growth. The protocol outlined below is based on those found on the iDISCO website (*see* **Note 2**) with some modifications.

2.1.1 Reagents

1. 1× PBS made in double-distilled water (ddH_2O).
2. 4% (w/v) Paraformaldehyde (PFA) in 1× PBS: Dissolve 4% (w/v) paraformaldehyde in 1× PBS in a fume hood under heat.
3. Bleaching solution: Methanol with 5% (v/v) of 30% hydrogen peroxide solution.
4. PTx.2: 1× PBS with 0.2% (v/v) Triton X-100.

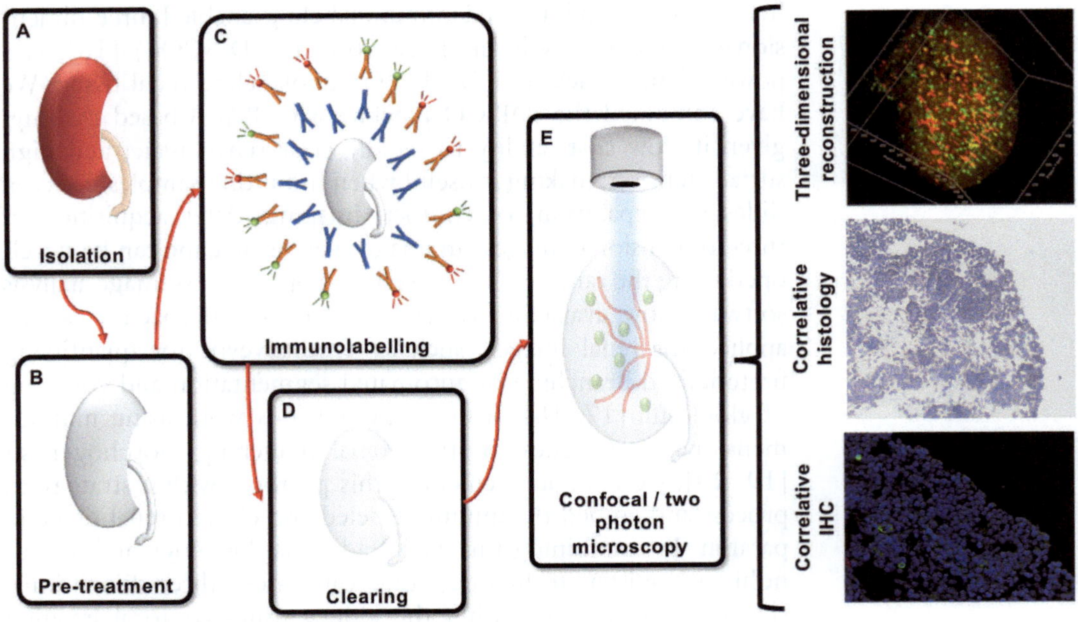

Fig. 1 Workflow for deep imaging of renal tissue. (**a**) Isolation of the mouse or human renal material. (**b**) Applying compounds such as DMSO to permeabilize, and hydrogen peroxide to bleach. (**c**) Immunolabeling using direct or indirect immunohistochemistry. (**d**) Clearing using solvent-based solutions, such as BABB. (**e**) Imaging using confocal microscopy with or without two-photon excitation. With this protocol, optional paraffin embedding and sectioning can be performed after confocal imaging to correlatively analyze confocal findings, by probing histology for disease phenotypes, or further characterizing confocal imaging using traditional fluorescence IHC. *IHC* immunohistochemistry

5. PTwH: 1× PBS with 0.2% (v/v) Tween-20 and 0.1% (v/v) heparin stock solution.
6. Blocking solution: PTx.2 with 10% (v/v) DMSO and 6% (v/v) serum. The choice of species from which serum is obtained, here and in the antibody solutions, must be selected carefully according to the antibody being used (*see* **Note 3**).
7. Heparin stock solution: ddH_2O with 1% (w/v) heparin sodium salt. We use heparin derived from porcine intestinal mucosa.
8. Methanol series: ddH_2O with 25%, 50%, or 75% (v/v) methanol.
9. Permeabilization solution: PTx.2 with 20% (v/v) DMSO and 2.3% (w/v) glycine.
10. Primary/secondary antibody solution: PTwH with 5% (v/v) DMSO, 3% (v/v) serum, and appropriate concentration of primary or secondary antibody (*see* **Note 3**).

2.1.2 Equipment

1. Plastic and/or glass Pasteur pipettes.
2. 2 mL, 1.5 mL, and/or 0.5 mL microcentrifuge tubes.

Table 1
Experimental reagents, storage conditions, and safety considerations

Reagent	Storage	Suggested safety considerations
4% PFA	Store at –20 °C for up to 1 year. We recommend storing in several small aliquots and defrosting when required. Avoid repeat freeze-thaw cycles, and once defrosted store at 4 °C for no longer than 1 week	PFA is an extremely hazardous chemical, is absorbed through the skin, and is toxic to mucus membranes. Make up in fume hood, and take precautions when handling. Dispose of as per departmental guidelines
Antibody solution	Make up fresh, storable for 1 week at 4 °C. Add antibodies immediately prior to use. For fluorophore-conjugated antibodies, protect from light with aluminum foil	Sodium azide is toxic, handle with care when making up PBS stock solution
BABB	Store in dark glass bottles, protected and away from light, at RT. We tend to make this fresh from benzyl alcohol and benzyl benzoate and store for 1 month at a time	BABB is toxic. Use with extreme caution under fume hood. When handling BABB, we recommend keeping a glass beaker filled with methanol to hand in case of spillage. BABB dissolves plastic and glue, so must be kept in glass containers at all times. Dispose of as per departmental guidelines
BABB:M	See BABB	See BABB
Bleaching solution	Make up fresh, use immediately. Store at 4 °C for up to 1 day	Hydrogen peroxide is corrosive, and skin contact and exposure to fumes should be minimized
Blocking solution	Make up fresh, storable for up to 1 week at 4 °C	Sodium azide is toxic, handle with care when making up PBS stock solution
Ethanol	Store ethanol series indefinitely at RT	Take care of flammability; be aware of local fire and safety guidelines
Histo-Clear II	Store indefinitely at RT	Take care of flammability; be aware of local fire and safety guidelines. Minimize skin contact and exposure to fumes. Dispose of as per departmental guidelines
Methanol	Store methanol series indefinitely at RT	Methanol is toxic; minimize skin contact and exposure to fumes. Take care of flammability; be aware of local fire and safety guidelines. Dispose of as per departmental guidelines
Paraffin	Store pellets indefinitely at RT	Take care when handling liquid paraffin, may cause burns
Permeabilization solution	If made up using 1× PBS with 0.02% sodium azide, this can be stored at RT for up to 1 month	Take care when handling due to high concentration of DMSO, which is readily absorbed into the skin and can carry toxic materials into the body. Avoid skin contact

(continued)

Table 1 (continued)

Reagent	Storage	Suggested safety considerations
1× PBS	If made up using 0.02% sodium azide, this can be stored at RT for up to 1 month	Sodium azide is toxic, handle with care when making up PBS stock solution
PTwH	If made up using 1× PBS with 0.02% sodium azide, this can be stored at RT for up to 1 month	Sodium azide is toxic, handle with care when making up PBS stock solution
PTx.2	If made up using 1× PBS with 0.02% sodium azide, this can be stored at RT for up to 1 month	Sodium azide is toxic, handle with care when making up PBS stock solution

3. Blunt forceps.
4. Carousel/rotator.
5. Aluminum foil.

2.2 Refractive Index Matching Reagents and Equipment

2.2.1 Reagents

1. BABB: Mix benzyl alcohol (BA) and benzyl benzoate (BB) in a 1:2 ratio (*see* **Note 4**).
2. BABB:M: Mix BABB and methanol in a 1:1 ratio.

2.2.2 Equipment

1. Plastic and/or glass Pasteur pipettes.
2. Blunt forceps.
3. FluoroDish Cell Culture Dish: There are different diameters available; for small kidneys we have found a 35 mm diameter to be suitable (*see* **Note 5**).
4. Large microscope slides and cover glasses: We use 102 × 76 mm large glass slides and 76 × 83 mm large cover glasses (thickness = 0.19–0.25 mm).
5. FKM Viton O-Rings (internal diameter: 30 mm, cross section: 1.5 mm): These are resistant to BA and BB (*see* **Note 6**).

2.3 Confocal Imaging with Single- or Dual-Photon Excitation

The confocal microscopy equipment will vary from institute to institute. As such, the individual setup should be tailored with the available resources for the desired application. In our department, we hold a Zeiss LSM 710 Inverted Confocal, with seven laser lines for excitation (405, 458, 488, 514, 561, 594, and 633 nm) and the following objectives: 10×/numerical aperture (NA) 0.45 (working distance 2000 μm), 20×/NA 0.8 Plan Apochromat (working distance 550 μm), and a 25×/NA 0.8 multi-immersion corrected (oil, glycerol, or water) Plan Apochromat (working distance 570 μm).

However, because of the longer working distances achievable with high NA water immersion objectives, for this application we use a Zeiss LSM 880 Upright Confocal Multiphoton. This has the same seven laser lines, but also has a SpectraPhysics Mai Tai eHP DeepSee multiphoton laser (690–1040 nm). Here, we use 10×/NA 0.5 or 20×/NA 1.0 W-Plan Apochromat water dipping objectives, with working distances of 3.7 mm and 2.4 mm, respectively. The latter confocal also has gallium arsenide phosphide (GaAsP) internal and external detectors for high sensitivity, making this confocal excellent for deep-tissue imaging. We recommend that the user contact their department's microscopy manager to optimize a setup for deep imaging of optically cleared tissue.

2.4 Paraffin Embedding

2.4.1 Reagents

1. Ethanol series: ddH_2O with 70%, 85%, or 95% (v/v) ethanol.
2. Histo-Clear II (National Diagnostics).
3. Pelleted paraffin.

2.4.2 Equipment

1. Embedding workstation and laboratory oven.
2. Glass vials.
3. Embedding cassettes.

3 Methods

3.1 Wholemount Immunofluorescence

This protocol assumes that renal tissue has already been isolated and collected. Our laboratory uses embryonic and adult mouse and human fetal kidneys. Ensure that the appropriate ethical regulations are followed regarding the handling and sacrifice of animals of the acquisition of human material (*see* **Note 7**). All incubation steps are performed in microcentrifuge tubes using a rotator, either at RT or at 4 °C. The precise timings of incubations should be optimized by the user for the desired application or tissue type. Between stages, transfer kidneys carefully between microcentrifuge tubes using equipment depending on the size of the kidney (*see* **Note 8**). If using the same microcentrifuge tube between different stages, carefully remove the previous solution using glass or plastic Pasteur pipettes, prior to adding the next solution, ensuring minimal contact with the tissue.

3.1.1 Fixation and Storage

1. After isolation, rinse kidneys 2–3 times briefly in ddH_2O prior to fixation to remove residual blood.
2. Incubate renal tissue in 4% PFA at 4 °C on a rotator for an appropriate duration of time. For mouse embryonic kidneys and slices of adult kidney, this can be performed overnight. For larger whole-adult kidneys up to 3 days may be required.

3. Rinse renal tissue in 2–3 changes of PBS, for 5 min each at RT. At this stage, tissue can be stored for several months until required.

3.1.2 Bleaching and Permeabilization

1. Collect kidneys in 1.5 mL microcentrifuge tubes. Incubate kidneys in increasing concentrations of methanol with ddH_2O at RT on a shaker. The following concentrations of methanol should be applied for 15–30 min each: 25%, 50%, 75%, and 100%.
2. Bleach kidneys by incubation in methanol with 5% H_2O_2 for 2 h at 4 °C. This reduces autofluorescence, particularly relevant when performing wholemount immunofluorescence of renal tissue due to the strong autofluorescence from the renal vasculature, tubules and erythrocytes. For large kidneys, such as mouse adult or human fetal, this step can be performed overnight.
3. Incubate kidneys in decreasing concentrations of methanol with ddH_2O at RT on a shaker, in reverse of **step 1**, with each incubation lasting for 15–30 min as follows: 75%, 50%, and 25%.
4. Incubate kidneys in 1× PBS for 30 min at RT. This is followed by two incubations in PTx.2 for 30 min per step at RT.
5. Permeabilize kidneys overnight at 4 °C by incubation in permeabilization solution. The high concentration of DMSO in this solution permeabilizes tissue and enables penetration and distribution of subsequent reagents throughout the kidneys.

3.1.3 Blocking and Antibody Incubation

1. Remove kidneys from permeabilization solution and incubate in blocking solution for 1 day at RT.
2. Incubate kidneys in primary antibody solution at 4 °C (*see* **Note 9**), with appropriate dilution of antibody for 1–3 days, depending on the size of kidney (*see* **Note 10**).
3. Remove kidneys from primary antibody solution and incubate six times in PTwH at RT for 30 min to 1 h per wash, to wash off all unbound primary antibodies. Use fresh PTwH for each incubation.
4. Incubate kidneys in secondary antibody solution at 4 °C, with appropriate dilution of antibody overnight (*see* **Note 10**).
5. Remove kidneys from secondary antibody solution and incubate six times in PTwH at RT for 30 min to 1 h per wash, to wash off all unbound secondary antibodies. Use fresh PTwH for each incubation.

3.2 Refractive Index Matching and Preparation for Imaging

During this step, the kidneys are dehydrated, followed by RI matching. For solvent-based, anhydrous RI solutions, this involves dehydration, prior to immersion in solutions such as BABB. Care should be taken during these steps, as solvent-based chemicals are often toxic. Preparation should be clean, as solvent-based solutions can cause considerable damage to confocal objectives (*see* **Note 4**).

3.2.1 Dehydration

1. Dehydrate stained kidneys through a series of increasing methanol concentrations as in Subheading 3.1.2, at RT with 15–30 min each per incubation: 25%, 50%, 75%, and 100%.

3.2.2 Tissue Clearing

1. Place the following reagents and equipment in a fume hood: BABB, BABB:M, glass Pasteur pipettes, FluoroDish, large glass slide, coverslip, BABB-resistant rubber ring, and glass container filled with methanol. *See* Table 1 for safety considerations when working with BABB.
2. The following steps vary depending on the size of the kidney. **Step 2** describes the setup for a small embryonic kidney. In our hands, this setup permits volume imaging of a maximum sample thickness of approximately 1 mm (Fig. 2a).
   (a) For small embryonic kidneys, place a prepared kidney, using glass Pasteur pipette, centrally in a FluoroDish, and remove excess methanol (*see* **Note 11**).
   (b) Carefully drop BABB:M solution onto the kidney using a new glass Pasteur pipette, until the kidney is immersed. For small embryonic kidneys this requires a few drops. Leave to clear for 5 min, or until the kidney is partially transparent.
   (c) Carefully remove the BABB:M solution with a glass Pasteur pipette, and dispose of the solution in a glass waste container. Ensure that there is no BABB:M solution remaining.
   (d) Add 1–2 drops of BABB on top of the kidney. The kidney will quickly turn transparent. When adding BABB, ensure that the solution is not close to the edges of the FluoroDish.
3. **Step 3** describes the setup for larger mouse embryonic, mouse adult, or human fetal kidneys. In our hands, this setup permits volume imaging of a maximum sample thickness of approximately 3 mm (Fig. 2a, b).
   (a) Using blunt forceps, place a larger kidney in a BABB:M solution in a small glass container. Leave for 10 min, or until the kidney has sunk to the bottom of the container.

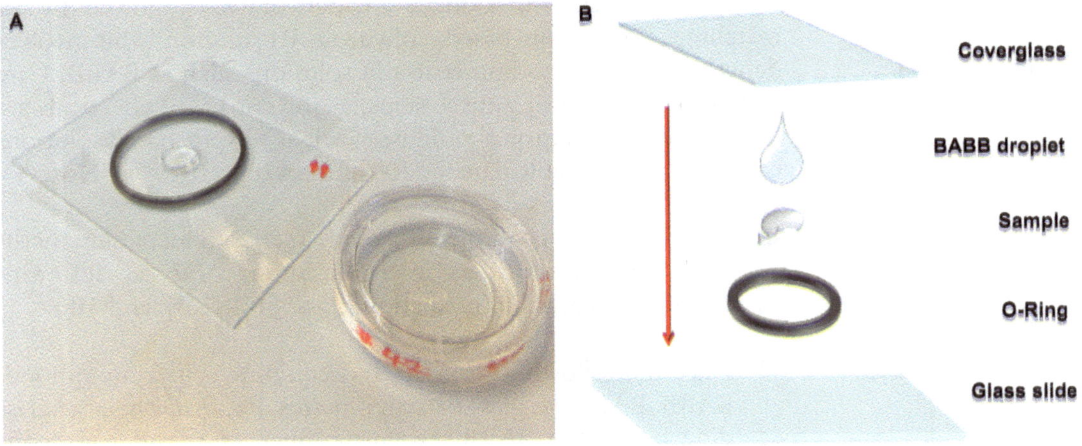

Fig. 2 Setup for upright confocal imaging of BABB-cleared tissue. (**a**) FluoroDish setup for small renal material (right), large cover glass and O-ring configuration for larger renal material (left). (**b**) The individual components of the cover glass/O-ring setup. Each component is applied in sequence, starting with the glass slide and finishing with the cover glass

(b) Remove the kidney with clean blunt forceps and transfer to the middle of a large glass slide. Remove excess BABB: M and place an O-ring around the kidney.

(c) Carefully place several drops of BABB onto the surface of the kidney, until it is immersed. The surface tension of the BABB holds the solution in a "mound" around the kidney.

(d) Place a large glass coverslip down upon the O-ring. With one finger, gently press the center of the coverslip until it "catches" the BABB solution. The tension between the BABB solution and the coverslip forms a "circular bridge," within which the kidney sits. Leave the BABB to render the kidney transparent for 1 h. For larger kidneys this may require longer.

3.3 Confocal Imaging with Single- or Two-Photon Excitation

The optically cleared kidneys are now ready for imaging with a confocal microscope. The setup for inverted confocal microscopy is relatively straightforward, so here we describe the setup for our Zeiss LSM 880 Upright Confocal Multiphoton microscope. The individual setup for different microscopes including Zeiss, Leica, Nikon, and Olympus varies; however the underlying principles remain the same (*see* **Note 12**).

3.3.1 Preparation and Setup for Upright Confocal Imaging

1. Switch on the confocal workstation as per the manufacturer's instructions (*see* **Note 13**).
2. Ensure that objective parfocality is set up, so the focus is correct when switching between objectives.

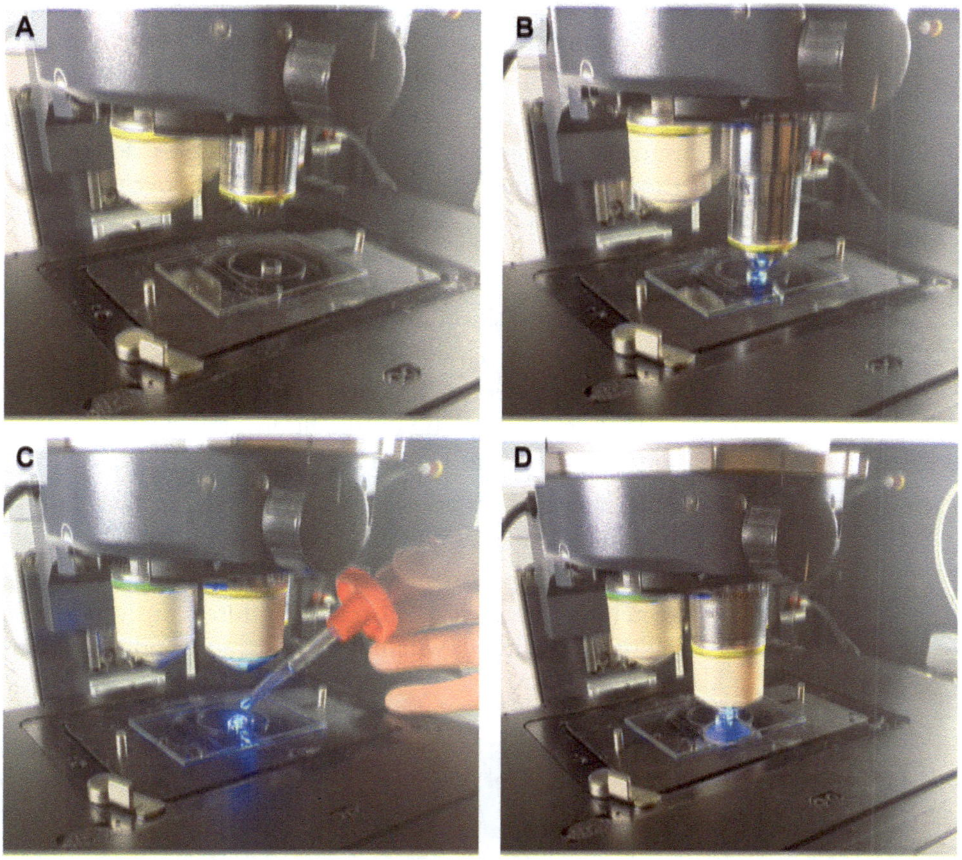

Fig. 3 Setting up and focusing the upright confocal objectives for imaging BABB-cleared tissue. (**a**) After placing the appropriate holder in the microscope stage and adjusting its height, carefully place the sample underneath a low-resolution air immersion objective. (**b**) Place the objective in the focused position and locate sample using eyepiece. (**c**) Remove objective from focused position and place a generous drop of distilled water on the cover glass, below which the BABB and the sample rest. (**d**) Change to a water immersion objective and carefully lower into the focused position, bringing the sample into clear view with sharp edges

3. Select and insert microscope stage appropriate for used sample preparations described in Subheading 3.2.2.
4. Adjust the height of microscope stage appropriate for sample preparation (*see* **Note 14**).
5. Insert sample, with caution (Fig. 3a). If a FluoroDish is being used, secure the lid and quickly invert the FluoroDish so that the BABB droplet containing the kidney is hanging from the uppermost surface of glass (*see* **Note 15**).
6. Carefully focus sample using eyepieces using 10× dry objective (Fig. 3b). This step is an approximation of subsequent focusing using a water immersion lens. Move the stage till kidney is in view and its edges are sharp (*see* **Note 16**).

7. Remove objective from focused position and, using a dropper, place a generous drop of ddH_2O on the FluoroDish or large glass coverslip (Fig. 3c).
8. Replace objective with 10× water immersion objective and return the objective to the focused position slowly, such that the lens is immersed in the drop of water above the level of, but in line with the BABB-cleared kidney (*see* **Note 17** and Fig. 3d).

3.3.2 Confocal Image Acquisition with Single-Photon Excitation

1. Turn on Acquisition Mode in software.
2. Set up confocal with appropriate configuration. The Zeiss software has a Smart Manager which automatically turns on appropriate lasers depending on the fluorophores you input into the software (*see* **Note 18** and Fig. 4).
3. Turn laser powers down, typically to 0.5% for standard photomultiplier tubes (PMT) and 0.05% for GaAsP PMT channels.
4. Choose an appropriate track switching strategy. We prefer line switching to visualize all tracks simultaneously during image capture, but frame switching may be more appropriate in some circumstances.

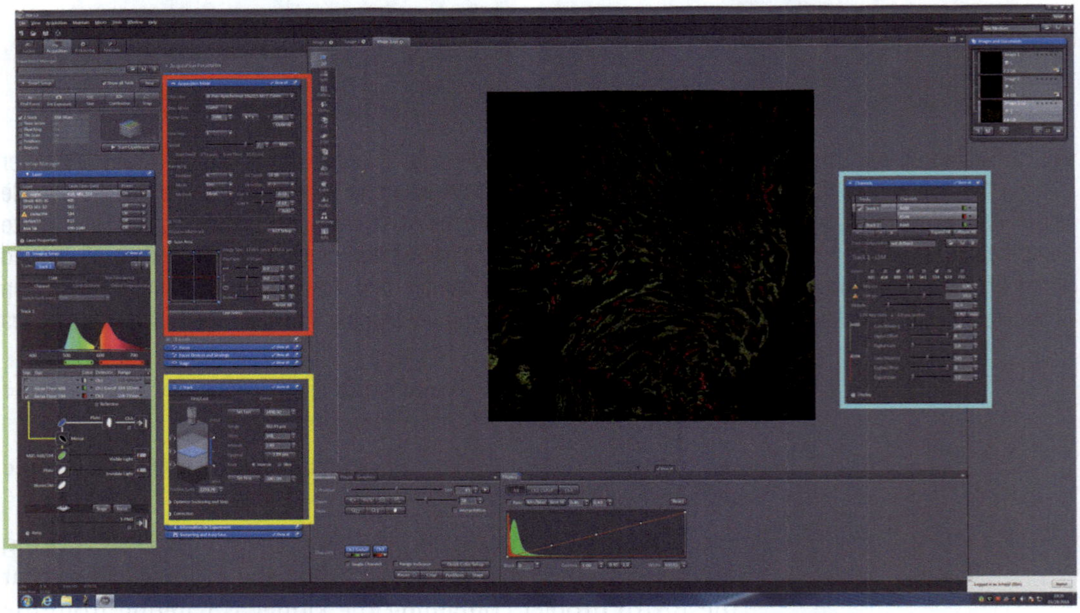

Fig. 4 Screenshot of the Zen confocal software. The Acquisition Mode, including dimensions, speed, pixel averaging, and scan area, is boxed in red. The Imaging Setup, above which the laser switches sit and within which the settings for the detectors and mirror sit, is boxed in green. The z-stack function, which must be activated by ticking the box in the top left of the screen, and with which the optical sectioning depth and bottom and top of the sample can be registered, is boxed in yellow. The Channels tool, with which laser powers, gain, and airy units can be set, is boxed in light blue. These tools and windows can be configured as the user prefers

5. Change "Airy Units" (AU) such that the channel of the longest wavelength corresponds to 1 AU (*see* **Note 19**).
6. Click "Live" and then turn on the Range Indicator. The sample may or may not appear in the acquisition window, as black or gray against the blue background.
7. Adjust laser power and detector gain such that structures in the sample are clearly displayed. Watch the image histogram and ensure that the maximum fluorescence intensity is not beyond the detector range (*see* **Note 20**).
8. Turn off Range Indicator and activate the software's z-stack function. Carefully focus through the sample, noting regions of interest, and indicating the top and the bottom of the sample in the z-stack window.
9. Each objective and wavelength has an optimal z-slice thickness. Select the optimal z-slice thickness for your setup. For our 10× water immersion objective, this is approximately 3 μm. This corresponds to the depth of each optical section in the *z*-axis (*see* **Note 21**).
10. Adjust the resolution of the image, the scanning speed, the degree of averaging, and the (bi-)directionality of the laser as required (*see* **Note 22**).
11. When ready, click "Start Experiment." The scan takes time to complete. With a resolution of 512 × 512 pixels scanning takes approximately 5 min for an embryonic day 14.5 mouse kidney. For larger kidneys, such as those from an embryonic day 18.5 mouse, this takes up to 15–20 min.
12. Remove sample, turn off lasers, and shut down microscope as per instructions provided by microscope manufacturer (*see* **Note 13**).

3.3.3 Confocal Image Acquisition with Two-Photon Excitation

1. Turn on Acquisition Mode in software. Ensure that the lid is securely placed on the imaging chamber to avoid any outside light hitting the detector (*see* **Note 23**).
2. Manually change mirror above imaging chamber such that the two-photon mirror is in place.
3. Set up confocal with two-photon configuration. Wait for the two-photon laser to heat up and switch on. Ideally the laser should run for 1 h before use.
4. Tune the laser to the appropriate wavelength [21]; we use a single-track acquisition with 800 nm for most fluorophores. Turn laser power down to 0.2%, switch on Range Indicator, Click "Live," and increase the Gain of each detector to locate sample as described in Subheading 3.3.2.
5. Proceed as per instructions 6–11 of Subheading 3.3.2.

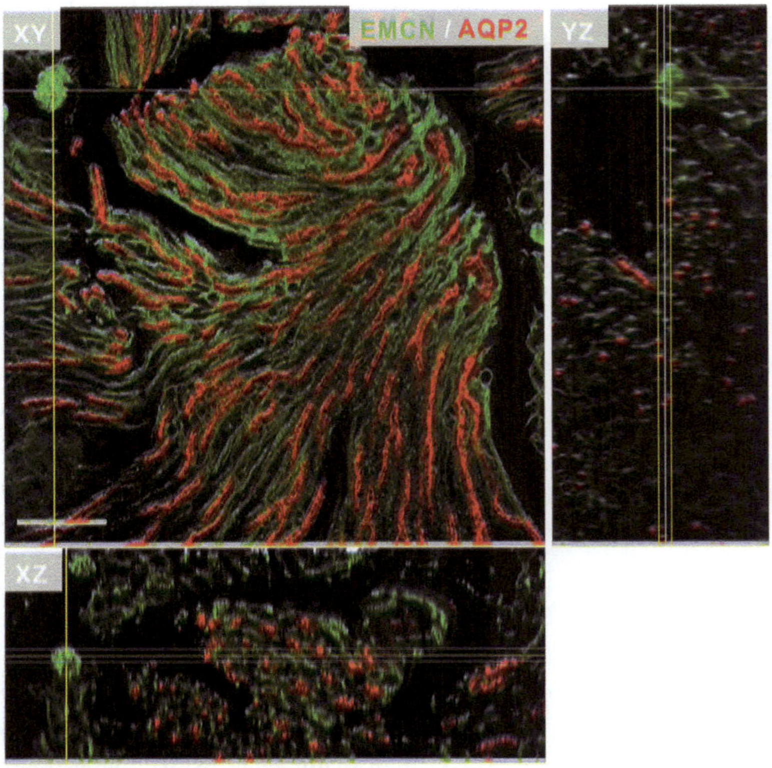

Fig. 5 Example of confocal imagery. The image is taken from an embryonic day 18.5 kidney, stained with rat anti-mouse endomucin (EMCN; 1:50; Santa-Cruz; sc-53941) and rabbit anti-mouse aquaporin 2 (AQP2; 1:50; Abcam; ab109926). A maximum intensity projection is shown, to display the continuity of $EMCN^{+}$ blood vessels and $AQP2^{+}$ collecting ducts. Orthogonal slices of the confocal scan are shown; letters in the top left of each image correspond to the plane of the image. The z-thickness of the optical section is 29 μm, and the orientation of optical sectioning is indicated using the white and yellow crosshairs. Scale bar, 200 μm

6. Perform post-image corrections if required (*see* **Note 24**). An example of a processed image is shown in Fig. 5.

3.4 Paraffin Embedding

Here, we describe the processing of renal tissue previously imaged using the confocal for traditional histology and immunohistochemistry. After rehydration in a methanol series, the ethanol dehydration, clearing, and paraffin embedding of the kidney are performed as standard. The length and repetition of these stages are particularly important for wax penetration, to make subsequent sectioning as easy as possible.

3.4.1 Paraffin Embedding

1. Immerse the BABB-cleared kidney in 100% methanol. For small kidneys, use a plastic Pasteur pipette to fill the FluoroDish with methanol, and wait for the kidney to become visible,

before transferring the kidney using a glass Pasteur pipette into a 1.5 mL microcentrifuge tube containing 100% methanol. For larger kidneys, remove the coverslip and use blunt forceps to transfer the kidney into a 1.5 mL microcentrifuge tube containing 100% methanol (*see* **Note 25**). Leave on a rotator at RT for 15–30 min.

2. Take the tissue through a series of decreasing methanol concentrations, diluted in water, down to PBS as follows, with 15–30 min per step, on a rotator at RT: 75%, 50%, 25%, PBS.
3. Incubate the kidneys in 70% ethanol in water at RT. At this stage, tissue can be stored at 4 °C up to 1 month.
4. Take the tissue through a series of increasing ethanol concentrations, diluted in water, with 1 h per step, on a rotator at RT as follows: 85%, 95%, 100%, 100%.
5. Transfer the dehydrated kidneys to a glass vial, and fill with Histo-Clear II. Leave to incubate at RT for 1 h.
6. Remove Histo-Clear II, replace with a 1:1 Histo-Clear II:liquid paraffin solution, and leave in an oven at 70 °C for 1 h.
7. Remove 1:1 Histo-Clear II:liquid paraffin solution, replace with liquid paraffin, and leave in an oven at 70 °C for 30 min.
8. Repeat liquid paraffin washes as above until 5–6 washes are complete, and then embed kidneys as per performed routinely. Leave paraffin to harden overnight at RT.
9. Thereafter, perform sectioning, staining, and microscopy as performed routinely (*see* **Note 26**). *See* Fig. 6 for an example of a confocal sample processed for histology and immunohistochemistry.

4 Notes

1. This is by no means an exhaustive list of all the safety information for reagents used in the protocol. Rather, this is a guide for users unfamiliar with the protocol and its reagents. Full safety information should be sought out via the local Control of Substances Hazardous to Health (COSHH) database, online, or through direction from your laboratory manager.
2. The iDISCO website is excellent, providing regular updates to the experimental protocol, a list of validated antibodies, useful tools such as guidance on three-dimensional analysis packages, and a question and answer and troubleshooting section. For the protocol presented in this chapter, we have modified and omitted certain steps. For example, we observed good immunolabeling at incubation times shorter than previously

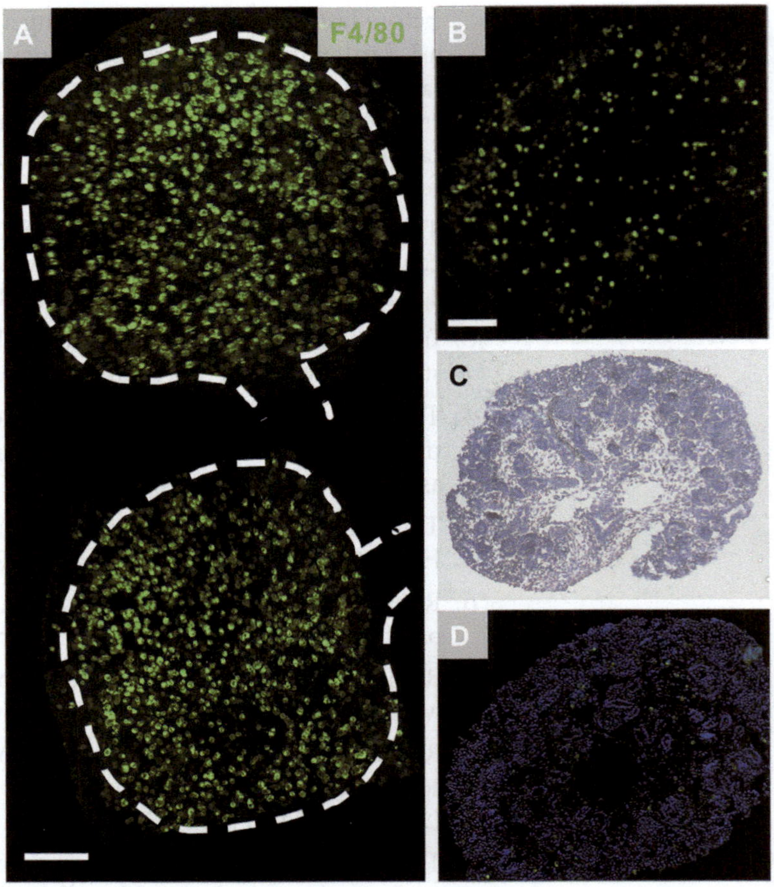

Fig. 6 Correlative histology and IHC of BABB-cleared material. (**a**) 3D reconstructions, performed in IMARIS (version 8.2, Bitplane) of an embryonic day 14.5 kidney stained with F4/80 (1:50; BioRad; MCAP497). The image was taken using a 25× multi-immersion objective. Two rotated views are provided, with white dashes delineating the metanephros and ureter for orientation. (**b**) An optical slice of the same kidney, using ImageJ/FIJI. (**c**) The same kidney, post-paraffin embedding, sectioning (at 5 μm) and staining with periodic acid-Schiff reagent. (**d**) An alternative section of the kidney processed with Hoechst and visualized under a fluorescence microscope. Scale bars, 100 μm

described, and removed steps using dichloromethane and dibenzyl ether. The website is accessible at https://idisco.info.

3. The choice of serum and primary and secondary antibody is crucial, and can be both tricky and frustrating to get right. The below guidance should be taken into consideration, and careful planning is required prior to starting each experiment, as antibodies are costly and the volume of each antibody solution required for this protocol is quite substantial, ranging from 500 μL for the smallest samples to 1–2 mL for larger ones. When a particular antibody combination works well, each

reagent should be noted down, in particular the catalog numbers of the primary and secondary antibodies. It is preferable that the serum should be raised in the same species as the secondary antibody, i.e., donkey serum with donkey secondary antibodies, but this is not always achievable. This can be avoided if the secondary antibodies are pre-adsorbed against the serum chosen for the experiment. Primary antibodies which work in other applications do not necessarily work in wholemount immunofluorescence, so the user will likely have to look at previous publications carefully and trial multiple antibodies with the same target to identify the best for this application. Many antibodies are not compatible with the methanol treatment and dehydration used in this protocol, but the original iDISCO protocol suggests incubation of PFA-fixed frozen tissue sections with or without methanol, prior to immunolabeling, to determine methanol compatibility. Fluorescent secondary antibodies must be selected with specificity for the primary antibodies in mind and also excitation and emission spectra. An example of a good choice of secondary conjugates for immunofluorescence would be 488, 546, and 633. In contrast, a 594 and 633 combination would cause considerable overlap between the spectra that may require post-imaging corrections. We tend to use Alexa Fluor secondary antibodies due to their good signal and photostability, the latter being important when imaging large volumes to avoid bleaching during image acquisition.

4. BABB is an extremely toxic material and should be handled with the utmost caution. Due to the solvent properties of BABB, it readily dissolves adhesives, such as those used to construct microscope objectives. It is for this reason that BABB should always be enclosed, and never come into contact with the objective or lens. The experimental setup provided in this chapter is a good solution, but improper handling of the sample, or lack of concentration when adjusting the focus of the confocal, is an extremely costly error. Leica Microsystems have also developed a 20× objective (NA, 0.95) which is designed for immersion in BABB, with a modest working distance of 1.95 mm. In any case, contact your confocal microscope manager prior to using BABB, and we recommend that the first few tries of this protocol should be performed under supervision.

5. The FluoroDish has a 0.17 mm thick coverslip base, which permits imaging from underneath the sample using an inverted confocal, or inversion of the dish and imaging using an upright confocal.

6. Screening for compounds which are resistant to BABB, we found that FKM Viton has minimal chemical reactivity with

BA and BB. FKM Viton rings, known as O-rings, can be purchased in a range of diameters and thicknesses. We recommend an internal diameter of 30 mm such that BABB does not come into contact with the edges of the ring. The cross-sectional size depends upon the size of the sample. Ideally, the sample should be as close to the coverslip as possible. For samples up to 1 mm in height, a 1 mm thick O-ring is suitable, as samples shrink during methanol dehydration. We have rings with depths ranging from 0.5 to 3.5 mm in 0.5 mm increments. As our 10×/NA0.5 W-Plan Apochromat objective has a working distance of 3.7 mm, we can confidently image the bottom of any sample in any of these O-rings without the objective contacting the uppermost coverslip. For our 20×/NA1.0 W-Plan Apochromat with a working distance of 2.4 mm, we only use O-rings up to 2 mm deep. A potential source of such O-rings is Polymax.

7. Animals should be sacrificed in accordance with national legislation. We have access to human fetal material through the Human Developmental Biology Resource, a UK-based resource for which any laboratory can apply to obtain material [22]. Clinical material and patient samples should be acquired with the relevant ethical approval. We have not tried this protocol with clinical material, but if optimized for this application has the potential to become a powerful tool for probing disease processes in human samples.

8. For small mouse embryonic kidneys we use a glass or plastic Pasteur pipette. Transfers of larger embryonic or adult mouse, or human fetal kidneys, are performed carefully with the use of a blunt forceps, working quickly to minimize the time that the samples are exposed to air, as drying of the samples can lead to artifact in imaging.

9. The original iDISCO+ protocol recommends several steps including permeabilization, blocking, and antibody incubation be performed at 37 °C. However we only have carousels at 4 °C or RT. There is evidence to suggest that increasing the temperature of incubation decreases the specificity of the antibody, increasing nonspecific binding [23, 24].

10. The concentration of antibody required for each experiment varies considerably. We find that most suitable primary antibodies for our applications appear to work well at a concentration of 1:100. However, some work better at 1:50, and others work best at lower concentrations of 1:200 or 1:500. We recommend starting at 1:100 and adjusting based on the signal to background achieved in the final image. We use all secondary antibodies at a concentration of 1:200. During antibody incubation stages, we transfer small kidneys into a 500 μL

microcentrifuge tube to minimize the volume of antibody used and avert the cost, and transfer samples back to larger 1.5 mL tubes after incubation is complete. This may not be achievable for larger samples. After the secondary antibody is applied, protect the samples from light by covering the tubes in aluminum foil.

11. At this stage, we recommend labeling the FluoroDish or glass slide with permanent marker, indicating details of the experiment, repeat number, and so on. After the protocol is completed and the kidney is virtually invisible, it becomes impossible to distinguish one sample from another.
12. Confocal microscopy can be relatively complicated for the uninitiated. Though incredible, journal cover-worthy images can be generated, it is easy to get wrong, and carelessness and lack of understanding of the principles of confocal can lead to poor image quality or interpretation, or damage to very expensive equipment. Instead of relying on the microscopy manager, we recommend that all users familiarize themselves with the concepts of confocal microscopy using the wealth of online resources available. One of our favorites is the Nikon MicroscopyU website, providing simple but detailed explanations of several topics in confocal and two-photon microscopy: https://www.microscopyu.com/techniques/confocal.
13. For our confocal microscope, setting up the system involves turning on the switches to the microscope and laser power supply, workstation computer, and components of computer in a particular sequence, after which the fluorescence lamp, Zen software, and lasers are switched on. There is also an appropriate sequence of instructions to shut down the microscope, to avoid damage to the system. Of note, some lasers, such as the 488 Argon laser, require several minutes to cool prior to shutting down. Consult your departmental microscopy expert or the microscope manufacturer for full details.
14. We always start with a 10× air objective, which is in focus when 5 mm above the coverslip or FluoroDish. This is used for both estimating the correct height to set the microscope stage and correctly focusing the sample prior to switching to water immersion lenses. Initial focusing with water immersion objectives is not advised as the distance between objective and coverslip is difficult to judge through the water. By setting objective parfocality on a safe (BABB-free) sample, focusing with the simple-to-use 10× air objective ensures that the water immersion objectives will automatically be in the correct focal plane.
15. Inverting the FluoroDish into a "hanging drop" configuration can be quite challenging. The droplet of BABB has to be

contained in the middle of the FluoroDish surface, as contact with the sides will cause the BABB to react with the adhesive used to construct the dish, forming a precipitate and making the kidney impossible to image. It requires a smooth and quick action to invert the FluoroDish while keeping the kidney central, and the high surface tension of BABB prevents the kidney from falling. The largest sample we have performed this successfully with was a whole kidney from an embryonic day 17.5 mouse fetus, bearing in mind that the BABB protocol and methanol dehydration cause the sample to shrink [5]. We advise a few practice runs with a drop of BABB alone. At the end of the imaging session, it is critical to re-invert the FluoroDish back to its original configuration for long-term storage.

16. When focusing the sample, a fluorescent bulb is active, so the fluorescent kidney comes into view, enabling alignment of the objective with the sample.

17. The air objectives on the confocal are changed to water immersion objectives to minimize the effects of RI mismatch. The RI of BABB is approximately 1.56 [1], whereas glass is 1.51, water is 1.33 and air is 1.0. When imaging samples with RI-mismatched objectives, an optical phenomenon termed spherical aberration leads to a loss of resolution and signal strength. As imaging depth increases so does the degree of spherical aberration, making imaging of deep tissue challenging. Most confocal software provides settings that adjust for spherical aberration by increasing the power of the laser as imaging depth increases, compensating for the loss of signal intensity. However, this does not restore the loss of resolution. Spherical aberration is more apparent with higher NA objectives, so if high resolution is required (therefore needing high NA) then it is vital to minimize the RI mismatch between BABB and the objective. Ideally imaging would be performed with an objective designed for high RI immersion media, such as an oil (RI ~1.51) immersion objective, as this is close to BABB (RI ~1.56) and therefore minimizes spherical aberration. However, oil immersion objectives have short working distances, with nothing longer than 570 μm currently available from Zeiss. Leica have developed a 20×/NA 0.95 BABB objective, designed for RI 1.56, but this is not compatible with Zeiss systems. Long-working-distance, high-NA water immersion objectives are a good compromise, providing high resolution with less aberration than high-NA air objectives. While the RIs in this setup are still not matched, we are able to image renal structures down to cellular resolution at depths beyond 1 mm. If details of sub-cellular structures, such as mitochondria, are required, using an oil immersion objective would be better. This is at the sacrifice of imaging depth, as

such objectives would have shorter working distances, so the renal tissue may have to be coarsely sliced using a vibratome prior to starting the protocol.

18. If using an argon laser to visualize a 488 fluorophore, wait for 5 min after switching the laser on, as it takes this time to warm up. Ideally argon lasers should be run on standby for an hour before imaging to stabilize the laser.

19. The defining feature of confocal microscopes is the use of a pinhole to ensure that only light from the plane of interest reaches the imaging detector, and out-of-focus light is excluded. Typically we set the pinhole diameter to match 1 AU for the longest wavelength channel, taking the view that axial resolution is determined by the longest wavelength (resolution decreases as wavelength increases). When the multiphoton laser is used, the pinhole is unnecessary due to the properties of two-photon excitation.

20. A higher laser power will photobleach the sample more quickly, whereas a higher gain will increase noise, leading to graininess of the image. The optimal image is a balance between these two components. When adjusting these, take into account the relative intensity of the signal to background and the image histogram. If fluorescence intensity is too high then the full range of fluorescence is "cropped," and this information is lost from the final image.

21. Distance is distorted when imaging into a sample with a different NA than the objective immersion media. The z-stack window has the option of inserting the refractive index ratio of the imaging material and objective immersion media. This then corrects the axial distance accordingly. We do not use this feature, but correct axial distance post-acquisition. Actual distance in the sample is the z-step distance multiplied by (RI sample/RI objective). For an air immersion objective using a BABB-cleared sample, a z-step of 1 μm gives a distance of $1\ \mu m \times 1.56/1.00 = 1.56\ \mu m$. The same sample using a z-step of 1 μm with a water immersion objective gives $1\ \mu m \times 1.56/1.33 = 1.165\ \mu m$.

22. As a principle, higher resolution, slower scanning speed, single directionality, and higher pixel averaging all result in better image quality, but increase the time taken to complete scanning. We tend to set the following parameters: resolution, 512×512 or 1024×1024; speed, 7–9; directionality, bidirectional; and averaging, 2. The same settings are applied for two-photon imaging, with a higher pixel averaging of 4 due to more noise with this imaging modality.

23. Two-photon imaging uses non-descanned detectors (no pinhole is present) so it must be performed in the dark to

prevent detection of ambient light. Exposure of the system to ambient light may damage the detectors.

24. Two-photon excitation harbors several potential advantages over standard confocal imaging for this application. In the context of fluorescence imaging of immunolabeled and cleared kidneys, the laser penetrates the sample better due to a higher wavelength, and captures more signal, given that out-of-focus light (produced as an effect of spherical aberration) is not obstructed by the presence of a pinhole. However, two-photon excitation generates considerably more autofluorescence from structures such as collagen and erythrocytes. This autofluorescence is greater at shorter wavelengths, and is particularly apparent in the green and yellow regions of the light spectrum. When imaging with multiple fluorophores, there is a greater chance of bleed through arising between fluorescence channels of the image as two-photon excitation at 800 nm often excites all fluorophores. Post-image corrections to automatically correct for this effect, such as spectral unmixing, may need to be performed as indicated by your local microscopy expert. Given this comparison of single- and two-photon excitation, the imaging modality we use depends on the desired application, and is influenced by the range of fluorophores used for each experiment.

25. Upon contact with 100% methanol, the BABB-cleared kidney starts to become white and opaque, which makes subsequent handling and transfers considerably easier.

26. Remarkably, fluorescence is preserved even after paraffin embedding, sectioning, and staining. We have omitted further detail of sectioning and staining as these are well-established protocols, and will likely be performed slightly differently in each laboratory. The key points here are that the duration of ethanol changes and length and frequency of liquid paraffin stages are critical to ensure satisfactory embedding of the kidney. Combes and colleagues suggest that unmasking using compounds such as citrate buffer is not necessary, as the BABB treatment appears to unmask antigens adequately [19]. We have not determined whether this protocol preserves RNA, but previous data of in situ hybridization patterns imaged using optical projection tomography appears to suggest that it does. Fluorescent proteins are not preserved by this protocol; however anti-fluorescent protein secondary antibodies may be used, or the protocol may be modified according to newer iterations to combine immunolabeling with detection of fluorescent protein expression [25, 26].

Acknowledgments

The authors would like to thank Drs. Karen Price, Maria Kolatsi-Joannou, Sarah Ivins, and Catherine Roberts and the rest of the Kidney Disease and Development Group and the Molecular Medicine Unit at UCL Great Ormond Street Institute of Child Health for their guidance, and the staff of the UCL Confocal Imaging Facility for their advice. We would also like to acknowledge Dr. Nicolas Renier (Institut du Cerveau et de la Moelle Epiniere), Dr. Alexander Combes, and Professor Melissa Little (Murdoch Children's Research Institute) for their email correspondence and clarifications of the methods used in their publications. DJ is supported by funding from the Child Health Research PhD Studentship at UCL Great Ormond Street Institute of Child Health and the UCL MB/PhD Programme. DAL's laboratory is supported by a Medical Research Council New Investigator Award (MR/J003638/1) and project grant (MR/P018629/1), project grants from Diabetes UK (13/0004763, 15/0005283), and Kidney Research UK (RP36/2015), and by the National Institute for Health Research (NIHR) Biomedical Research Centre (BRC) at Great Ormond Street Hospital (GOSH) for Children NHS Foundation Trust and University College London. Microscopy was performed at the Light Microscopy Core Facility at UCL Great Ormond Street Institute of Child Health, also supported by the NIHR BRC at GOSH (17DD08).

References

1. Richardson DS, Lichtman JW (2015) Clarifying tissue clearing. Cell 162:246–257
2. Tainaka K, Kuno A, Kubota SI, Murakami T, Ueda HR (2016) Chemical principles in tissue clearing and staining protocols for whole-body cell profiling. Annu Rev Cell Dev Biol 32:713–741
3. Puelles VG, Moeller MJ, Bertram JF (2017) We can see clearly now: optical clearing and kidney morphometrics. Curr Opin Nephrol Hypertens 26:179–186
4. Richardson DS, Lichtman JW (2017) SnapShot: tissue clearing. Cell 171:496–496
5. Hama H, Kurokawa H, Kawano H, Ando R, Shimogori T, Noda H, Fukami K, Sakaue-Sawano A, Miyawaki A (2011) Scale: a chemical approach for fluorescence imaging and reconstruction of transparent mouse brain. Nat Neurosci 14:1481–1488
6. Hama H, Hioki H, Namiki K, Hoshida T, Kurokawa H, Ishidate F, Kaneko T, Akagi T, Saito T, Saido T, Miyawaki A (2015) ScaleS: an optical clearing palette for biological imaging. Nat Neurosci 18:1518–1529
7. Kuwajima T, Sitko AA, Bhansali P, Jurgens C, Guido W, Mason C (2013) ClearT: a detergent- and solvent-free clearing method for neuronal and non-neuronal tissue. Development 140:1364–1368
8. Dodt HU, Leischner U, Schierloh A, Jährling N, Mauch CP, Deininger K, Deussing JM, Eder M, Zieglgänsberger W, Becker K (2007) Ultramicroscopy: three-dimensional visualization of neuronal networks in the whole mouse brain. Nat Methods 4:331–336
9. Puelles VG, van der Wolde JW, Schulze KE, Short KM, Wong MN, Bensley JG, Cullen-McEwen LA, Caruana G, Hokke SN, Li J, Firth SD, Harper IS, Nikolic-Paterson DJ, Bertram JF (2016) Validation of a three-dimensional method for counting and sizing podocytes in whole glomeruli. J Am Soc Nephrol 27:3093–3104
10. Lindström NO, McMahon JA, Guo J, Tran T, Guo Q, Rutledge E, Parvez RK, Saribekyan G,

Schuler RE, Liao C, Kim AD, Abdelhalim A, Ruffins SW, Thornton ME, Basking L, Grubbs B, Kesselman C, McMahon AP (2018) Conserved and divergent features of human and mouse kidney organogenesis. J Am Soc Nephrol 29:785–805

11. Ertürk A, Becker K, Jährling N, Mauch CP, Hojer CD, Egen JG, Hellal F, Bradke F, Sheng M, Dodt HU (2012) Three-dimensional imaging of solvent-cleared organs using 3DISCO. Nat Protoc 7:1983–1995
12. Renier N, Wu Z, Simon DJ, Yang J, Ariel P, Tessier-Lavigne M (2014) iDISCO: a simple, rapid method to immunolabel large tissue samples for volume imaging. Cell 159:896–910
13. Renier N, Adams EL, Kirst C, Wu Z, Azevedo R, Kohl J, Autry AE, Kadiri L, Umadevi Venkataraju K, Zhou Y, Wang VX, Tang CY, Olsen O, Dulac C, Osten P, Tessier-Lavigne M (2016) Mapping of brain activity by automated volume analysis of immediate early genes. Cell 165:1789–1802
14. de Chaumont F, Dallongeville S, Chenouard N, Hervé N, Pop S, Provoost T, Meas-Yedid V, Pankajakshan P, Lecomte T, Le Montagner Y, Lagache T, Dufour A, Olivo-Marin JC (2012) Icy: an open bioimage informatics platform for extended reproducible research. Nat Methods 9:690–696
15. Peng H, Bria A, Zhou Z, Iannello G, Long F (2014) Extensible visualization and analysis for multidimensional images using Vaa3D. Nat Protoc 9:193–208
16. Royer LA, Weigert M, Günther U, Maghelli N, Jug F, Sbalzarini IF, Myers EW (2015) ClearVolume: open-source live 3D visualization for light-sheet microscopy. Nat Methods 12:480–481
17. Short K, Hodson M, Smyth I (2013) Spatial mapping and quantification of developmental branching morphogenesis. Development 140:471–478
18. Klingberg A, Hasenberg A, Ludwig-Portugall-I, Medyukhina A, Männ L, Brenzel A, Engel DR, Figge MT, Kurts C, Gunzer M (2017) Fully automated evaluation of Total glomerular number and capillary tuft size in nephritic kidneys using lightsheet microscopy. J Am Soc Nephrol 28:452–459
19. Combes AN, Short KM, Lefevre J, Hamilton NA, Little MH, Smyth IM (2014) An integrated pipeline for the multidimensional analysis of branching morphogenesis. Nat Protoc 9:2859–2879
20. Brzóska HL, d'Esposito AM, Kolatsi-Joannou-M, Patel V, Igarashi P, Lei Y, Finnell RH, Lythgoe MF, Woolf AS, Papakrivopoulou E, Long DA (2016) Planar cell polarity genes *Celsr1* and *Vangl2* are necessary for kidney growth, differentiation, and rostrocaudal patterning. Kidney Int 90:1274–1284
21. Mütze J, Iyer V, Macklin JJ, Colonell J, Karsh B, Petrášek Z, Schwille P, Looger LL, Lavis LD, Harris TD (2012) Excitation spectra and brightness optimization of two-photon excited probes. Biophys J 102:934–944
22. Gerrelli D, Lisgo S, Copp AJ, Lindsay S (2015) Enabling research with human embryonic and fetal tissue resources. Development 142:3073–3076
23. Güven E, Duus L, Lydolph MC, Jørgensen CS, Laursen I, Houen G (2014) Non-specific binding in solid phase immunoassays for autoantibodies correlates with inflammation markers. J Immunol Methods 403:26–36
24. Ward JM, Rehg JE (2014) Rodent immunohistochemistry: pitfalls and troubleshooting. Vet Pathol 51:88–101
25. Schwarz MK, Scherbarth A, Sprengel R, Engelhardt J, Theer P, Giese G (2015) Fluorescent-protein stabilization and high-resolution imaging of cleared, intact mouse brains. PLoS One 10:e0124650. https://doi.org/10.1371/journal.pone.0124650
26. Pan C, R1 C, Quacquarelli FP, Ghasemigharagoz A, Lourbopoulos A, Matryba P, Plesnila N, Dichgans M, Hellal F, Ertürk A (2016) Shrinkage-mediated imaging of entire organs and organisms using uDISCO. Nat Methods 13:859–867

Part IV

Assessing the Function and Pathophysiological Properties of the Diabetic Kidney

Chapter 9

Transcutaneous Measurement of Glomerular Filtration Rate in Rodents

Cristina Daniele, Daniela Nardozi, Angelo Torelli, Arif ul Maula Khan, and Norbert Gretz

Abstract

Glomerular filtration rate (GFR) is considered the gold standard to test kidney function. However, the serial blood and/or urine sample collection required for the calculation of the GFR is stressful for the animal and time consuming for the experimenter. Here, we describe a transcutaneous assessment of renal function in conscious animals that does not require plasma or urine sampling and/or deep anesthesia. For the measurement, we use a near-infrared (NIR) device that records the excretion kinetic of the renal marker ABZWCY-HPβCD. ABZWCY-HPβCD is a new hydrophilic, stable, and nontoxic NIR fluorescent agent that can be used as a renal marker as it is filtrated and completely excreted through the kidneys into the urine without reabsorption or secretion and without accumulation in the skin. The data recorded in the device are then analyzed with "GFRmeasure," an open-source, freely downloadable, and user-friendly software.

Key words Glomerular filtration rate, GFR marker, Transcutaneous measurement, Half-life calculation, Renal function evaluation, User-friendly software

1 Introduction

The assessment of glomerular filtration rate (GFR) is the traditional and widely adopted way to test kidney function and determine the stage of kidney disease. It is often calculated from the results of blood creatinine tests, taking into account the age, body size, and gender of the patient.

In animal experiments, calculation of GFR is based on the urinary or plasma clearance of exogenous renal markers [1]. It requires the collection of serial blood and/or urine samples, which is very stressful for the animals; in addition posterior laboratory assays for their analysis are time consuming for the experimenter.

Even though several alternative approaches have been developed to simplify the classical procedures to determine GFR, urine and plasma sampling [2–5] still remains an indispensable step in

Luigi Gnudi and David A. Long (eds.), *Diabetic Nephropathy: Methods and Protocols*, Methods in Molecular Biology, vol. 2067, https://doi.org/10.1007/978-1-4939-9841-8_9, © Springer Science+Business Media, LLC, part of Springer Nature 2020

both the infusion and the bolus GFR. Additionally, most of the time these techniques also require deep anesthesia [6, 7], which can influence renal hemodynamics and thus renal function [8, 9].

To overcome these issues, recently Herrera Pérez et al. [10] described a transcutaneous methodology to assess renal function in conscious animals which does not require plasma or urine sampling and/or deep anesthesia.

Briefly, a small electronic device [11] is used to monitor the excretion of the exogenous renal marker fluorescein isothiocyanate (FITC)-sinistrin transcutaneously. The device has an optical part which consists of two light-emitting diodes (LEDs) and a photodiode. When the renal marker is intravenously administrated to the animal, it is excited by the LEDs and the emitted fluorescence is detected by the photodiode. The data are recorded and stored in the internal memory of the device and are used to generate the elimination kinetics curve of the marker. The device is easily attachable on the shaved back of the animals by simply using an adhesive black patch. Animals are awake and freely moving for the whole recording period, which is around 2 h in mice and rats. This simple and fast method represents a noninvasive technique that allows performing sequential measurements in the same animal [12].

Nevertheless, the strong intrinsic autofluorescence background from living tissue is a parameter that has to be taken into account when using a marker with an emission wavelength shorter than 600 nm, such as FITC-sinistrin, since it can interfere with the accuracy of the measurement [13]. Furthermore, the penetration depth increases with increasing wavelength. For these reasons, it would be preferable to use markers with a higher emission wavelength, such as in the NIR region (650–900 nm). Huang et al. [14] developed a novel zwitterionic NIR fluorescent agent (ABZWCY-HPβCD) that can be used in combination with the aforementioned device.

Here, we describe a transcutaneous assessment of renal function in conscious, freely moving animals by using a NIR device and the ABZWCY-HPβCD renal marker. For the analysis of the data, we also propose an open-source freely available software named "GFRmeasure" based on MATLAB.

This user-friendly graphical user interface (GUI) is required to evaluate the half-life of the fluorescent agent ABZWCY-HPβCD. "GFRmeasure" describes the excretion kinetic of ABZWCY-HPβCD by fitting the signal measured by the device to 1–3-compartment models. This software is freely downloadable, very intuitive, and easy to use even for new users.

2 Materials

2.1 Device

1. Transdermal GFR monitor (IRxxx), charger, rechargeable battery, and double-sided adhesive patch (MediBeacon GmbH, Mannheim, Germany).

2.2 ABZWCY-HPβCD Renal Marker Preparation and Administration

1. ABZWCY–HPβCD fluorescent agent (CYANAGEN S.r.l, Bologna, Italy).
2. Deltajonin Physiologic solution.
3. Intravenous cannula.
4. 1 mL Syringe.

2.3 Animal Preparation and Fixation of the Device

1. Isoflurane 1 mg/mL.
2. Electric shaver.
3. Black plastic foil.
4. Tubular elastic net bandage.
5. Black double-sided adhesive tape.

2.4 Software

1. Basic PC software (MediBeacon GmbH, Mannheim, Germany) is required to read the data out from the device. A basic evaluation of half-life using one- and two-compartment models is also provided in the software.
2. The open-source software "GFRmeasure" for advanced evaluation (three-compartment model) can be downloaded with usage instructions under https://github.com/AngeloTorelli/GFRmeasure.

3 Methods

In order to reduce the time of the anesthesia, it is recommended to prepare the dose of ABZWCY-HPβCD and to mount the device and the battery on the patch in advance. Once the animal is under anesthesia, the whole process of the fixation of the device on the animal and the ABZWCY-HPβCD administration usually lasts for approximately 5 min.

3.1 ABZWCY-HPβCD Preparation

1. Dissolve ABZWCY-HPβCD powder in Deltajonin to prepare a stock solution at a concentration of 160 mg/mL for rats and 60 mg/mL for mice. The suggested administration dose is 15 mg/100 g body weight for rats and 30 mg/100 g body weight for mice.

   Note: Stock solution can be prepared in advance and stored at −20 °C, protected from the light.
2. Weigh the animal and calculate the appropriate ABZWCY-HPβCD volume of injection.

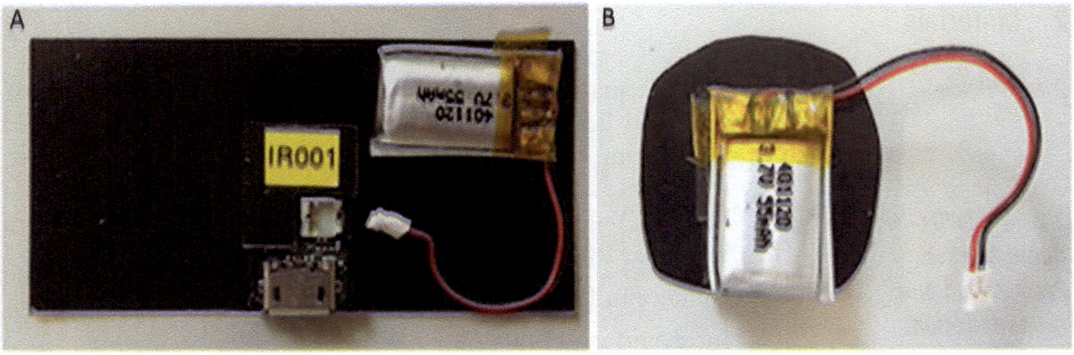

Fig. 1 Device and battery preparation. The device is placed on the adhesive patch. (**a**) In rats the battery can be placed next to the device. (**b**) In smaller rodents, due to the reduced space, the battery must be placed on top of the device and the size of the patch has to be reduced

3.2 Device Preparation

1. Place the device on one of the two faces of the double-sided adhesive patch, keeping the protective foil on the opposite side intact. Take care that one side of the patch is stickier than the other one. The device has to be placed on the stickier side, carefully putting the optical part exactly above the clear window.
2. Place the battery on the same adhesive patch side where the device has been attached. When working with rats, the battery can be positioned next to the device. In case of mice, reduce the size of the patch and put the battery on the device by using a small piece of double-sided adhesive patch (Fig. 1a, b).

3.3 Animal Preparation and Anesthesia

1. Anesthetize the animal using 5% isoflurane at 3 L/min airflow. When the animal is properly anesthetized, decrease the anesthesia to 2% isoflurane at 1.5 L/min airflow (*see* **Note 1**).
2. By using an electric shaver, remove the fur on the back of the animal. It is recommended to shave an area slightly bigger than the area of the adhesive patch to be attached.

3.4 Fixation of the Device on the Animal

1. Cut a piece of tubular elastic bandage approximately 1 cm bigger than the width of the double-side adhesive patch.
2. Connect the battery to the device and cover it with a piece of plastic black foil approximately two times the size of device (*see* **Note 2**). Remove the protective foil from the patch and ensure that the battery is properly connected (LED on the device starts blinking if attached properly).
3. Place the patch with device and battery on the shaved area on the back of the animal, and then carefully fix it by using the elastic bandage, trying to avoid the pressure on the device (Fig. 2).

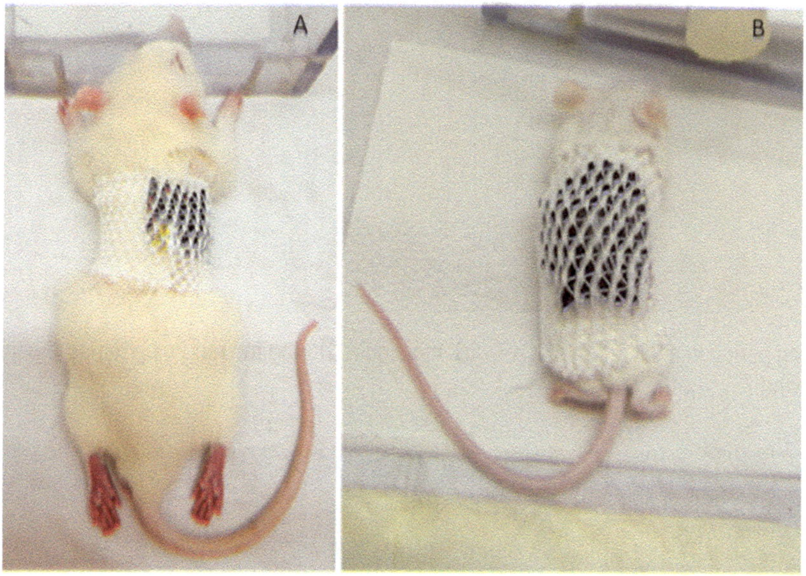

Fig. 2 Fixation of the device on a SD rat (**a**) and a Swiss mouse (**b**). Once the device is placed on the shaved back of the animal, it is covered with the black plastic foil and fixed to the animal by using the elastic tubular bandage. The bandage should cover the double-sided adhesive patch without interfering with the free movement of the animal

4. Stretch the bandage properly so that the animal is free to move.
5. To fix the device in a much better way, apply two strips of adhesive tape.

3.5 ABZWCY-HPβCD Administration

1. Inject through tail vein the right amount of ABZWCY-HPβCD solution. Make sure that all the solution is administrated intravenously and not subcutaneously (*see* **Note 3**).
2. Put the animal in a cage in order to avoid abrupt movements and pressure on the device. The animal must stay awake and alone in a quiet place (*see* **Note 4**) (Fig. 3).
3. Perform the measurement for at least 2 h.

3.6 Device Removal

1. After the recording period, remove the device from the animal without using anesthesia (*see* **Note 5**) by cutting the tape and then the tubular bandage.
2. Return the animal to its home cage.

3.7 Data Reading

1. Carefully remove the black plastic foil, then disconnect the battery from the device, and remove it from the adhesive patch.
2. Connect the device to a PC using an USB cable and download the data using the basic software (Fig. 4a, b). The output file is saved as a .csv file (*see* **Note 6**).

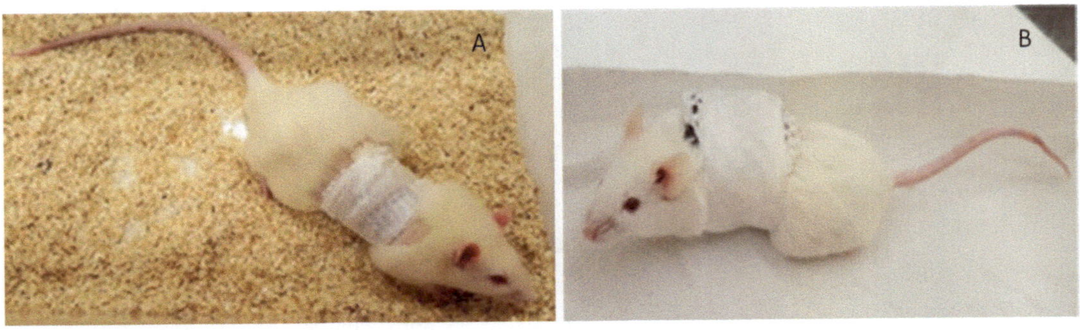

Fig. 3 Recording period in a SD rat (**a**) and a Swiss mouse (**b**). During the recording period the animal is awake and freely moving

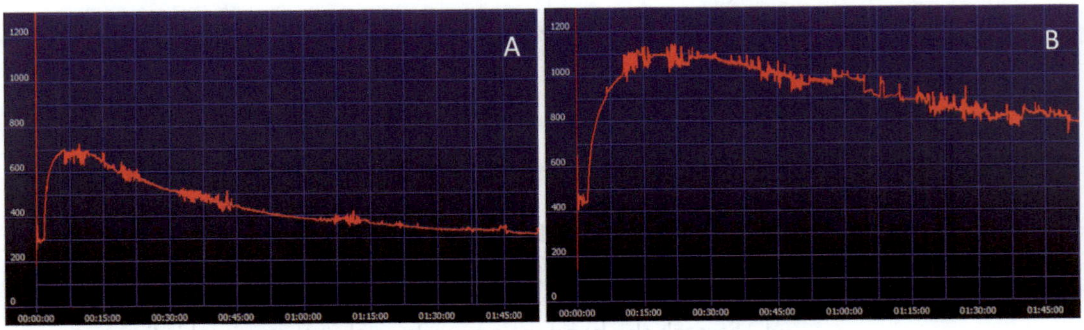

Fig. 4 Representative graphs of excretion curves of ABZWCY-HPβCD in a healthy (**a**) and cisplatin-induced kidney failure in (**b**) Sprague-Dawley rat, respectively. The signal emitted by ABZWCY-HPβCD is transcutaneously detected by the device and stored in its internal memory. The recorded data are read by the basic software that generates curves as shown in the images. *Y*-axis represents the fluorescence intensity emitted by the injected ABZWCY-HPβCD marker, while *X*-axis shows the duration of the measurement in time. These curves can be evaluated using 1–2-compartment models provided by the software

3.8 Data Analysis

1. Open software "GFRmeasure" (*see* **Note 7**) and add the ".csv" or ".xlsx" file containing the signal values over time for one experiment using the tab "Add table and calculate." This loads the signal as a function of time as a graph in the graphical user interface.
2. Select the number of compartments using "No. of compartments" tab. The corresponding model equation would be displayed in "Model equation" space. A three-compartment model is selected by default.
3. A reasonable initial guess for curve fitting is already provided. However, if the model does not fit well and residual error is high, the initial parameters could be changed using "Initial guesses" tab.
4. Manually click (single left click of mouse) on the injection point displayed in the graph. Similarly, cutoff point is also selected using double click (left). A good selection of injection and

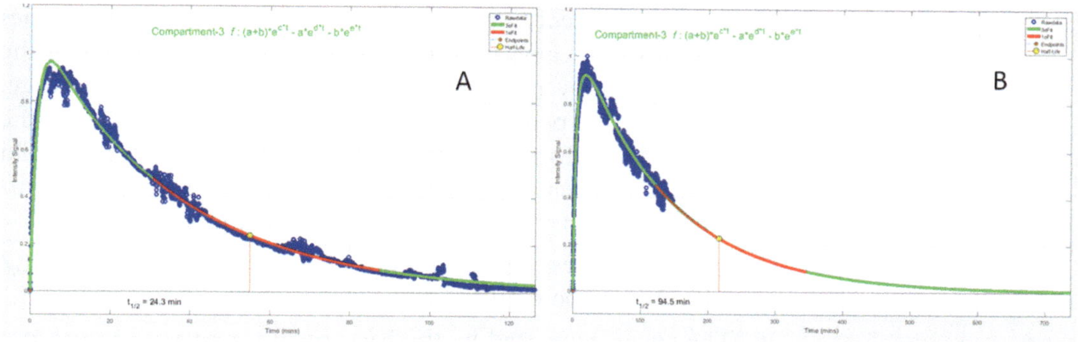

Fig. 5 Curve fitting to a three-compartment model using the representative graphs is shown in Fig. 4. The data are analyzed with the "GFRmeasure" software. It performs curve fitting showing the half-life of the substance injected in a healthy (**a**) and cisplatin-induced kidney failure in (**b**) Sprague-Dawley rat, respectively. *Y*-axis represents the fluorescence intensity emitted by the injected ABZWCY-HPβCD marker, while *X*-axis shows the duration of the measurement in time

cutoff points is required in order to evaluate the half-life in an efficient way. An automatic selection of the injection and cutoff points is also possible (*see* **Note 8**).

5. The model fitting process will be performed and fitting parameters along with the half-life calculations are obtained in the output window at the bottom right. One-exponent and three-exponent half-life values are displayed in minutes. Residual error of the three-exponent fit is also displayed.
6. The results are saved as images and .csv files in the user-selected folder (Fig. 5a, b).

4 Notes

1. During the anesthesia, it is recommended to put the animal on a heating plate to compensate the hypothermia due to the isoflurane.
2. Since the ABZWCY-HPβCD emission is in the near-infrared spectrum, a black plastic foil must be put on top of the device to prevent ambient light to induce noise. Avoid the use of aluminum foil since it interferes with the proper functioning of the device by short-circuiting that deletes the data recorded in the device.
3. For a better visualization of the tail vein, it is recommended to warm the tail up with warm tap water or to place the animal in a heating chamber for approximately 10 min before starting with the anesthesia. Additionally, instead of using a normal needle, an intravenous cannula could be used in order to easily inject the solution intravenously.

4. During the recording period, it is possible that the animal tries to remove the device from its back by biting or scratching the bandage or by rubbing its back against the lid of the cage. Putting some pellet food in the cage is a good way to give the animal some distraction. Furthermore, it is better to put the lid of the cage upside down. Avoiding all those abrupt movements can reduce noise in the signal during the measurement.
5. In certain cases, a short anesthesia with 5% isoflurane at 3 L/min O_2 may be required while removing the device.
6. The curve generated by the basic software gives an initial idea of the data quality. It is important to pay attention to the shape of the curve and, above all, to the maximum value of the peak on the *Y*-axis, which represents the fluorescence intensity emitted by the injected ABZWCY-HPβCD marker.

   The curves with the maximum peak values between ~400 and ~2000 are considered the optimum, while curves lower than ~400 and higher than ~2000 are not considered usable and have to be discarded.

   In the latter cases, the curves have to be considered implausible because at values ~400 it is not possible to discriminate the signal from the background, whereas at values higher than ~2000 the device saturation point was reached. Additionally, for curves between ~1500 and ~2000, the effect of quenching has to be taken into account.

   This first analysis of the curves is absolutely user dependent and is essential for discriminating the data and selecting only the usable ones.

   Choosing the appropriate ABZWCY-HPβCD dose for the animal we are working with is the first important step for having good and trustable curves.
7. The open software "GFRmeasure" is a stand-alone application based on MATLAB for which the user does not have to buy MATLAB license. A runtime compiler is however required that is freely available at https://www.mathworks.com/products/compiler/matlab-runtime.html.
8. The manual selection of the injection and cutoff points is a crucial step for an efficient evaluation of the half-life. During the recording period, the animal is awake and freely moving; hence, abrupt movements made by the animal can disturb the measurement and generate noisy curves. Therefore, when possible, it is convenient to exclude such artifacts from the analysis. For instance, if a curve ends with a noisy part, a cutoff point immediately before it should be selected. For an accurate determination of half-life value, it is way better to select a shorter but a smoother portion of the curve instead of a longer and noisy one. However, not much can be done if movement artifacts are

generated around the peak of the signal. In such a case, nothing can be done to exclude this part from the analysis. Therefore, it is very important to handle the animal very carefully after the injection in order to avoid artifacts in the read signal.

References

1. Stevens LA, Levey AS (2009) Measured GFR as a confirmatory test for estimated GFR. J Am Soc Nephrol 20(11):2305–2313. https://doi.org/10.1681/asn.2009020171
2. Katayama R, Yamaguchi N, Yamashita T, Watanabe S, Satoh H, Yamagishi N, Furuhama K (2010) Calculation of glomerular filtration rate in conscious rats by the use of a bolus injection of iodixanol and a single blood sample. J Pharmacol Toxicol Methods 61 (1):59–64. https://doi.org/10.1016/j.vascn.2009.10.002
3. Reinhardt CP, Germain MJ, Groman EV, Mulhern JG, Kumar R, Vaccaro DE (2008) Functional immunoassay technology (FIT), a new approach for measuring physiological functions: application of FIT to measure glomerular filtration rate (GFR). Am J Physiol Renal Physiol 295(5):F1583–F1588. https://doi.org/10.1152/ajprenal.90354.2008
4. Rieg T (2013) A high-throughput method for measurement of glomerular filtration rate in conscious mice. J Vis Exp 75:e50330. https://doi.org/10.3791/50330
5. Shmarlouski A, Schock-Kusch D, Shulhevich Y, Buschmann V, Rohlicke T, Herdt D, Radle M, Hesser J, Stsepankou D (2016) A novel analysis technique for transcutaneous measurement of glomerular filtration rate with ultralow dose marker concentrations. IEEE Trans Biomed Eng 63(8):1742–1750. https://doi.org/10.1109/tbme.2015.2501544
6. Wang E, Sandoval RM, Campos SB, Molitoris BA (2010) Rapid diagnosis and quantification of acute kidney injury using fluorescent ratiometric determination of glomerular filtration rate in the rat. Am J Physiol Renal Physiol 299(5):F1048–F1055. https://doi.org/10.1152/ajprenal.00691.2009
7. Yu W, Sandoval RM, Molitoris BA (2007) Rapid determination of renal filtration function using an optical ratiometric imaging approach. Am J Physiol Renal Physiol 292(6): F1873–F1880. https://doi.org/10.1152/ajprenal.00218.2006
8. Colson P, Capdevilla X, Cuchet D, Saussine M, Séguin JR, Marty-Anè C, Roquefeuil B (1992) Does choice of the Anesthetic influence renal function during Infrarenal aortic surgery? Anesth Analg 74(4):481–485
9. Fusellier M, Desfontis JC, Madec S, Gautier F, Debailleul M, Gogny M (2007) Influence of three anesthetic protocols on glomerular filtration rate in dogs. Am J Vet Res 68(8):807–811. https://doi.org/10.2460/ajvr.68.8.807
10. Herrera Perez Z, Weinfurter S, Gretz N (2016) Transcutaneous assessment of renal function in conscious rodents. J Vis Exp 109:e53767. https://doi.org/10.3791/53767
11. Schreiber A, Shulhevich Y, Geraci S, Hesser J, Stsepankou D, Neudecker S, Koenig S, Heinrich R, Hoecklin F, Pill J, Friedemann J, Schweda F, Gretz N, Schock-Kusch D (2012) Transcutaneous measurement of renal function in conscious mice. Am J Physiol Renal Physiol 303(5):F783–F788. https://doi.org/10.1152/ajprenal.00279.2012
12. Scarfe L, Rak-Raszewska A, Geraci S, Darssan D, Sharkey J, Huang J, Burton NC, Mason D, Ranjzad P, Kenny S, Gretz N, Levy R, Kevin Park B, Garcia-Finana M, Woolf AS, Murray P, Wilm B (2015) Measures of kidney function by minimally invasive techniques correlate with histological glomerular damage in SCID mice with adriamycin-induced nephropathy. Sci Rep 5:13601. https://doi.org/10.1038/srep13601
13. Huang J, Gretz N, Weinfurter S (2016) Filtration markers and determination methods for the assessment of kidney function. Eur J Pharmacol 790:92–98. https://doi.org/10.1016/j.ejphar.2016.06.060
14. Huang J, Weinfurter S, Daniele C, Perciaccante R, Federica R, Della Ciana L, Pill J, Gretz N (2017) Zwitterionic near infrared fluorescent agents for noninvasive real-time transcutaneous assessment of kidney function. Chem Sci 8(4):2652–2660. https://doi.org/10.1039/c6sc05059j

Chapter 10

An In Vitro Method to Analyze Glucose Uptake in Podocytes

Abigail C. Lay and Richard J. Coward

Abstract

Podocytes are terminally differentiated, insulin-sensitive cells of the glomerular filtration barrier, with a central role in filtration barrier maintenance. Podocyte injury is one of the earliest features observed in diabetic nephropathy (DN) and plays a key role in the development of albuminuria. Several factors are associated with diabetes-mediated podocyte injury, including dysregulated metabolic pathways and insulin sensitivity (Lay & Coward, Nephrol Dial Transplant 29:1127–1133, 2014); thus, reliable assays to study these responses are key in understanding podocyte alterations in DN. Here, we detail an in vitro method to analyze glucose uptake in conditionally immortalized human podocytes (Saleem, J Am Soc Nephrol 13:630–638, 2002; Coward, Diabetes 54:3095–3102, 2005); this assay is useful for detecting changes in podocyte metabolism, nutrient sensing, and insulin sensitivity.

Key words Podocyte, Glucose uptake, Insulin signaling, In vitro

1 Introduction

Assaying the cellular uptake of glucose is important in the study of many metabolic disorders, reflecting changes in cellular metabolism, nutrient-sensing pathways, and insulin sensitivity. Podocytes are terminally differentiated, insulin-sensitive cells of the glomerular filtration barrier, crucial in the prevention of albuminuria. Podocyte injury plays a central role in the early stages of diabetic nephropathy (DN); thus, studying podocyte metabolism in the context of diabetes is critical for understanding the mechanisms behind DN progression.

Podocytes express many glucose transporters, including the insulin-sensitive transporters GLUT1 and GLUT4, and rapidly uptake glucose in response to insulin [1–3]. Importantly, both the expression of glucose transporters and insulin-sensitive glucose uptake are dysregulated in podocytes in DN, playing pathogenic roles in podocyte damage [4–7].

This section outlines a method for studying insulin-stimulated glucose uptake into podocytes in vitro, by measuring the

Luigi Gnudi and David A. Long (eds.), *Diabetic Nephropathy: Methods and Protocols*, Methods in Molecular Biology, vol. 2067,
https://doi.org/10.1007/978-1-4939-9841-8_10, © Springer Science+Business Media, LLC, part of Springer Nature 2020

intracellular accumulation of radiolabeled glucose in conditionally immortalized human podocytes [8]. This method can be adapted to study podocyte glucose transport in response to other molecules and stimuli, including diabetic mediators and to use primary culture podocytes.

2 Materials

2.1 Podocyte Culture

Prepare and store all cell culture materials under sterile conditions.

1. RPMI-1640 medium containing L-glutamine and $NaHCO_3$, stored at 4 °C.
2. Fetal bovine serum (FBS), stored at 4 °C or –20 °C long term.
3. Biological safety cabinet suitable for human cell culture.
4. CO_2 cell culture incubators set at 5% CO_2, 33 °C and 37 °C.
5. Cell-culture-coated plasticware, typically T-75 cm^2 flasks for cell stocks and 6-well or 12-well plates.

2.2 Glucose Uptake

Prepare all solutions using sterile, deionized water and analytical grade reagents. Prepare reagents at room temperature and store at 4 °C, unless otherwise stated. Special care should be taken when handling radioactive material, ensuring that all guidelines for the storage, handling, and disposal of radioactive waste are followed.

1. Calcium-free KREBS salts: 1.36 M NaCl, 47 mM KCl, 125 mM $MgSO_4.7H_2O$.
2. Sodium phosphate buffer: 10 mM NaH_2PO_4, 10 mM Na_2HPO_4. Titrate to pH 7.4.
3. Krebs Ringer phosphate (KRP): Prepare on the morning of use. 2.5 mL Ca-free KREBS solution (as above), 12.5 mL sodium phosphatase stock solution (as above), 1.25 mM $CaCl_2$, 2 mM $NaHCO_3$, 25 mM HEPES. Make up to 25 mL.
4. Insulin.
5. Tritiated 2-deoxy-D-glucose (e.g., [3H] 2-deoxy-D-glucose, *see* **Note 1**).
6. Radiolabeled glucose solution: 0.5 mM Deoxy-D-glucose, 5-10 μCi [3H] 2-deoxy-D-glucose, diluted to 1 mL in KRP.
7. Phosphate-buffered saline (PBS), sterile-filtered.
8. Sterile-filtered PBS containing 1% Triton X-100.
9. Scintillation fluid, such as Ultima Gold™ liquid scintillation cocktail.
10. Multipurpose scintillator counter.
11. Polyethylene scintillation vials.

12. Vortex mixer.
13. Water bath, set at 37 °C.

3 Methods

3.1 Podocyte Culture

Perform all routine cell culture under sterile conditions, using an appropriate biological safety cabinet and maintain conditionally immortalized human podocytes (as previously characterized [8]) in RPMI containing 5% FBS.

1. Plate podocytes onto 12-well cell culture plates (*see* **Note 2**) and grow to 80% confluence at 33 °C in 5% CO_2.
2. Transfer the experimental plates to 37 °C in 5% CO_2 and allow to differentiate for 10–14 days (*see* **Note 3**), changing the cell culture media twice a week.

3.2 Cellular Glucose Uptake

Ensure that each experimental condition is carried out in duplicate or triplicate. Regulations for the storage, handling, and disposal of radioactive material should be followed. Appropriate measures for radiation monitoring should be employed at the end of the assay.

1. Serum-starve podocytes 2–4 h prior to the glucose uptake assay by washing the cells twice in RPMI-1640 medium without FBS and incubating with this serum-free medium (*see* **Notes 4–6**).
2. At room temperature, wash the cells three times in filter-sterilized PBS, and then add 450 μL of KRP solution to each well (*see* **Note 7**).
3. Transfer the plates to a water bath set at 37 °C, submerging the bases of the wells, and incubate for 15 min (*see* **Note 8**).
4. Where required, add the appropriate dose of insulin in a maximum volume of 5 μL and incubate for 15 min (*see* **Note 9**).
5. To each well, add 50 μL of radiolabeled glucose solution (*see* **Note 10**) and incubate for 5 min.
6. Remove the plate from the water bath and place on ice. Wash the cells three times in ice-cold PBS (*see* **Note 11**). After the third wash, aspirate the PBS and permeabilize the cells in 500 μL of sterile-filtered PBS containing 1% Triton X-100. Incubate for a minimum of 10 min.
7. Collect the cell supernatant (*see* **Note 12**) and add to scintillation vials containing 2 mL of scintillant fluid.
8. Briefly vortex the samples and measure the amount of radiolabeled glucose by scintillation counting (*see* **Note 13**).

4 Notes

1. 2-Deoxyglucose is a non-metabolized glucose analog, which accumulates inside cells as 2-deoxyglucose-6-phosphate once it is transported and phosphorylated. We generally use [3H] 2-deoxy-D-glucose with a specific activity of 5-10 Ci (185-370GBq)/mmol.
2. Cells can alternatively be grown in 6-well tissue culture plates if appropriate for the conditions being tested.
3. Maintaining the cells at 37 °C inactivates the heat-sensitive SV40 transgene, allowing the podocytes to differentiate, as previously characterized in detail [8].
4. Before and during the incubation with serum-free media, cells may be pre-treated with any drugs or conditions that are required.
5. If required, glucose transporters can be inhibited with a 30-min preincubation with cytochalasin B at a concentration of 10 μmol/L [9, 10].
6. At this point, podocytes can be counted so that the radiochemical results can be normalized to cell number.
7. If cells are grown in 6-well tissue culture plates, 900 μL of KRP solution should be added to each well.
8. This assay can also be performed at room temperature, but the changes observed will be much smaller and slower.
9. We have found that insulin concentrations of 10–100 nmol/L for 15 min successfully increase glucose uptake. Alternatively, other stimuli or inhibitors of glucose transport could be added here. In control (unstimulated) wells, a vehicle solution should be added.
10. If 6-well plates are being used, 100 μL of radiolabeled glucose solution should be added, to achieve a final concentration of 0.5–1 μCi/well [3H] 2-deoxy-D-glucose and 50 μM deoxy-D-glucose (unlabeled).
11. This wash in ice-cold PBS terminates the reaction. Care should be taken when removing radioactive waste (and in subsequent wash steps), ensuring that all local guidelines are followed.
12. Tilt the plate and pipette the triton/PBS solution over the cells a few times to ensure that the solubilized suspension (containing radioactive deoxyglucose) collects at the bottom of each well.
13. To calculate the number of moles of radiolabeled glucose transported into cells, values must first be converted from dpm (disintegrations per minute) to curie, which can then be converted into moles using the specific activity of the batch of [3H] 2-deoxy-D-glucose used in the assay.

References

1. Coward RJ et al (2005) The human glomerular podocyte is a novel target for insulin action. Diabetes 54(11):3095–3102
2. Schiffer M et al (2005) Localization of the GLUT8 glucose transporter in murine kidney and regulation in vivo in nondiabetic and diabetic conditions. Am J Physiol 289(1): F186–F193
3. Lennon R et al (2009) Rosiglitazone enhances glucose uptake in glomerular podocytes using the glucose transporter GLUT1. Diabetologia 52(9):1944–1952
4. Guzman J et al (2014) Podocyte-specific GLUT4-deficient mice have fewer and larger podocytes and are protected from diabetic nephropathy. Diabetes 63(2):701–714
5. Lennon R et al (2009) Saturated fatty acids induce insulin resistance in human podocytes: implications for diabetic nephropathy. Nephrol Dial Transplant 24(11):3288–3296
6. Lay AC et al (2017) Prolonged exposure of mouse and human podocytes to insulin induces insulin resistance through lysosomal and proteasomal degradation of the insulin receptor. Diabetologia 60(11):2299–2311
7. Lay A, Coward RJ (2014) Recent advances in our understanding of insulin signalling to the podocyte. Nephrol Dial Transplant 29 (6):1127–1133
8. Saleem MA et al (2002) A conditionally immortalized human podocyte cell line demonstrating nephrin and podocin expression. J Am Soc Nephrol 13(3):630–638
9. Czech MP, Lynn DG, Lynn WS (1973) Cytochalasin B-sensitive 2-deoxy-D-glucose transport in adipose cell ghosts. J Biol Chem 248 (10):3636–3641
10. Jung CY, Rampal AL (1977) Cytochalasin B binding sites and glucose transport carrier in human erythrocyte ghosts. J Biol Chem 252 (15):5456–5463

Chapter 11

Glomerular Endothelial Cells: Assessment of Barrier Properties In Vitro

Raina D. Ramnath and Simon C. Satchell

Abstract

Endothelial cells form the inner lining of all blood vessels and play a vital role in regulating vascular permeability. This applies to the circulation in general and also to specific capillary beds including the renal glomerular capillaries. Endothelial dysfunction, including increased permeability, is a key component of diabetes-induced organ damage. Endothelial cells together with their glycocalyx, grown on porous membranes, provide an excellent model to study endothelial permeability properties. Here we describe the measurement of two characteristics of glomerular endothelial cell (GEnC) monolayers: electrical resistance and macromolecular passage. Trans-endothelial electrical resistance provides a measure of small-pore pathways across the endothelium and provides an index of monolayer confluence and cell-cell junction integrity. Measurement of macromolecular passage provides an index of large-pore pathways and use of labeled albumin provides direct relevance to the clinically important parameter of albuminuria. The combination of the two approaches provides a fantastic tool to elucidate endothelial barrier function in vitro including in response to cytokines, pathological stimuli, and potential therapeutic agents.

Key words Glomerular endothelial cells (GEnC), Macromolecular permeability, Trans-endothelial electrical resistance, Porous membrane

1 Introduction

The permeability characteristics of the glomerular capillary wall depend on its unique three-layer structure, consisting of endothelial cells on the luminal side of the capillaries, the basement membrane in the middle, and podocytes on the urinary side. Together, they form the glomerular filtration barrier, which is highly permeable to water and small molecules but has low permeability to macromolecules. The glomerular filtration barrier functions as a whole with disruption of the permeability properties of any one layer, including the endothelium, affecting the overall permeability.

Glomerular endothelial cells are characterized by fenestrations, circular transcellular pores 60–80 nm in diameter, essential for water permeability. The presence of fenestrations has meant that

Luigi Gnudi and David A. Long (eds.), *Diabetic Nephropathy: Methods and Protocols*, Methods in Molecular Biology, vol. 2067, https://doi.org/10.1007/978-1-4939-9841-8_11, © Springer Science+Business Media, LLC, part of Springer Nature 2020

the glomerular endothelium has been considered to contribute little to the barrier to macromolecules. However, it is now widely accepted that the luminal surface of the glomerular endothelium is covered with a glycocalyx which constitutes a significant permeability barrier [1–5].

The glycocalyx is a negatively charged hydrated mesh of cell surface-anchored proteoglycans and adsorbed proteins and glycosaminoglycans in dynamic equilibrium with the plasma. Because of the ubiquitous nature of the endothelial glycocalyx, damage to the endothelial glycocalyx alters the permeability of multiple capillary beds: in the glomerulus this is clinically apparent as albuminuria [6], the presence of plasma albumin in the urine. Albuminuria is the most reliable sign of development of diabetic kidney disease and is a powerful predictor of both renal and cardiovascular disease progression [1, 7].

Trans-endothelial electrical resistance (TEER) is a measure of pathways across the endothelium including small-pore pathways accessible only to water, small molecules, and ions. In a sub-confluent layer of cells, the resistance is related to the fractional area covered by the cells. In a confluent monolayer it provides a measure of cell-cell junction integrity. It can therefore be used to confirm the presence of a cell monolayer before using the cells to measure macromolecular passage. The measurement of macromolecular permeability (e.g., of fluorescence-labeled albumin) across glomerular endothelial cell monolayer provides a simple and robust measure of trans-endothelial solute flux. As endothelial glycocalyx restricts passage of albumin but provides relatively little hindrance to ions differential changes in TEER and macromolecular passage can be used to infer changes in glycocalyx. With both measurements cells can be treated with exogenous agents to measure their effects on permeability properties. Cyclic AMP and thrombin provide useful controls which are expected to decrease and increase endothelial permeability parameters, respectively [8]. Tumor necrosis factor alpha (TNFα) provides an example of an inflammatory mediator elevated in diabetic milieu which tends to increase endothelial permeability [3].

2 Materials

Prepare all solutions using sterile, deionized water and analytical grade reagents. Prepare reagents at room temperature and store at 4 °C. Special care should be taken to follow waste disposal regulations.

2.1 Solutions

1. EGM-2MV Bullet Kit (CC-3202; Lonza, Basel, Switzerland) consists of EBM2 basal medium (CC-3156) and singlequots (CC-4147) which contains growth factors, antimicrobials, and

serum. EGM-2MV is used in the following experiments (*see* **Note 1**).

2. 5 mL EBM2 basal medium is added to 50 mg of fluorescein isothiocyanate-conjugated bovine serum albumin (FITC-BSA) to make 10 mg/mL stock FITC-BSA. 1 mL FITC-BSA is added to 9 mL EBM2 basal medium to make 1 mg/mL FITC-BSA. To remove free dye, the solution is spun at 2934× *g* for 20 min in a 10 kD ultrafiltration device. Following reconstitution in 10 mL EBM2 basal medium, the solution is sterilized by passing through a 0.2 μm filter.
3. 10 mg Unlabeled bovine serum albumin (BSA) is dissolved in 10 mL EBM2 basal medium to make 1 mg/mL unlabeled BSA. The solution is sterilized by passing through a 0.2 μm filter.
4. A solution of a cell membrane-permeable cAMP analog, 8-(4-chlorophenylthio) (pCPT)-cAMP (300 μM) in combination with a cAMP-specific phosphodiesterase inhibitor, RO-20-1724 (20 μM) in EGM-2MV (cAMP medium), and sterilized by passing through a 0.2 μm filter.
5. 1 U/mL Thrombin is made up in EGM-2 V and sterilized by passing through a 0.2 μm filter.
6. Vehicle: Phosphate-buffered saline, pH 7.4, containing 0.1% BSA, sterilized by passing through a 0.2 μm filter.
7. 10 ng/mL TNFα is prepared from a 10 μg TNFα stock, dissolved in the vehicle (above).

2.2 Equipment

1. Epithelial voltohmmeter (EVOM).
2. EndOhm 12 chamber (World Precision Instruments) is suitable for 12 mm culture cup.
3. Polycarbonate cell culture inserts and carrier plates; pore size, 0.4 μm; pore density, pores/cm^2 < 0.85 × 108; culture area, 0.47 cm^2.
4. Tissue culture incubator: 5% CO_2: 95% air, set at 37 °C.

3 Methods

3.1 Tissue Culture Insert Preparation

1. Human conditionally immortalized glomerular endothelial cells (GEnC), previously characterized in detail [9, 10], are cultured in EGM-2MV containing 5% fetal calf serum and growth factors as supplied (*see* **Note 2**).
2. The cells are seeded at a density of 100,000 cells/cm^2 in a volume of 0.5 mL EGM-2MV onto polycarbonate porous membranes in tissue culture inserts (*see* **Note 3**).

3. 0.5 mL of EGM-2MV is also added to blank inserts without cells.
4. Inserts are placed in 24-well plates and 0.5 mL EGM-2MV is added to the wells.
5. The plate is placed in the 37 °C incubator and media are changed three times per week.

3.2 Trans-Endothelial Electrical Resistance (TEER) (See Note 4)

1. The experimental apparatus used to measure TEER is shown in Fig. 1.
2. The EVOM and the EndOhm 12 chamber are sterilized with 70% ethanol before placing them in the laminar flow hood.
3. The EVOM power button is turned on.
4. The function switch on the EVOM is set to Ohms (*see* **Note 5**).

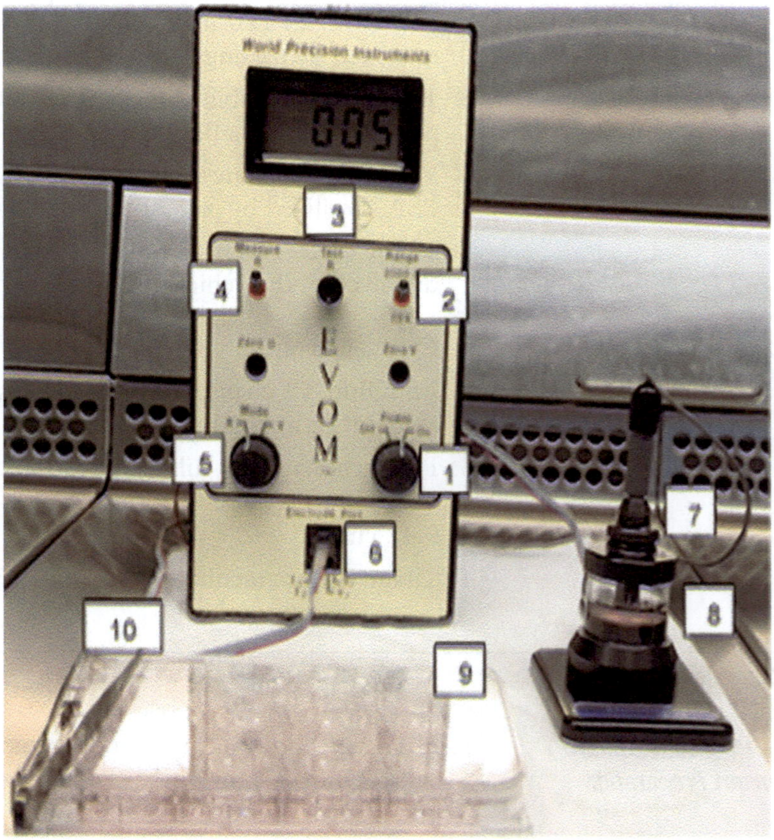

Fig. 1 The setup used to carry out TEER on endothelial cells. (*1*) Power switch on/off. (*2*) Range toggle switch. (*3*) Test R pushbutton. (*4*) Measure R pushbutton (EVOM). (*5*) Mode switch R/V. (*6*) Electrode port. (*7*) Cap containing the top electrode. (*8*) Chamber containing the bottom electrode. (*9*) 12-Well plate containing the inserts. (*10*) Forceps

5. 2 mL of EGM-2MV medium is added to the EndOhm chamber.
6. The 24-well plate containing the inserts is moved from the 37 °C incubator to the laminar flow hood. The inserts are transferred sequentially from the well to the EndOhm chamber by a pair of forceps.
7. The cap is placed on the chamber so that the top electrode is centered and 1–2 mm above the cell layer (*see* **Note 6**).
8. After 20 s of stabilization, the resistance of the blank insert (no cells) is recorded.
9. Similar procedure is carried out to measure the resistance of the GEnC-seeded inserts.
10. The resistance of a blank insert is subtracted from that of the GEnC-containing inserts to obtain the resistance attributable to the GEnC monolayer.
11. The resistance of the monolayer is multiplied by the effective growing area to obtain the electrical resistance of the endothelial monolayer (Ohms.cm^2).

3.3 Trans-Endothelial Permeability to Macromolecules

1. 50 μL of medium from inserts and wells is pipetted out (discarded) and replaced with 50 μL of 1 mg/mL FITC-labeled BSA or unlabeled BSA, respectively.
2. After 1-, 2-, and 3-h incubation at 37 °C, 100 μL aliquots are removed from the wells (for measurement) and replaced with 100 μL of media containing unlabeled BSA (100 μg/mL).
3. During the incubation time, prepare 6 μg/mL FITC-labeled BSA standard using 100 μg/mL unlabeled BSA. Set up 7 points of diluted standard such as 6 μg/mL, 3 μg/mL, 1.5 μg/mL, 0.75 μg/mL, 0.375 μg/mL, 0.1875 μg/mL, and 0.0938 μg/mL, and the last one is the 0 μg/mL blank (*see* **Notes**).
4. Add 100 μL of each dilution of standards (in duplicate) and samples into a 96-well clear flat-bottom plate.
5. Measure the fluorescence using a fluorescence plate reader set at an excitation wavelength of 495 and an emission wavelength of 520.
6. Average the duplicate readings for each standard and construct a standard curve by plotting fluorescence intensity against concentration.
7. The amount of FITC-labeled BSA passing through the monolayer is calculated by reference to the BSA standard curve and then the cumulative amount at each hour calculated and plotted against time.

3.4 Effects of Exogenous Agents

1. Cell monolayers on polycarbonate inserts are treated with cAMP medium, thrombin, or control (EGM-2MV) for 1 h at 37 °C by replacement of the medium in the insert and well with the above solutions, prior to measurement of TEER or the albumin passage assay.
2. The cells on the polycarbonate inserts are stimulated with 10 ng/mL TNFα or vehicle for 2 h at 37 °C prior to measurement of TEER or the albumin passage assay.

4 Notes

1. Other endothelial media (e.g., ScienCell, catalog number 1001) can be used if shown to be suitable for culture of endothelial cells studied.
2. Other endothelial cells can be used in the same assay. We have successfully used it with primary culture human glomerular endothelial cells and human cardiac microvascular endothelial cells. Optimal seeding densities will need to be determined for each cell type.
3. Commercially available treated polycarbonate membranes are used to promote cell attachment and they have high pore density to allow more exchange through the membrane.
4. TEER is used to test the quality of the endothelial cell barrier using an EndOhm chamber. The EndOhm chamber and cap each contains a pair of concentric electrodes. TEER is determined by the resistance against the flow of ions between the two compartments. Since ions flow easily through the porous membrane but not cells, high TEER values indicate successful establishment of a cell monolayer for albumin permeability study. The formation of a cell barrier can take several days as the cells must grow to confluence and form cell-cell junctions.
5. To test if the EVOM is working properly, press the Test R button. Pressing this pushbutton when the meter is in the R mode will connect the circuit to an internal 1000 Ω standard resistor whose resistance will then be measured. If the display shows a value close to 1000 Ω (± 1%), then the meter's resistance measurement is acceptable.
6. The height setting of the top electrode of the EndOhm can be adjusted by loosening the locking nut on the cap assembly, so that the top electrode is immersed in the apical media. Once set, the height of the top electrode should not be changed; otherwise it can change the TEER readings. With the cap in place, the height of the EGM-2MV medium in the chamber (approximately 2 mL) should be at the same level as inside the insert (approximately 500 μL) to avoid hydrostatic pressure on

the membrane. Also, care should be taken to avoid air bubbles being trapped between the top electrode and the surface of the medium by tilting the top electrode slightly as it is replaced.

References

1. Satchell SC, Tooke JE (2008) What is the mechanism of microalbuminuria in diabetes: a role for the glomerular endothelium? Diabetologia 51:714–725
2. Satchell SC (2012) The glomerular endothelium emerges as a key player in diabetic nephropathy. Kidney Int 82:949–951
3. Ramnath R, Foster RR, Qiu Y, Cope G, Butler MJ, Salmon AH, Mathieson PW, Coward RJ, Welsh GI, Satchell SC (2014) Matrix metalloproteinase 9-mediated shedding of syndecan 4 in response to tumor necrosis factor alpha: a contributor to endothelial cell glycocalyx dysfunction. FASEB J 28(11):4686–4699
4. Haraldsson B, Nystrom J, Deen WM (2008) Properties of the glomerular barrier and mechanisms of proteinuria. Physiol Rev 88:451–487
5. Curry FE, Adamson RH (2012) Endothelial glycocalyx: permeability barrier and mechanosensor. Ann Biomed Eng 40:828–839
6. Salmon AH, Satchell SC (2012) Endothelial glycocalyx dysfunction in disease: albuminuria and increased microvascular permeability. J Pathol 226:562–574
7. Heerspink HJ, Holtkamp FA, de Zeeuw D, Ravid M (2011) Monitoring kidney function and albuminuria in patients with diabetes. Diabetes Care 34(Suppl 2):S325–S329
8. Satchell SC, Anderson KL, Mathieson PW (2004) Angiopoietin 1 and vascular endothelial growth factor modulate human glomerular endothelial cell barrier properties. J Am Soc Nephrol 15:566–574
9. Singh A, Ramnath RD, Foster RR, Wylie EC, Friden V, Dasgupta I, Haraldsson B, Welsh GI, Mathieson PW, Satchell SC (2013) Reactive oxygen species modulate the barrier function of the human glomerular endothelial glycocalyx. PLoS One 8:e55852
10. Satchell SC, Tasman CH, Singh A, Ni L, Geelen J, von Ruhland CJ, O'Hare MJ, Saleem MA, van den Heuvel LP, Mathieson PW (2006) Conditionally immortalized human glomerular endothelial cells expressing fenestrations in response to VEGF. Kidney Int 69:1633–1640

Chapter 12

Methods to Detect Endoplasmic Reticulum Stress and Apoptosis in Diabetic Nephropathy

Khurrum Shahzad, Sanchita Ghosh, Akash Mathew, and Berend Isermann

Abstract

A variety of pathophysiological cellular dysfunctions stress the endoplasmic reticulum (ER), promoting an accumulation of unfolded proteins in the ER lumen. The latter is sensed by intrinsic ER transmembrane proteins: IRE1α (inositol-requiring protein-1α), PERK (protein kinase RNA (PKR)-like ER kinase), and ATF6 (activating transcription factor 6) which when activated trigger the unfolded protein response (UPR), which includes an inhibition of protein translation while inducing specific transcription factors that induce genes aiming to relieve the ER stress response. Collectively, this reduces the burden of unfolded proteins within the ER, eventually restoring ER homeostasis and thus promoting cell survival and adaptation. However, under unresolvable ER stress conditions, the UPR promotes cell death. Diabetic nephropathy (dNP), a leading cause of end-stage renal disease in industrialized countries, is mechanistically closely linked with ER stress and renal cell death. Here, we describe methods (both in vivo and in vitro) for monitoring ER stress, UPR signaling, and cell death in renal cells by analyzing proteins and protein-protein interactions serving as markers of ER stress or cell death. These methods include visualization of interactions of UPR regulators by proximity ligation assay on renal tissue and cells and methods to detect cell death based on DNA fragmentation or fluorochrome substrates for caspases. We include two selected in vivo models to manipulate ER stress regulators and thus the UPR in murine models of dNP. Collectively, these analyses allow assessment of the activation of ER stress-induced signaling pathways and cell death in dNP and manipulation of the UPR in vivo, enabling researchers to probe for causality.

Key words Endoplasmic reticulum, Unfolded protein response, Activated protein C, Apoptosis, Cell death, Diabetic nephropathy

1 Introduction

The endoplasmic reticulum (ER) is primarily recognized as the site of synthesis and folding of secreted, membrane-bound, and some organelle-targeted proteins [1]. The efficient functioning of the ER is essential for most cellular activities and survival. Conditions that interfere with ER function lead to the accumulation and aggregation of unfolded proteins—a condition referred to as ER stress. The latter is sensed by intrinsic ER transmembrane proteins: IRE1α (inositol-requiring protein-1α), PERK (protein kinase RNA

Luigi Gnudi and David A. Long (eds.), *Diabetic Nephropathy: Methods and Protocols*, Methods in Molecular Biology, vol. 2067, https://doi.org/10.1007/978-1-4939-9841-8_12, © Springer Science+Business Media, LLC, part of Springer Nature 2020

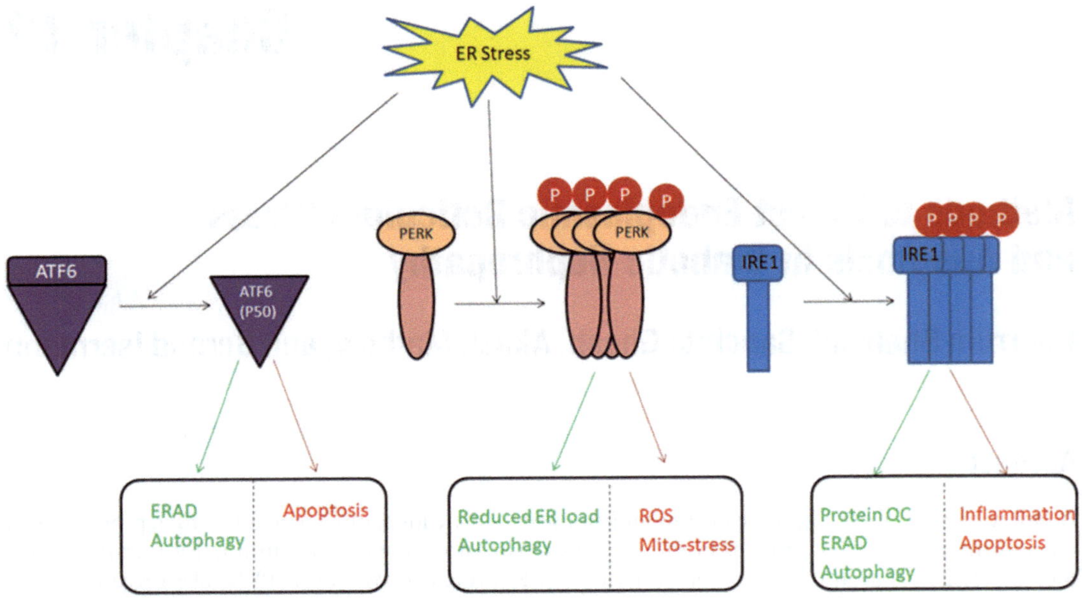

Fig. 1 A brief schematic of the double-edged nature of the ER stress response. The conversion of the ER stress sensors from the inactive to their active signaling state is indicated here by arrows moving from left to right. Text in green is representative of cytoprotective functions (adaptive ER stress response), while red text is indicative of detrimental functions (maladaptive ER stress response) initiated by signaling of each ER stress arm. *ERAD* endoplasmic reticulum-associated protein degradation, *ROS* reactive oxygen species, *Protein QC* protein quality control, *mito-stress*, mitochondrial stress

(PKR)-like ER kinase), and ATF6 (activating transcription factor 6, Fig. 1) [2, 3]. Activation of each of these stress sensors leads to a series of corrective actions known as the unfolded protein response (UPR, shown in green in Fig. 1). The UPR relieves ER stress by several mechanisms, including inhibition of protein translation, which decreases the load of proteins entering the ER, and induction of chaperone molecules, which promotes proper protein folding. ATF6, PERK, and IRE1 form complexes with immunoglobulin-binding protein (BiP), a resident chaperon of the ER, through their luminal domains. On sensing ER stress, BiP dissociates from PERK and IRE1, allowing them to form oligomers, trans-autophosphorylate, and activate further signaling. Dissociation from BiP allows ATF6 to translocate to the Golgi apparatus, where it is cleaved by site-1 and -2 proteases [3, 4]. A cleaved cytoplasmic domain of the ATF6 then translocates to the nucleus to activate target genes such as BiP and C/EBP homologous protein (CHOP) [5]. While the PERK arm globally halts protein translation to reduce ER protein load (but selectively induces the transcription of ATF4), ATF6 and IRE1 activate downstream chaperones and enzymes that facilitate protein folding and maturation [1]. Upon accumulation of unfolded proteins in the ER lumen, activated IRE1 cleaves the mRNA encoding X-box-binding protein-1 (XBP1), resulting in a shift of the reading frame and a higher molecular weight protein, which is referred to as spliced XBP1 (sXBP1). sXBP1 relocates to the nucleus to induce the transcription of essential UPR genes such as ER chaperones and ER-associated degradation regulators, thus effectively increasing the ER folding capacity and expanding the ER membrane surface area (adaptive ER stress response, shown in green in Fig. 1). As a result, proteins retained in the ER are properly folded or delivered to the cytosol for ubiquitin-proteasomal degradation (ERAD, endoplasmic reticulum-associated protein degradation). The nuclear translocation of sXBP1 depends on its interaction with the regulatory subunits of the class IA phosphatidylinositol 3-kinase (PI3K), p85α, and p85β [6].

Perturbations in ER homeostasis due to prolonged accumulation of misfolded proteins or increased protein synthesis trigger UPR-mediated cell death, probably via programmed cell death (apoptosis), characterized by cell shrinkage, chromatin condensation, and DNA fragmentation (shown in red in Fig. 1). ER stress and cell death are thought to contribute to the pathogenesis of many diseases including diabetic nephropathy (dNP), atherosclerosis, cardiac hypertrophy, and fatty liver disease [1, 7–10].

Various methods are established for monitoring the activation of ER stress and cell death pathways in dNP [11, 12]. Here we add to the repertoire by introducing methods for the visualization of proteins involved in ER stress and cell death in dNP. Furthermore, we describe in vivo murine models for manipulation of ER stress in dNP.

2 Materials

2.1 Proximity Ligation Assay Using Tissue Sections

2.1.1 Equipment Required

(a) Incubator at 65 °C for dewaxing.

(b) Incubator at 37 °C.

(c) Fluorescence microscope with appropriate filters, camera, and software for image acquisition.

(d) Orbital shaker (100 rpm).

2.1.2 Reagents Required

(a) Xylene for dewaxing.

(b) Ethanol dilutions for rehydration of tissue sections: 100%, 95%, 80%, 70%, 50%, and 30% ethanol solutions made in high-purity filtered water.

(c) 1× Phosphate-buffered saline (PBS): Dissolve 8 g of NaCl, 0.2 g of KCl, 1.44 g of Na_2HPO_4, and 0.24 g of KH_2PO_4 in 800 mL of distilled water. Adjust pH to 7.4 with HCl and make up to 1000 mL.

(d) Antigen-retrieval buffer consisting of 10 mM sodium citrate buffer, pH 6.0, and 0.05% Tween-20: Dissolve 2.94 g of trisodium citrate (dihydrate) in 800 mL of distilled water. Adjust pH to 6.0 with 1 N HCl, add 0.5 mL of Tween 20, dissolve, and make up to 1000 mL.

(e) 100% Acetone (ice cold).

(f) 100% Methanol (ice cold).

(g) Blocking solution: 2% Donkey serum made in 1× PBS + 0.5% Tween 20 + 0.2% Triton X-100.

(h) Two primary antibodies raised in different species: For example, anti-XBP1 antibody raised in rabbit and anti-PI3 kinase, p85α antibody raised in mouse.

(i) Hydrophobic pen.

(j) Staining jars and plastic cuvettes.

(k) Humidied chamber for incubating tissue sections.

(l) Forceps.

(m) Coverslips compatible with fluorescence microscopy.

(n) Vectashield mounting media containing DAPI (4′,6-diamidino-2-phenylindole, dihydrochloride).

(o) Duolink PLA probes 5× (PLUS and MINUS probes stored at 4 °C).

(p) Antibody diluent (provided in the Duolink kit, stored at 4 °C).

(q) Duolink Fluorescence detection reagent kit (contains 5× ligation buffer, ligase enzyme, 5× amplification buffer, and polymerase stored at −20 °C).

(r) Wash buffers for fluorescence (A and B; Duolink): Prepared by dissolving the contents of one pouch in 1000 mL of high-purity water as per instructions and stored at 4 °C.

(s) 0.01× Wash buffer B: Prepared by diluting wash buffer B 1:100 in high-purity water.

(t) FITC-phalloidin (diluted in DMSO to a stock concentration of 1 mg/mL and stored at −20 °C).

2.2 Proximal Ligation Assay Using Paraffin-Fixed Cells (Additional Material Required)

(a) Glass coverslips or chamber slides coated with collagen.

(b) 3.7% Paraformaldehyde solution: Warm up 1× PBS to 60 °C in a ventilated hood under constant stirring, add 37 g of paraformaldehyde powder, and continue stirring. Slowly raise the pH by adding 1 N NaOH dropwise until the solution becomes clear. Once the paraformaldehyde is dissolved and the solution is cooled, recheck the pH and adjust it to approximately 6.9 with small amounts of HCl. Adjust the volume to 1000 mL with 1× PBS.

2.3 Assessment of Cell Death Using TUNEL Fluorescein Assay

2.3.1 Equipment Required

(a) Incubator at 37 °C.

(b) Light microscope with appropriate filters, camera, and software for image acquisition.

(c) Humidified chamber for incubating coverslips.

2.3.2 Reagents Required

1. TUNEL detection kit (this follows Roche Diagnostic reagents).
   (a) For analyses of samples add 15 μL enzyme (terminal deoxynucleotidyl transferase) solution to 285 μL nucleotide mixture in reaction buffer (1:20 dilution). This is a 1:2 dilution of the recommended concentration (1:10), which works well and tends to give less background. It is highly recommended to prepare this solution fresh.
   (b) For negative control use 100 μL label solution only.
   (c) Anti-fluorescein antibody, Fab fragment from sheep, conjugated with peroxidase.
2. DAB Substrate Kit for Peroxidase: Prepare fresh DAB working solution: Take 5 mL dH_2O, add two drops of buffer stock solution, mix, add four drops of DAB stock solution, mix, add two drops of H_2O_2 solution, and mix well. Prepare directly before using.
3. Roti Histo-Kit II (Roth): Comparable assays are available from different providers.
4. Xylene.
5. Hematoxylin counterstain (e.g., Gill's formula): The stock solution can be used multiple times provided that the solutions are clear and kept covered. It is recommended to filter the solution before each use to remove oxidized particle.
6. Ethanol: Dilute pure ethanol with distilled water to prepare 100%, 95%, 80%, 70%, 50%, and 30%. These ethanol solutions can be used multiple times provided that the solutions are clear and kept closed to avoid evaporation of ethanol.
7. PBS: Prepare PBS stock (10×) by adding 80 g NaCl, 2 g KCl, 14.4 g Na_2HPO_4, and 2.4 g KH_2PO_4. Dissolve in 800 mL dH_2O and adjust the pH to 7.4. Adjust volume to 1 L.
8. PBS containing 0.1% Triton and 0.1% sodium citrate.
9. Acid rinse solution (take 2 mL of glacial acetic acid and add 98 mL of dH_2O): The solution can be used for multiple times provided that the solutions are clear and kept covered. It is recommended to filter the solution before each use to remove oxidized particle.

10. Bluing solution (take 1.5°mL NH_4OH and add 98.5°mL of 70% EtOH). The solution can be used multiple times provided that the solutions are clear and kept covered. It is recommended to filter the solution before each use to remove particle.
11. Hydrophobic pen.

2.4 In Situ Caspase-3/7 Activity Assay

2.4.1 Reagents Required

(a) FAM-FLICA® Caspase-3/7 Assay Kit: Prepare 3× FLICA™ working solution (by diluting 150× stock solution into 1:50 in PBS); protect from light.

(b) PBS: Prepare 10× stock by adding 80 g NaCl, 2 g KCl, 14.4 g Na_2HPO_4, and 2.4 g KH_2PO_4. Dissolve in 800 mL dH_2O and adjust the pH to 7.4. Adjust volume to 1 L.

(c) Blocking solution: 20% Aqua-block in media with 0.2% Tween 20.

(d) Distilled water (dH_2O).

(e) Hydrophobic pen.

(f) Vectashield mounting medium with DAPI.

(g) Fluorescent microscope.

3 Methods

3.1 Proximity Ligation Assay on Paraffin-Embedded Sections

Proximity ligation assay (PLA) may be employed to visualize and thus localize activation of ER stress in different cells and tissues. Unlike other methods in molecular biology such as fluorescence resonance energy transfer (FRET), PLA allows one to visualize both stable and transient interactions of endogenous proteins without requiring the overexpression of plasmids or genetic manipulation of cells or animals. While FRET can detect stable protein-protein interactions in live cells, PLA can be used to study protein-protein interactions in fixed tissues or cells. In PLA, the interaction of two proteins can be seen only when a pair of oligonucleotide-labeled antibodies (PLA probes) are used to generate an amplified signal within close proximity (<40 nm) of each other. While FRET allows for the detection of proteins within 1–10 nm range, it requires external illumination to initiate fluorescence transfer that can lead to background noise from direct excitation of the acceptor or to photobleaching. PLA is highly specific since the two antibodies are probed with two specific oligonucleotides reducing false positives.

PLA is compatible with all fixations suitable for immunofluorescence (IF) and immunohistochemistry (IHC). The choice of fixative may vary depending on the sample type (cells or tissue), primary antibodies, and targeted protein (*see* **Note 1**). Below, we outline a protocol of PLA for paraffin-embedded human and

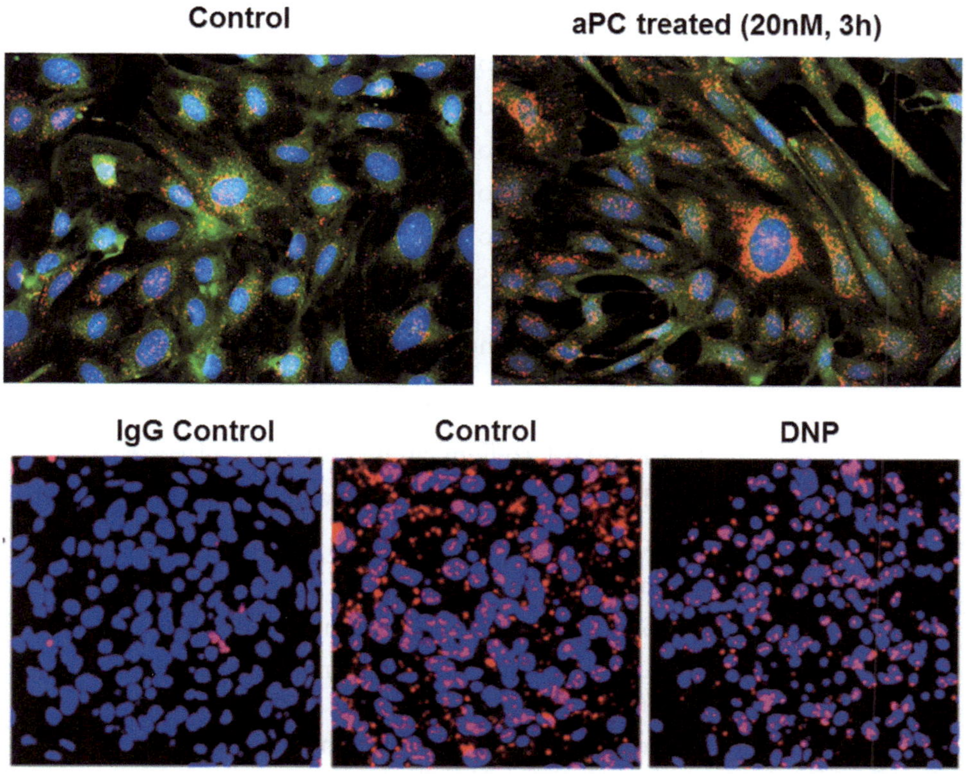

Fig. 2 Proximity ligation assay in mouse podocytes plated on collagen-coated coverslips and paraformaldehyde fixed (top), and in paraffin-embedded human kidney sections (bottom). The red dots are the PLA-positive signals indicating the increased sXBP1-p85α and sXBP1-p85β interactions in podocytes [8, 9] (DNP: diabetic nephropathy)

mouse kidney sections (3–5 μm thick). Tissue samples originate from control and 24-week hyperglycemic age-matched mice (streptozotocin-induced model of type 1 diabetes mellitus) as well as human renal biopsies obtained from type 2 diabetic patients.

To determine the activation of ER stress pathways one can detect and quantify the interaction between spliced XBP1 and p85α or p85β in the nucleus and cytoplasm of cells (e.g., podocytes) within the glomerulus or tubular compartment [8, 9]. The protocol below can be used to determine whether the interaction between sXBP1 and p85α or p85β in the nucleus and cytoplasm of podocytes is increased or reduced under hyperglycemia (Fig. 2).

3.1.1 Dewaxing Tissue Sections

1. Incubate paraffin slides for 30 min at 65 °C.
2. 10 min Xylene.
3. 10 min Fresh xylene.
4. 2 min in 100% ethanol.

3.1.2 Rehydrating Tissue Sections

1. 20 s 100% Ethanol.
2. 20 s 95% Ethanol.
3. 20 s 85% Ethanol.
4. 20 s 70% Ethanol.
5. 20 s 50% Ethanol.
6. 20 s 30% Ethanol.
7. 2× 5 min in PBS.

3.1.3 Postfixing

1 min in 4 ° C acetone:MeOH (1:1), followed by 5 min in 1× PBS.

3.1.4 Antigen Retrieval

1. Boil 800 mL distilled water in a 2 L glass beaker.
2. Add 60 mL sodium citrate buffer to a plastic cuvette.
3. Add the slides to the cuvette and cover with a glass lid.
4. Store the cuvette safely in the boiling 2 L glass.
5. Cover with aluminum foil.
6. Boil the cuvette for 30 min in the 2 L glass.
7. Remove the cuvette containing the glass slides to room temperature and allow them to cool down for 20 min.
8. Rinse slides twice for 2 min in high-purity water.

3.1.5 Blocking

1. Briefly dry the glass slides with tissue without drying out the tissue sections and circle around the tissues with a hydrophobic pen to delimit the reaction areas (*see* **Note 2**).
2. Block tissues with blocking solution (homemade preparation) at room temperature in a humidified chamber.

3.1.6 Primary Antibodies

1. Shake off the blocking solutions and incubate sections with anti-XBP1 and anti-PI3 kinase antibody, p85α antibodies diluted 1:200 appropriately diluted in the antibody diluent (Duolink) overnight at 4 °C in a humidified chamber (*see* **Note 3**).
2. Tap off the primary antibodies and wash with buffer A twice for 5 min each (*see* **Note 4**).

3.1.7 PLA Probes

1. Dilute the PLA probes (PLUS and MINUS) 1:5 in the antibody diluent provided in the kit.
2. Incubate the slides in a preheated humidity chamber for 1 h at 37 °C.

3.1.8 Ligation

1. Dilute the ligation stock 1:5 in high-purity water and mix.
2. Tap off the PLA probe solution from the slides and wash in 1x wash buffer A for 2 × 5 min under gentle agitation in a plastic cuvette.

3. Remove the ligase (provided in the Duolink fluorescence detection reagent kit) from the freezer using a freezing block (−20 °C). Add ligase to the ligation mix at a 1:40 dilution and vortex.
4. Add the ligation-ligase solution to each sample and incubate slides in a preheated humidity chamber for 30 min at 37 °C.

3.1.9 Amplification

1. Dilute the amplification stock 1:5 in high-purity water and mix (*see* **Note 5**).
2. Tap off the ligation-ligase solution from the slides and wash them in 1× wash buffer A twice for 2 min under gentle agitation.
3. Remove the polymerase from the freezer using a freezing block (−20 °C). Add the polymerase to the amplification solution at a 1:80 dilution and vortex.
4. Add the amplification-polymerase solution to each sample and incubate the slides in a preheated chamber for 100 min at 37 °C in the dark.

3.1.10 Actin Cytoskeleton Staining

1. Dilute FITC-phalloidin to a working concentration of 50 μg/mL in 1× PBS.
2. Tap off the amplification-polymerase solution from the slides and add the phalloidin to each sample. Incubate at 37 °C for 1 h at room temperature in a dark, humid chamber.

3.1.11 Final Wash

1. Tap off the FITC-phalloidin solution from the slides.
2. Wash the slides in 1× wash buffer B twice for 10 min in the dark.
3. Wash the slides in 0.01× wash buffer B for 1 min in the dark.
4. Let the slides dry at room temperature in the dark.

3.1.12 Prepare Samples for Imaging

1. Once the sections are dry, mount your slides using a minimal volume of vectasheild mounting media containing DAPI. Ensure that no air bubbles get trapped under the coverslips.
2. Nail polish can be used to seal the edges.
3. Wait for approximately 15–30 min before imaging in a fluorescence or confocal microscope. Slides can be stored at 4 °C in the dark up to 72 h without a relevant loss of fluorescent signal.

3.1.13 Quantification of PLA Signals

1. Keep the exposure settings and gain of laser the same for each condition imaged (i.e., for control and diabetic sections).
2. To get representative results, 30 fields per slide need to be acquired, on the same focal plane.

3. Before beginning analysis, images should be converted to 8-bit images on ImageJ-Fiji. A threshold range needs to be set to distinguish the objects of interest from the background.
4. Automated particle analysis can be used to detect the nuclei count. To exclude "noise" the size of particles is ideally defined between 150 and infinity pixels^2 and roundness values are limited to 0.00–1.00.
5. The accumulative counts for each cell type appear in the Counters menu. After counting the cells within the ROI (region of interest), the size of the ROI can be calculated and used to identify the number of cells labeled per image.
6. To count the PLA-positive signals, *Point Picker* plug-in can be used. The Point List dialog enables the calculation of PLA-positive signals in the nucleus and cytoplasm.

3.2 Proximal Ligation Assay Using Paraffin-Fixed Cells

Below, we outline a protocol of PLA in mouse podocytes plated on collagen-coated glass coverslips and fixed in 3.7% paraformaldehyde solution. The choice of fixative may vary depending on the sample type (cells or tissue), primary antibodies, and targeted protein (*see* **Note 1**). In in vitro experiments, mouse podocytes were treated with activated protein C (aPC) to determine whether aPC promotes and increases the interaction between sXBP1 and p85α or p85β (Fig. 2).

3.2.1 Culture and Fixation of Cells for Immunofluorescence

1. Differentiated mouse podocytes are plated on collagen-coated glass coverslips and fixed in 3.7% PFA (*see* **Note 6**).
2. Coverslips were washed thrice in PBS + 0.2% Triton X-100 for 10 min each and blocked in the blocking buffer (homemade) for 1 h at room temperature in a humidified chamber.

Primary Antibodies

1. Shake off the blocking solutions and incubate sections with anti-XBP1 and anti-PI3 kinase antibody, p85α antibodies diluted 1:200 appropriately diluted in the antibody diluent provided in the Duolink kit (*see* **Note 3**) overnight at 4 °C in a humidified chamber.
2. Tap off the primary antibodies and wash with buffer A twice for 5 min each (*see* **Note 4**).
3. The protocol for PLA can be continued from PLA probes as mentioned previously for tissue sections.

3.3 Assessment of Cell Death in Diabetic Nephropathy Using TUNEL Fluorescein Assay

Apoptosis is a programmed form of cell death and repeatedly has been linked with dNP when present in glomerular cells. The most widely used method to detect apoptosis is the TUNEL (TdT-mediated dUTP-X nick-end labeling) assay [13–15]. This method is based on one of the hallmarks of apoptosis being DNA fragmentation, which in early stages yields double-stranded and single-stranded DNA breaks (nicks). Both types of breaks can be detected by labeling the free 3′-OH termini with modified nucleotides in an enzymatic reaction. The enzyme terminal deoxynucleotidyl transferase (TdT) catalyzes the template-independent polymerization of deoxyribonucleotides to the 3′-end of single- and double-stranded DNA. The TUNEL method is a precise, fast, and simple nonradioactive technique to detect and quantify cell death at the single-cell level by fluorescence microscopy in tissue sections and fixed cells [13, 16]. The TUNEL assay on kidney sections is frequently associated with high background, which may result in falsely elevated cell death numbers. Therefore, it is highly recommended to carefully conduct control experiments to avoid falsely elevated counts due to a high background. Freshly prepared frozen kidney tissue is also preferred for the TUNEL assay. For this purpose, it is recommended to perfuse the mouse with PBS only and not with paraformaldehyde. It is also advised to cut the kidney tissue on the same day of prepping the mouse tissue. Prolonged freezing intervals disrupt the morphology of the tissue.

3.3.1 Dewaxing

1. Incubate paraffin slides for 30 min at 65 °C.
2. 10 min Xylene.
3. 10 min Xylene.
4. 2 min in 100% ethanol.

3.3.2 Rehydrating Tissues

1. 20 s 100% Ethanol.
2. 20 s 95% Ethanol.
3. 20 s 85% Ethanol.
4. 20 s 70% Ethanol.
5. 20 s 50% Ethanol.
6. 20 s 30% Ethanol.
7. 2 × 5 min in PBS.

3.3.3 TUNEL

1. Circle the entire tissue section with a hydrophobic pen.
2. Wash sections with freshly prepared PBS (containing 0.1% Triton, 0.1% sodium citrate) for 5–10 min at room temperature.
3. Add 50–100°μL of freshly prepared TUNEL reaction mix per section.
4. Incubate the sections for 60 min at 37 °C in a humidified chamber.
5. Wash the slides in PBS, three times, each for 2 min at room temperature.
6. Add 50–100 μL per section of anti-fluorescein antibody, Fab fragment from sheep, conjugated with peroxidase.

7. Incubate the sections for 30 min at 37 °C.
8. Wash the slides twice with PBS, each for 2 min at room temperature.
9. Add 50–100 μL of freshly prepared DAB stain.
10. Wipe bottom of the slides clean, and observe development of brown color under microscope. When negative control starts to develop color, wash all slides immediately in PBS. It takes 3–10 min to develop color, depending on the tissue type and antigen/antibody concentration. It is strongly recommended to first optimize your protocol using some extra and less important slides and then staining the desired experimental tissues.

3.3.4 Counterstain (Hematoxylin)

1. If desired to counterstain your tissue sections, immerse the slides in vector hematoxylin counterstain. Incubate at room temperature for 1–2 min.
2. Rinse/wash in running tap water until water is clear.
3. Immerse the slides by dipping ten times in acid rinse solution.
4. Immerse the slides ten times in dH_2O.
5. Incubate the slides in bluing solution for 1 min.
6. Immerse the slides ten times in dH_2O.
7. Dehydrate the slide using serial ethanol dilutions (30–100% EtOH).
8. After 100% ethanol step, immerse the slides in xylol for 5–10 min.
9. Let the slides air-dry for short time and wipe off liquid or any dirt around the section.
10. Add 20–30 μL of Roti Histo-Kit II mounting and cover the slides with a coverslip carefully by avoiding any air bubbles.
11. Take images using a microscope and count the frequency of TUNEL-positive cells (in percentage) (Fig. 3a, b).

3.4 In Situ Caspase-3/7 Activity Assay

Recent studies have indicated that TUNEL is not specific for apoptosis, but likewise detects other forms of cell death like pyroptosis [17, 18]. Apoptosis can be more precisely characterized by caspase-3 activation; therefore an alternative way to assess apoptosis of glomerular cells constitutes the caspase-3/7 FLICA™ assay [16, 19]. The caspase-3/7 FLICA™ assay measures apoptosis by detecting active caspases in whole, living cells. The methodology is based on a cell-permeable and noncytotoxic reagent called the fluorochrome inhibitor of caspases (FLICA). The FLICA™ reagent contains a caspase inhibitor sequence linked to a green (carboxyfluorescein, FAM) fluorescent probe. A probe specific for caspase-3 is currently not available. This assay does not determine DNA

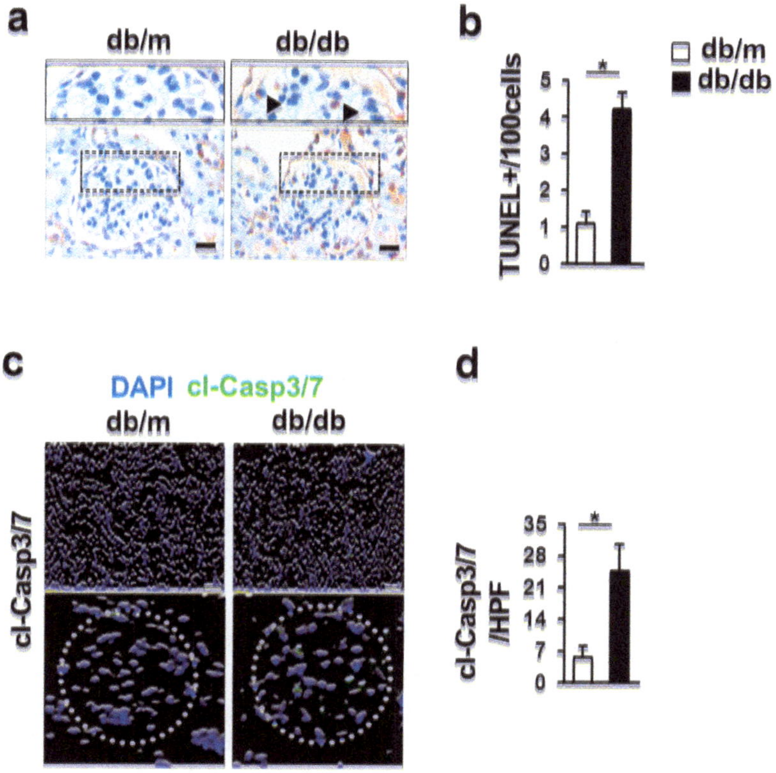

Fig. 3 Detection of glomerular cell death (apoptosis) by TUNEL and FLICA assay. Cell death as detected by TUNEL assay (**a**) in *db/db* mice. Higher magnification (top) of glomeruli indicated by black dotted lines and TUNEL-positive cells indicated by black arrowheads (**a**) detected by HRP-DAB reaction, brown; hematoxylin counterstain, blue and bar graph summarizing results of integrated optical density (IOD) of positive DAB stain (**b**). Increased caspase-3/7 activity in *db/db* mice compared to *db/m* (control), as detected by FLICA assay, for FLICA (green), DAPI counterstain (blue, **c**, **d**). Mean value ± SEM (**b**, **d**) of at least six mice in each group; representative TUNEL-stained glomeruli (**a**, size bar: 20 μm); representative images of frozen sections incubated with FLICA probes: overviews (**c**, size bar: 20 μm) and higher (4×) magnification of glomeruli (glomeruli indicated by white dotted circles) (**c**); $*P < 0.05$, *t*-test

fragmentation, but rather the activity of caspase-3/7, which are required for apoptotic cell death. Because the FAM probe becomes covalently coupled to the active enzymes, it is retained within the cell, while any unbound FAM probe diffuses out of the cell and is washed away. The remaining green fluorescent signal is a direct measure of the active caspase 3 and 7 enzyme activity present in the cell at the time the reagent was added. Cells that contain the bound FLICA can be analyzed by a fluorescence microscopy. Freshly prepared frozen kidney tissues are preferred for the FLICA assay. For this purpose, it is recommended to perfuse the mouse with PBS only and not with paraformaldehyde. It is also advised to cut the kidney tissue on the same day of prepping the mouse tissue. Prolonged freezing intervals disrupt the morphology of the tissue.

3.4.1 Methods

1. Prepare frozen kidney tissue sections, 3–5 μM thick, and allow to air-dry (for 10 min at room temperature).
2. Fix the slides in ice-cold acetone (100%) for 5–8 min at room temperature.
3. Rehydrate tissue by washing (twice for 5 min) in PBS containing 0.01% Tween (PBSt) at room temperature.
4. Circle each tissue section with a hydrophobic pen.
5. Block each section with 50–100 μL of blocking solution containing 20% aqua-block in media with 0.2% Tween 20 for 30 min at room temperature.
6. Shake off the blocking solution, add 50–100 μL of 3× FLICA™ working solution per section, and incubate at room temperature for 1–2 h, protected from light.
7. Remove FLICA™ solution and wash sections three times in wash buffer for 5 min each.
8. Mount the tissue with 20–30 μL of Vectashield mounting medium (if desired containing DAPI) and cover the tissue section with a coverslip carefully by avoiding any air bubbles.
9. Take fluorescent images using a microscope and count the FLICA-positive cells (Fig. 3c, d).

3.5 In Vivo Models for ER Stress Studies

There are several tools that have been used to study ER stress in vitro. These tools have been effectively used to delineate key mechanisms underlying the UPR. With the advent and refinement of modern mouse genetic techniques there has been significant progress in the generation of in vivo models to study the UPR.

This section highlights two such models that have been used to study the in vivo UPR and have important implications for future ER stress research in the context of dNP.

3.5.1 TETATF6 Mouse

Background

ATF6 initiates one of the three primary signaling arms of the UPR in the ER. As is the case with its contemporaries (PERK and IRE1α), ATF6 is anchored to the ER and comprises an ER luminal domain, a transmembrane domain, and a cytoplasmic domain. Activation of ATF6 involves the release of ATF6 from the ER membrane, followed by transport to the Golgi, where it is further processed to its transcriptionally active p50 fragment [8].

In terms of function, ATF6 plays a dual role in the ER stress response, regulating protective functions such as chaperone upregulation, as well as regulating the expression of XBP1, an important cytoprotective component of the ER stress response [20]. On the other hand, ATF6 has also been shown to promote the expression of C/EBP homologous protein (CHOP), a transcription factor conveying pro-apoptotic effects within the kidney [8].

Description

In order to delineate the effects of ATF6 a mouse model with inducible active ATF6 was generated. This model allows for the tissue-specific control of the transcriptionally active ATF6 fragment, and also incorporates a visual marker, β-galactosidase, to monitor the activity of drug-induced ATF6 [8].

This tool consists of two genetic inserts. The first insert comprises a bidirectional promoter designed with a *tetO* site flanked by a *LacZ* gene and a gene coding for the active p50 fragment of ATF6, respectively, along with individual cytomegalovirus (CMV) promoter sequences [8] that further enhance expression in the presence of the VP1 transcription factor (Fig. 4).

The second genetic insert includes a *rTeta-VP16* insert which codes for a modified version of the conventional tetracycline repressor element. The modification was first described in 1995 by Grossen et al. and involves the alteration of four amino acid residues from the native TtA protein [21]. The VP16 component is an essential transcriptional activator of the CMV promoter region (Fig. 4).

The native TtA protein functions by binding to a 19-nucleotide sequence in the absence of tetracycline, or an analog of the same, and thus prevents the transcription of proximal DNA elements. The

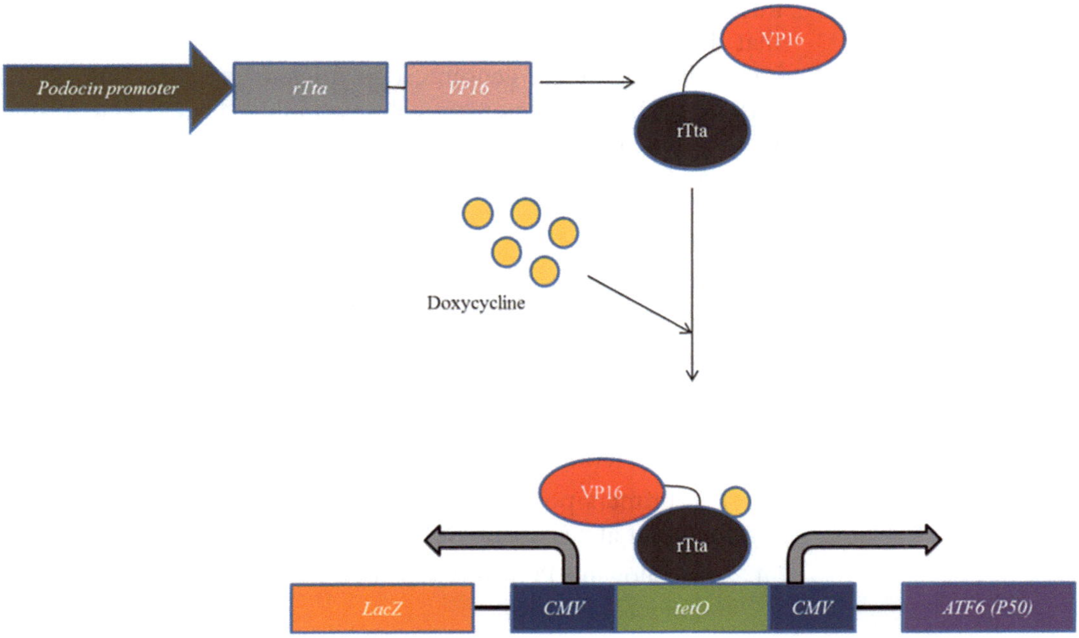

Fig. 4 Schematic of the TETATF6 mouse. All boxes have been appropriately labeled as seen in the figure and represent either protein or gene names

mutant variant used in the model has an opposing effect; that is, in the presence of tetracycline it induces rather than suppresses the expression of genes proximal to the *tetO* sites by promoting the binding of the *rTtA-VP16* construct to these sites [21], thereby activating the expression of any genes downstream of the included CMV regions present in the second insert.

The *rtTA-VP16* cassette can be inserted along with a tissue-specific promoter (like the podocin receptor if podocyte-specific expression is required) or can be constitutively expressed by inserting it within the ROSA26 locus along with a constitutive promoter.

The insert containing the tet-operator/CMV-driven ATF6-P50 and *LacZ* gene cassette was initially introduced into a wild-type background via random insertion. This transgenic mouse can then be crossed with a line containing the rtTA-VP16 insert to generate the desired mouse line containing both constructs.

Induction of ATF6 P50 can be achieved by addition of a tetracycline analog such as doxycycline into the drinking water. The desired level of expression can be achieved by altering the concentration of doxycycline [8]. Madhusudhan et al. reported increasing expression in podocytes at doxycycline concentrations ranging from 0.2 to 2.0 mg/mL in the drinking water, when the *rtTa* construct is combined with a podocyte-specific promoter. The level of expression can then be monitored by the level of β-galactosidase activity in the desired tissue.

This was successfully used by Madhusudhan et al. in 2015 to show the detrimental effect of ATF6 expression in the podocytes of mice with an experimental model of dNP [8]. In order to confirm that the desired mutations have been introduced into the correct loci within the mouse genome, a polymerase chain reaction (PCR) was used. The following protocol was employed with tissue lysates. In this case, two sets of primers, one set flanking the TETATF6 insert and another flanking the podocin-*rtTA* gene construct, were employed sequentially.

Genotyping Protocol for the TETATF6 Construct

1. Tail-DNA extracts from transfected mice were subjected to PCR with primers flanking the ATF6-P50 insert (Fig. 5a).
2. The forward primer was designed to cover a sequence area containing fragment from the pBI-G vector backbone and the ATF6-p50 insert, and the reverse primer was designed to bind to the 3′ terminal of the ATF6-p50 insert (Fig. 5b).
3. The primers post-amplification were calculated to produce a fragment at a size of 576 base pairs.
4. The following PCR mix was used for the amplification of this fragment:
   (a) For 25 μL reaction volumes:
   (b) Nuclease-free water: 18.25 μL.

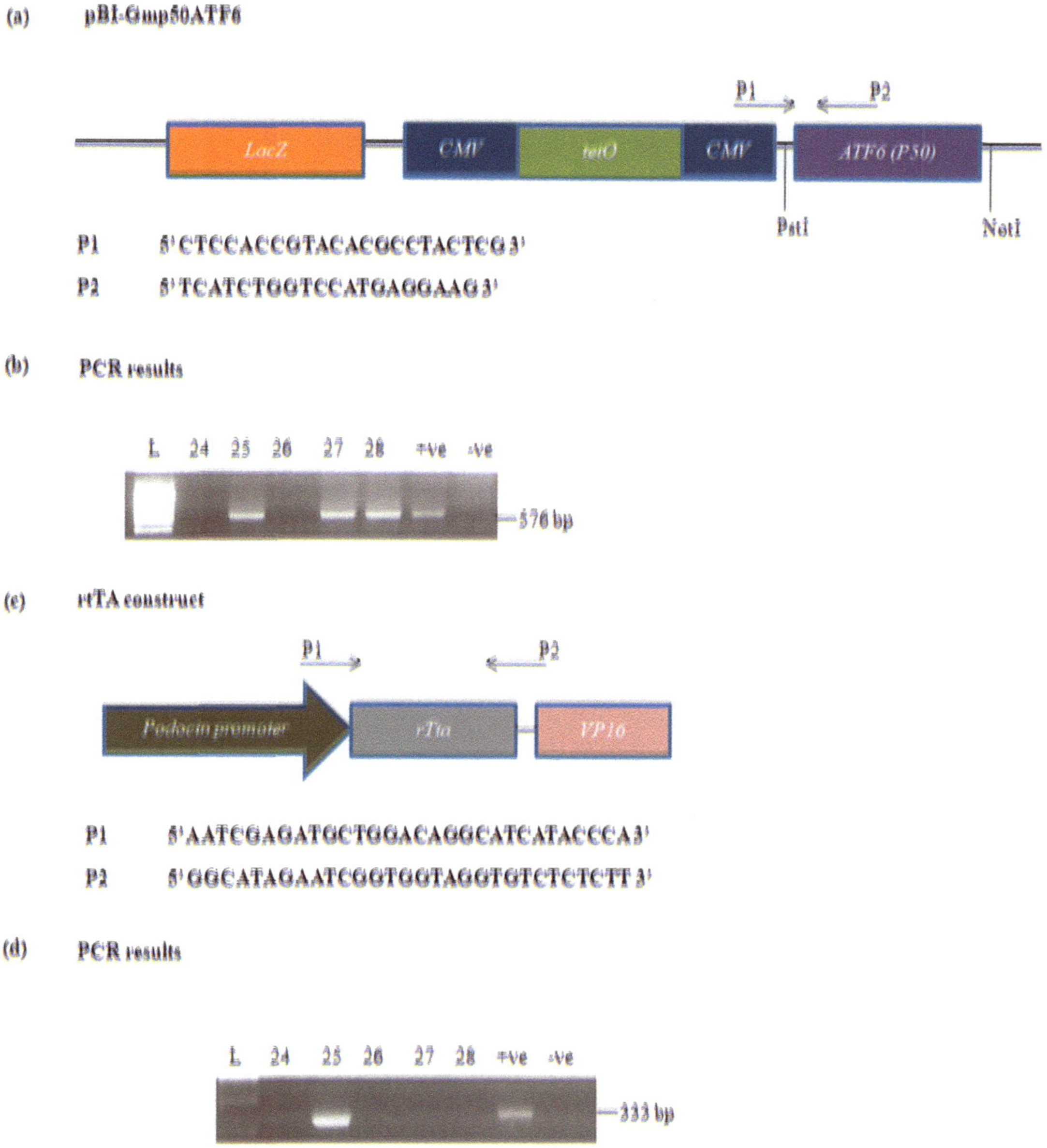

Fig. 5 Scheme of PCRs for confirmation of transgenic modifications. (**a**) Schematic of primary construct employed for the TETATF6 mouse, along with primer-binding sites; P1 and P2, as well as sequences of both primers. (**b**) Results showing relevant band, from left to right; lane "L" represents DNA size marker, while lanes labeled 25–28 are representative of PCRs conducted from test mouse samples. Lanes "+ve" and "−ve" represent the positive and negative controls, respectively. (**c**) Schematic of secondary construct used in the TETATF6 mouse, comprising the Tet-on promoter (rtTA) with the primer-binding sites P3 and P4. Sequences of both primers are also provided in the figure. (**d**) Results showing relevant band, abbreviations, and symbols for lane names are the same as those described for Fig. 5b

   (c) Reaction buffer: 5 μL.
   (d) dNTPs (25 mM): 0.5 μL.
   (e) Forward primer (1.25 pM): 0.5 μL.
   (f) Forward primer (1.25 pM): 0.5 μL.
   (g) Phusion Taq polymerase: 0.025 μL.
   (h) DNA extract: 0.2 μL.
5. In addition to test samples, appropriate positive (highly diluted cloning vectors) and negative controls (wild-type DNA) were also included.
6. The PCR was set up for 24 cycles with the following conditions:
   (a) Hot start: 94 °C for 3 min.
   (b) Denaturation: 94 °C for 45 s.
   (c) Annealing: 60 °C for 60 s.
   (d) Extension: 72 °C for 1 min.
7. On completion of 24 cycles, a final extension step at 72 °C was applied for 2 min, and samples were stored at 4–10 °C before being run in a 0.5% agarose gel (Fig. 5b).
8. Samples that displayed a band at 576 bp as seen in the positive control were then taken forward and subjected to the next PCR step to confirm the presence of the podocin-*rtTA* construct.
9. Steps 1–8 were repeated as such, with a different set of primers flanking the *rtTA* insert, and including a small portion of the podocin promoter (Fig. 5c).
10. Samples that resulted in a 333 bp fragment were then presumed to contain the podocin-*rtTA* construct (Fig. 5d).
11. Those samples that were positive (displayed the appropriate-size PCR fragments) were then presumed to have come from mice that contained both inserts required for the TETATF6 mouse and were subject to further in vivo studies (immunostaining and histology) to confirm successful generation of a complete TETATF6 mouse.

3.5.2 TREXBP1s

Background

X-box-binding protein-1 or XBP1 is an integral part of the cytoprotective UPR. Under basal conditions, the *XBP1* mRNA is not spliced due to the presence of an unconventional splice site which is incompatible with the cellular spliceosome. However, on activation of inositol-requiring enzyme-1 (IRE1), one of the preliminary signaling components of the UPR, the *XBP1* mRNA, is spliced by a unique RNase domain present in IRE1 to produce the mRNA coding for spliced XBP1 protein (sXBP1) which is transcriptionally active and promotes the expression of further ER stress elements [8].

This construct has been successfully used to study the effects of sXBP1 under physiological stressors. Employing these mice would be an important tool to better understand the role of sXBP1 in the context of dNP [8, 9, 20].

Description

The TREXBP1s system comprises three individual transgenes (Fig. 6). The first construct consists of a spliced *Xbp1* gene (the active form) along with a Tet-binding cassette which was first described by Deng et al. in 2013 [7]. This allows for drug-induced expression of *sXbp1*.

As in the case of the TETATF6 transgene this system also provides a high degree of spatiotemporal control over the expression of *sXbp1*. This gene is directly incorporated into the genome via random insertion [8].

The second construct includes an *rTta* element located downstream of a stop codon flanked by *LoxP* sites which is incorporated into the ROSA26 locus of the mouse genome. The *rTta* transgenic mouse is then crossed with a mouse expressing the third construct, a *Cre* recombinase under the control of a tissue-specific promoter (such as *Nphs2* to induce podocyte-specific expression or a constitutive promoter as required) [8, 22].

The resulting offspring containing all desired modifications are then crossed with the TREXBP1s mice to generate a line that actively expressed *rTta* in specific tissues. Expression of XBP1s can be induced by treatment with tetracycline or an analog like doxycycline [7] (Fig. 6; see also notes above for the TET-ATF6 mice). It is recommended that control group mice consist of age-matched mice expressing the tissue-specific *Cre* and thus *rTta*, but not the TREXBP1s transgene [7].

Successful mice can then be selected via PCRs designed in the same vein as described in the case of the TETATF6 mice, discussed earlier, along with immunohistochemistry against the XBP1 protein in the appropriate tissue.

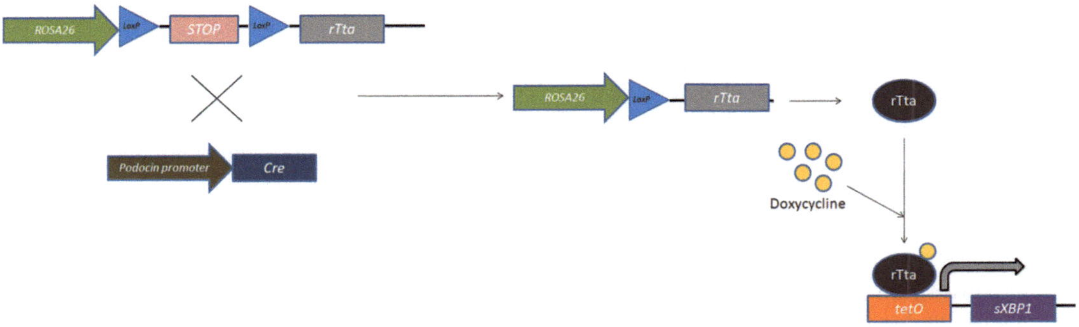

Fig. 6 Schematic of the TETXBP1s mouse. All boxes have been appropriately labeled as seen in the figure and represent either protein or gene names

4 Notes

1. Proximity ligation assay is compatible with all fixations suitable for IF and IHC. The choice of fixative may vary depending on the sample type (cells or tissue), primary antibodies, and protein target. Different fixatives can influence the antigenicity, and thus the performance, of primary antibodies. If there is no recommended fixation for the selected primary antibodies, this must be optimized by the user.
2. Two technical controls should be included for each PLA experiment. One negative control each for the primary antibodies is used where one of the two primary antibodies will be omitted and a second negative control where both primary antibodies have been omitted.
3. The dilution of the antibodies has to be optimized for IF/IHC in different fixations before proceeding with the PLA. The duration of incubation and ideal temperature for incubation should also be optimized for both the antibodies used. Moreover, if one of the primary antibodies have been raised in mouse and the section or cells being stained also originate from mice, it would be advisable to block and dilute primary antibodies in the blocking solution and antibody diluent provided in the M.O.M. kit (Mouse on Mouse), respectively.
4. The wash buffers need to be brought down to room temperature before use.
5. All steps following the ligation require the use of light-sensitive reagents. Therefore, it is of utmost importance to make sure that containers for washing are wrapped in aluminum foil and that all steps are taken to protect samples from white light.
6. Cells can be fixed in 100% ice-cold methanol for PLA. As mentioned previously, the fixation has to be optimized for the cell or tissue type as well as for the proteins of interest.

References

1. Szegezdi E, Logue SE, Gorman AM, Samali A (2006) Mediators of endoplasmic reticulum stress-induced apoptosis. EMBO Rep 7 (9):880–885
2. Oakes SA, Papa FR (2015) The role of endoplasmic reticulum stress in human pathology. Annu Rev Pathol 10:173–194
3. Walter P, Ron D (2011) The unfolded protein response: from stress pathway to homeostatic regulation. Science 334(6059):1081–1086
4. Liu Z, Lv Y, Zhao N, Guan G, Wang J (2015) Protein kinase R-like ER kinase and its role in endoplasmic reticulum stress-decided cell fate. Cell Death Dis 6:e1822
5. Sano R, Reed JC (2013) ER stress-induced cell death mechanisms. Biochim Biophys Acta 1833(12):3460–3470
6. Park SW, Zhou Y, Lee J, Lu A, Sun C, Chung J et al (2010) The regulatory subunits of PI3K, p85alpha and p85beta, interact with XBP-1 and increase its nuclear translocation. Nat Med 16(4):429–437
7. Deng Y, Wang ZV, Tao C, Gao N, Holland WL, Ferdous A et al (2013) The Xbp1s/GalE

axis links ER stress to postprandial hepatic metabolism. J Clin Invest 123(1):455–468
8. Madhusudhan T, Wang H, Dong W, Ghosh S, Bock F, Thangapandi VR et al (2015) Defective podocyte insulin signalling through p85-XBP1 promotes ATF6-dependent maladaptive ER-stress response in diabetic nephropathy. Nat Commun 6:6496
9. Madhusudhan T, Wang H, Ghosh S, Dong W, Kumar V, Al-Dabet MM et al (2017) Signal integration at the PI3K-p85-XBP1 hub endows coagulation protease activated protein C with insulin-like function. Blood 130 (12):1445–1455
10. Ozcan L, Tabas I (2012) Role of endoplasmic reticulum stress in metabolic disease and other disorders. Annu Rev Med 63:317–328
11. Kennedy D, Samali A, Jager R (2015) Methods for studying ER stress and UPR markers in human cells. Methods Mol Biol 1292:3–18
12. Ron D, Walter P (2007) Signal integration in the endoplasmic reticulum unfolded protein response. Nat Rev Mol Cell Biol 8(7):519–529
13. Isermann B, Vinnikov IA, Madhusudhan T, Herzog S, Kashif M, Blautzik J et al (2007) Activated protein C protects against diabetic nephropathy by inhibiting endothelial and podocyte apoptosis. Nat Med 13 (11):1349–1358
14. Meyer TW, Bennett PH, Nelson RG (1999) Podocyte number predicts long-term urinary albumin excretion in Pima Indians with Type II diabetes and microalbuminuria. Diabetologia 42(11):1341–1344
15. Susztak K, Raff AC, Schiffer M, Bottinger EP (2006) Glucose-induced reactive oxygen species cause apoptosis of podocytes and podocyte depletion at the onset of diabetic nephropathy. Diabetes 55(1):225–233
16. Shahzad K, Bock F, Al-Dabet MM, Gadi I, Kohli S, Nazir S et al (2016) Caspase-1, but not caspase-3, promotes diabetic nephropathy. J Am Soc Nephrol 27(8):2270–2275
17. Brennan MA, Cookson BT (2000) Salmonella induces macrophage death by caspase-1-dependent necrosis. Mol Microbiol 38 (1):31–40
18. Fink SL, Cookson BT (2005) Apoptosis, pyroptosis, and necrosis: mechanistic description of dead and dying eukaryotic cells. Infect Immun 73(4):1907–1916
19. Nazir S, Gadi I, Al-Dabet MM, Elwakiel A, Kohli S, Ghosh S et al (2017) Cytoprotective activated protein C averts Nlrp3 inflammasome-induced ischemia-reperfusion injury via mTORC1 inhibition. Blood 130 (24):2664–2677
20. Yoshida H, Matsui T, Yamamoto A, Okada T, Mori K (2001) XBP1 mRNA is induced by ATF6 and spliced by IRE1 in response to ER stress to produce a highly active transcription factor. Cell 107(7):881–891
21. Gossen M, Freundlieb S, Bender G, Muller G, Hillen W, Bujard H (1995) Transcriptional activation by tetracyclines in mammalian cells. Science 268(5218):1766–1769
22. Moeller MJ, Sanden SK, Soofi A, Wiggins RC, Holzman LB (2003) Podocyte-specific expression of cre recombinase in transgenic mice. Genesis 35(1):39–42

- Nextera XT DNA Library Preparation Kit (Illumina, Inc.) or equivalent.

Sample Preparation for Proteomics

- Urea solution: 6 M Urea, 10 mM arginine, 50 mM citrate buffer, pH 3.5.
- Benchtop rocker.
- HFDa system.
- Distilled water.
- Protein low-binding tubes.

3 Methods

3.1 Urine Sampling

Many studies have used either spot urine (first morning) or 24-h urine collection samples.

This is an important practical decision point and considerations here include storage capacity availability and the scope of research to be conducted. The use of HFD appears to provide a practical solution in *concentrating sample volume* from 1 to 2 L/24 h to a representative 2–3 mL useful for any downstream application. This easily solves the issue of storage capacity especially for large biobank sample collections. However, the need of protease inhibitors or prevention of bacterial growth for each setting is an important consideration and ways to their management are presented below.

Where first morning voids are *collected at the clinic*, the protocol is as follows (*see* **Notes 1** and **2**):

1. Gently invert urine container 8–10 times to resuspend any sediment that may have settled.
2. Add protease inhibitors.
3. Pour contents of container into 50 mL Falcon tubes.
4. Balance sample per your site's centrifuge protocol and handling policy.
5. Centrifuge Falcon tubes at 2000 × *g* for 30 min at room temperature without brake.
6. Remove the sample from the centrifuge taking care not to disturb the separated contents.
7. Transfer supernatant to clean 50 mL Falcon tubes.
8. Store all samples at −80 °C (*see* **Note 3**).

3.2 Thawing the Urine Samples

1. Place the urine samples in a +37 °C water bath until samples have almost thawed (*see* **Note 4**).
2. Check progress of thaw regularly to ensure that samples remain cold.

3. Melt the remaining ice by agitating the tube by flicking or vortex gently.
4. Place thawed urine samples on ice.
5. Tubes should be dried thoroughly before opening.
6. Prepare appropriate number of aliquots for each sample.
7. Keep the remaining sample volume in the original tube.
8. Store at −80 °C as appropriate until measurement.
9. Record the volume of original sample and the number of full-volume aliquots and partial-volume aliquots if appropriate.

3.3 Procedures for Extracellular Vesicle Isolation

When there is particular interest in exosomes, microvesicles, apoptotic bodies, or any other subfraction of EVs, specific isolation methods (e.g., ultracentrifugation, ultrafiltration, size-exclusion chromatography (SEC), sucrose gradient, or any other combinations or specific device for each) should be consulted. Practical instructions can be found in Refs. [3, 10, 12, 13]. However, for most practical diagnostic, prognostic, and biomarker search purposes, the hydrostatic filtration dialysis has shown to be the method of choice as it does not lose important EV classes. Its capacity covers volumes up to 2 L (or more) at a time; it is not affected by protein content (proteinuria), urinary salts or urine concentration, pigments, or naturally occurring proteins like Tamm-Horsfall glycoprotein [14].

Thus, the *generic method for HFD* is presented below (*see* Figs. 1 and 2):

1. Centrifuge fresh samples at 2000 × *g* for 30 min at room temperature (RT) without braking (*see* **Note 5**).
2. Inhibition of bacterial growth: after thawing the sample, add 0.1 mg silver chloride, 4.5 mg troclosene sodium per tablet per liter of urine.
3. *Perform filtration-concentration-dialysis* (HFD) using a cellulose ester dialysis membrane with molecular weight cutoff (MWCO) of 1000 kDa creating a gentle hydrostatic pressure of the urine in the funnel to push the solvent through the dialysis membrane together with all the analytes below the selected MWCO.
4. After concentration of sample to around 5 mL, add 200 mL of distilled water into the funnel to allow removal of possible residual material with a molecular weight smaller than the MWCO of the membrane.
5. Collect samples after the volume is reduced to less than 5 mL (HFDa) (*see* **Note 6**).
6. Aliquot the samples in low-protein or DNA-binding tubes for downstream applications.

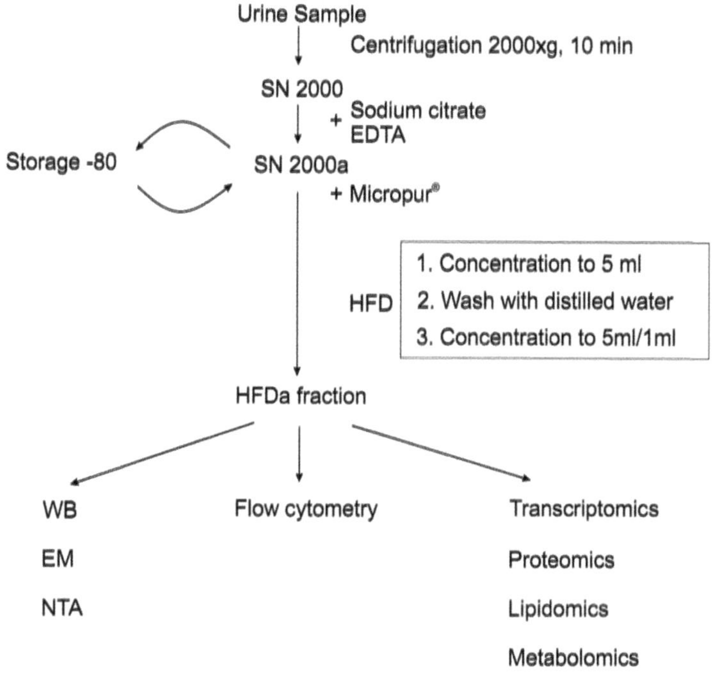

Fig. 1 General protocol for hydrostatic filtration dialysis. *EM* electron microscopy, *WB* Western blot, *NTA* nanoparticle tracking analysis

3.4 Available Techniques for Downstream EV Analysis

There are a number of standard downstream applications and uses for the isolated EVs [17–21], which are to be selected based on the study needs. Some standard first procedures are presented below to first characterize the vesicle harvest, its purity, and size variation of the vesicle yield.

For initial characterization of EVs collected, a short procedure for nanoparticle tracking, Western blotting, and transmission electron microscopy (TEM) is presented. For detailed protocols, respective protocols should be consulted:

3.4.1 Nanoparticle Tracking Analysis (NTA)

NTA is a useful and fast method to determine concentration and size distribution of EV samples. For example Nanosight series instruments can measure particles in the size range of 10–2000 nm (*see* Fig. 3 for a typical NTA profile of HFDa samples). There are some important tips given by the manufacturer to take into consideration when using Nanosight instruments (*see* **Note** 7).

3.4.2 Western Blot

Western blotting is one of the most widely used methods to characterize EVs. There are several available markers for the EV yield [22] and the respective antibodies for use. Here we present a simple protocol to prepare HFDa samples for SDS-PAGE and blotting to detect tumor susceptibility gene 101 (TSG-101), a marker of exosomes.

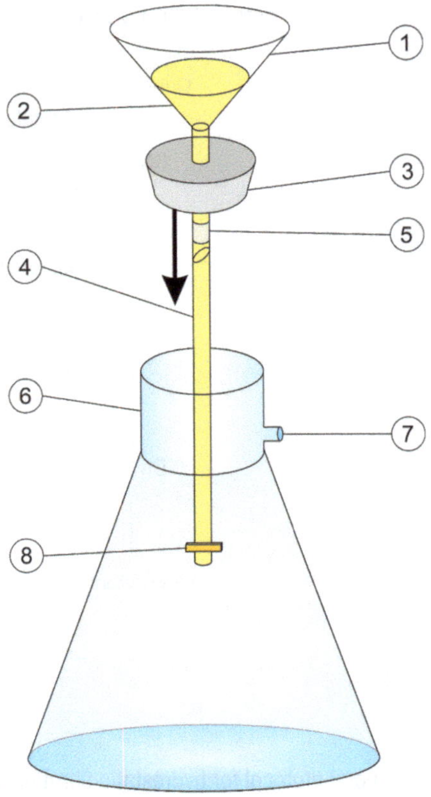

Fig. 2 Basic setup to perform hydrostatic filtration dialysis. (1) Funnel or separating funnel; (2) urine (supernatant 2000 *g*, 30 min); (3) rubber stopper; (4) Biotech CE Dialysis Tubing 1000 kD MWCO; (5) Parafilm® M to hold the membrane to the funnel stem; (6) Büchner flask; (7) side arm to connect the system to a vacuum pump; (8) dialysis tubing closure

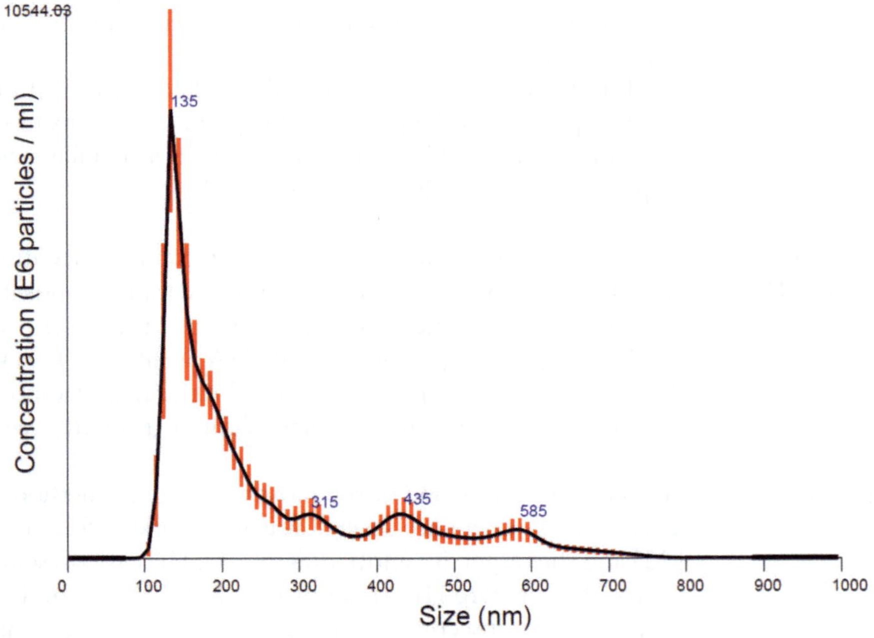

Fig. 3 Typical NTA analysis results of urinary extracellular vesicles isolated using HFD

1. Measure the protein concentration using micro BCA or Bradford Ultra methods (*see* **Note 8**).
2. Thaw samples on ice.
3. Add 5× Laemmli buffer.
4. Incubate for 5 min at +95 °C and spin down the samples.
5. Load the samples 5–10 μg (*see* **Note 9**) to 4–20% gradient SDS-PAGE gels. Run the gel at 150 V 1 h.
6. Transfer to PVDF membrane at 100 V, 90 min.
7. Block the membrane with 3% BSA in TBS, 1 h, at room temperature.
8. Incubate with primary mouse antibody TSG-101 diluted in 3% BSA in 0.1% Tween-20 in TBS (TTBS).
9. Wash the membranes in TTBS.
10. Incubate with secondary antibody rabbit anti-mouse diluted in 3% BSA in TTBS.
11. Wash the membrane in TTBS and a final wash in TBS.
12. Detect signals using chemiluminescence.

3.4.3 Transmission Electron Microscopy

Negative Staining for Transmission Electron Microscopy [23]

1. Slowly thaw EV samples on ice.
2. Pipette a drop (5 μL) of EVs on parafilm. Dilute with PBS (*see* **Note 10**) if needed (target a concentration of 1e+11 particles/mL; measured by NTA).
3. Place pioloform (or formvar) and carbon-coated glow-discharged copper grids on the drops for a total time of 5–60 min to load EVs.
4. Wash in three drops of 0.1 M $NaPO_4$ buffer with pH close to the original pH of samples.
5. Fix in freshly made (keeps up to 2 weeks refrigerated) 2% paraformaldehyde (PFA) in 0.1 M $NaPO_4$ buffer for 10 min.
6. Wash in three drops of 0.1 M $NaPO_4$ buffer.
7. Wash in five drops of distilled water, 2 min each, with two last washes on ice.
8. Contrast stain using 2% neutral uranyl acetate for 10–15 min, in the dark, on ice.
9. Rinse quickly by transferring the grid through a drop of deionized water on ice.
10. Embed in 1.8% methyl cellulose (25ctp)/0.4% uranyl acetate in distilled water on ice and incubate for 10 min in the dark.
11. Pick up the grid with forceps and remove excess liquid from the side of the grid using filter or Whatman paper. Dry the grid sample side facing up.

3.4.4 RNA Isolation and Measurement

1. Thaw EV samples on ice.
2. As guidance follow Table 1 to achieve good yields of RNA using HFD vacuum method.
3. Lyse the samples using TRIzol-LS instead of Qiazol reagent when working with volumes ≥200 μL.
4. Extract total EV-RNA. Depending on the starting material you may use with miRNeasy Mini columns Kit (available commercially) according to the manufacturer's instructions for purification of total RNA including small RNAs from animal cells.
5. RNA samples should be analyzed for example with 2100 BioAnalyzer using BioAnalyzer Pico kit. A characteristic peak of small RNAs <200 nucleotides and sometimes small ribosomal peaks is visible (Fig. 4).

3.4.5 RNA Sequencing (RNA-Seq)

1. 1 ng of RNA is needed for the sample preparation.
2. cDNA library to be prepared using ultralow amount protocol:
   (a) Smart-Seq v4 Ultra Low Input Kit (Takara Bio) or equivalent.
   (b) Nextera XT DNA Library Preparation Kit (Illumina, Inc.) or equivalent.
3. RNA-seq using Hiseq 2000 (Illumina, Inc.) pair-end (2 × 100) protocol or equivalent.

Table 1
Reference volumes for total RNA extraction using EVs isolated by HFD

Concentration ratio (mL)	HFDa volume for RNA extraction (μL)
150:1	200
50:1	800

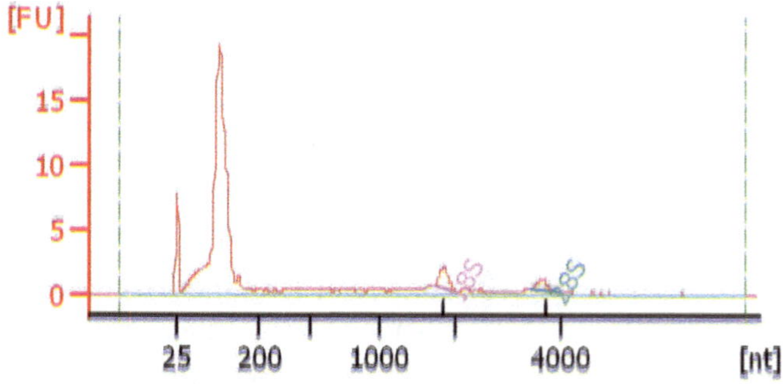

Fig. 4 Typical Pico 6000 RNA Chip electropherogram run in Agilent 2100 BioAnalyzer for RNA extracted from urinary EVs isolated using HFD

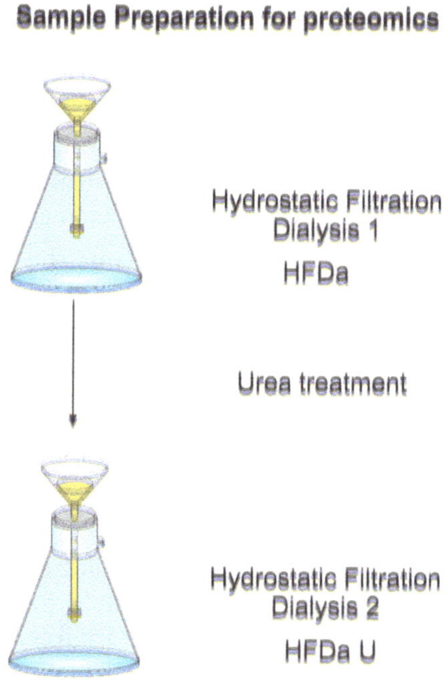

Fig. 5 Workflow of sample preparation for proteomics analysis

4. Align reads to human reference genome and count using GENCODE gene annotations.
5. Use gene length-normalized values FPKM (fragments per kilobase of exon per million) as expression measurement for genes.

RNA-seq data will be stored in FASTQ format and alignments to genomic sequence in compressed binary (BAM) format. As for microarray data, associated metadata will be stored together with the data files to ensure that it can be analyzed together with other data types during the project and following project completion.

3.4.6 Sample Preparation for Proteomics

Tamm-Horsfall Denaturation for Proteomics

1. Treat 1 mg of HFDa with 5 mL (final volume) of a solution made of 6 M urea in 50 mM citrate buffer, pH 3.5, and 10 mM arginine.
2. Mix in end-over-end agitation (40 revolutions per minute) for 1 h at RT.
3. Place the mix in the HFD system using a 1000 kDa MWCO dialysis membrane (Fig. 5).
4. Wash with 50 mL of the same buffer followed by 200 mL of distilled water to remove all the proteins below the MWCO.
5. Collect samples after the volume is reduced to less than 5 mL (HFDaU).

Store HFDaU samples in low-protein-binding tubes at −80 °C.

4 Notes

1. Practical urine sample collection:
   (a) First/second morning voids should be collected for vesicle isolation and carefully labeled for their intended use on the vials as in any supporting documentation.
   (b) Participants should be instructed to provide a minimum of 50 mL in container containing protease inhibitor (*see* **Note 2**).
   (c) Samples can be stored at room temperature or preferentially at +4 °C for up to a maximum of 6 h before processing.
2. For home collection of samples, the key points to observe are the following:
   (a) Home-collected samples must be refrigerated (+4 °C) immediately following collection and throughout until samples are freezing and processing can be started within 6 h. Participants should be instructed of this.
   (b) A mix of protease inhibitors should be provided to the patient so it can be added to the urine collection device as soon as the collection starts.
   (c) A cooling box should be used for transfer to the clinical site.
   (d) Once the sample is at the clinical site proceed from **step 3**, Subheading 3.1.
3. If samples will be further processed in another facility, ship the samples in dry ice.
4. (a) Should a water bath be used for thawing, care must be taken to ensure that labels will not come off the tubes and also that inks on tubes or labels will not deteriorate.
   (b) Samples should not be submerged in the water and care should be taken to prevent tube caps from being wet.
   (c) Water should be circulating to ensure an even rate of sample thaw.
5. If samples will be frozen before performing HFD, add sodium citrate and ethylenediaminetetraacetic acid (EDTA) to supernatant (final concentration of 50 mM and 8 mM, respectively) to chelate divalent cations and therefore to prevent calcium oxalate crystal formation. Moreover, the citrate-EDTA helps to resolubilize the cryo-precipitate formation when stored at −80 °C until further processed.
6. HFD can also be performed under vacuum, to accelerate the filtration rate. A pressure of −40 kPa reduces the filtration time

in 1/4 compared with no vacuum conditions. Moreover, better concentration ratios can be obtained. We recommend not to reduce the HFDa volume more than 1 mL because it may be difficult to recover smaller volumes from the membrane.

7. Avoid particles bigger than $\geq$10 μm:
   (a) If such particles are in the samples, remove them by centrifugation, and filtration of settling.

   Dilution of the sample:

   (a) The instrument can measure sample concentrations in the range of 10^6 and 10^9 particles/mL (optimal concentration of 1–25 × 10^8 particles/mL).

   Repeat the measurement 2–5 times for accurate results.
8. If using micro BCA method, dilute the samples and standard curve in 2% SDS to eliminate interference from lipids.
9. When using HFD method without vacuum and depending on the initial volume, it may be difficult to achieve 10 μg of protein in a reasonable volume to load the gels for protein electrophoresis. In such a case, after determining the protein concentration it is advisable to make aliquots depending on the quantity of proteins of interest and vacuum dry the samples using freeze dryer or speed vacuum.
10. Except 1.8% methyl cellulose (25ctp)/0.4% uranyl acetate in distilled water, the rest of the solutions used for EM should be filtered using 0.2 μm PES syringe-driven filters.

References

1. Kourembanas S (2015) Exosomes: vehicles of intercellular signaling, biomarkers, and vectors of cell therapy. Annu Rev Physiol 77:13–27. https://doi.org/10.1146/annurev-physiol-021014-071641
2. Barteneva NS, Fasler-Kan E, Bernimoulin M, Stern JN, Ponomarev ED, Duckett L, Vorobjev IA (2013) Circulating microparticles: square the circle. BMC Cell Biol 14:23. https://doi.org/10.1186/1471-2121-14-23
3. Erdbrugger U, Le TH (2016) Extracellular vesicles in renal diseases: more than novel biomarkers? J Am Soc Nephrol 27(1):12–26. https://doi.org/10.1681/asn.2015010074
4. van der Pol E, Boing AN, Gool EL, Nieuwland R (2016) Recent developments in the nomenclature, presence, isolation, detection and clinical impact of extracellular vesicles. J Thromb Haemost 14(1):48–56. https://doi.org/10.1111/jth.13190
5. Zhao H, Achreja A, Iessi E, Logozzi M, Mizzoni D, Di Raimo R, Nagrath D, Fais S (2018) The key role of extracellular vesicles in the metastatic process. Biochim Biophys Acta Rev Cancer 1869(1):64–77. https://doi.org/10.1016/j.bbcan.2017.11.005
6. Seo N, Akiyoshi K, Shiku H (2018) Exosome-mediated regulation of tumor immunology. Cancer Sci 109(10):2998–3004. https://doi.org/10.1111/cas.13735
7. Huang-Doran I, Zhang CY, Vidal-Puig A (2017) Extracellular vesicles: novel mediators of cell communication in metabolic disease. Trends Endocrinol Metab 28(1):3–18. https://doi.org/10.1016/j.tem.2016.10.003
8. Wang Y, Wang Q, Wei X, Shao J, Zhao J, Zhang Z, Chen Z, Bai Y, Wang N, Wang Y, Li M, Zhai X (2017) Global scientific trends on exosome research during 2007–2016: a bibliometric analysis. Oncotarget 8(29):48460–48470. https://doi.org/10.18632/oncotarget.17223
9. Raimondo F, Morosi L, Chinello C, Magni F, Pitto M (2011) Advances in membranous

vesicle and exosome proteomics improving biological understanding and biomarker discovery. Proteomics 11(4):709–720. https://doi.org/10.1002/pmic.201000422

10. Merchant ML, Rood IM, Deegens JKJ, Klein JB (2017) Isolation and characterization of urinary extracellular vesicles: implications for biomarker discovery. Nat Rev Nephrol 13 (12):731–749. https://doi.org/10.1038/nrneph.2017.148

11. Turturici G, Tinnirello R, Sconzo G, Geraci F (2014) Extracellular membrane vesicles as a mechanism of cell-to-cell communication: advantages and disadvantages. Am J Physiol Cell Physiol 306(7):C621–C633. https://doi.org/10.1152/ajpcell.00228.2013

12. Lotvall J, Hill AF, Hochberg F, Buzas EI, Di Vizio D, Gardiner C, Gho YS, Kurochkin IV, Mathivanan S, Quesenberry P, Sahoo S, Tahara H, Wauben MH, Witwer KW, Thery C (2014) Minimal experimental requirements for definition of extracellular vesicles and their functions: a position statement from the International Society for Extracellular Vesicles. J Extracell Vesicles 3:26913. https://doi.org/10.3402/jev.v3.26913

13. Liu X, Chinello C, Musante L, Cazzaniga M, Tataruch D, Calzaferri G, James Smith A, De Sio G, Magni F, Zou H, Holthofer H (2015) Intraluminal proteome and peptidome of human urinary extracellular vesicles. Proteomics Clin Appl 9(5-6):568–573. https://doi.org/10.1002/prca.201400085

14. Musante L, Tataruch D, Gu D, Benito-Martin-A, Calzaferri G, Aherne S, Holthofer H (2014) A simplified method to recover urinary vesicles for clinical applications, and sample banking. Sci Rep 4:7532. https://doi.org/10.1038/srep07532

15. Musante L, Tataruch DE, Holthofer H (2014) Use and isolation of urinary exosomes as biomarkers for diabetic nephropathy. Front Endocrinol 5:149. https://doi.org/10.3389/fendo.2014.00149

16. Barreiro K, Holthofer H (2017) Urinary extracellular vesicles. A promising shortcut to novel biomarker discoveries. Cell Tissue Res 369 (1):217–227. https://doi.org/10.1007/s00441-017-2621-0

17. Rupert DLM, Claudio V, Lasser C, Bally M (2017) Methods for the physical characterization and quantification of extracellular vesicles in biological samples. Biochim Biophys Acta 1861(1 Pt A):3164–3179. https://doi.org/10.1016/j.bbagen.2016.07.028

18. Zaborowski MP, Balaj L, Breakefield XO, Lai CP (2015) Extracellular vesicles: composition, biological relevance, and methods of study. Bioscience 65(8):783–797. https://doi.org/10.1093/biosci/biv084

19. Puhka M, Takatalo M, Nordberg ME, Valkonen S, Nandania J, Aatonen M, Yliperttula M, Laitinen S, Velagapudi V, Mirtti T, Kallioniemi O, Rannikko A, Siljander PR, Af Hallstrom TM (2017) Metabolomic profiling of extracellular vesicles and alternative normalization methods reveal enriched metabolites and strategies to study prostate cancer-related changes. Theranostics 7 (16):3824–3841. https://doi.org/10.7150/thno.19890

20. Rosa-Fernandes L, Rocha VB, Carregari VC, Urbani A, Palmisano G (2017) A perspective on extracellular vesicles proteomics. Front Chem 5:102. https://doi.org/10.3389/fchem.2017.00102

21. Kreimer S, Belov AM, Ghiran I, Murthy SK, Frank DA, Ivanov AR (2015) Mass-spectrometry-based molecular characterization of extracellular vesicles: lipidomics and proteomics. J Proteome Res 14(6):2367–2384. https://doi.org/10.1021/pr501279t

22. Colombo M, Raposo G, Thery C (2014) Biogenesis, secretion, and intercellular interactions of exosomes and other extracellular vesicles. Annu Rev Cell Dev Biol 30:255–289. https://doi.org/10.1146/annurev-cellbio-101512-122326

23. Puhka M, Nordberg ME, Valkonen S, Rannikko A, Kallioniemi O, Siljander P, Af Hallstrom TM (2017) KeepEX, a simple dilution protocol for improving extracellular vesicle yields from urine. Eur J Pharm Sci 98:30–39. https://doi.org/10.1016/j.ejps.2016.10.021

Chapter 14

Examining Cell-Cell Interactions in the Kidney Using AFM Single-Cell Force Spectroscopy

Eleftherios Siamantouras, Claire E. Hills, Kuo-Kang Liu, and Paul E. Squires

Abstract

The ability of individual cells to synchronize activity is a basic feature of efficient and appropriate tissue function. Central to this is the physicochemical binding between cells through multiprotein complexes that functionally mediate adhesion. Importantly, the direct connection of physical properties and intercellular signaling is of great importance to certain pathologies including diabetes. Atomic force microscopy (AFM) single-cell force spectroscopy (SCFS) is a high-resolution technique that provides a statistically reliable measurement of the minute forces involved in cell tethering and membrane dynamics. Detection of altered nanoscale forces underlying the loss of adhesion in early tubular injury is pivotal for the development of novel therapeutic strategies for diabetic nephropathy. Here we describe the step-by-step use of an integrated AFM-SCFS system designed to measure functional force-displacement in separating renal tubular epithelial cells. Parameters such as unbinding forces, detachment energy, and distance to complete separation can be obtained from force-displacement (*F-d*) curves and are critical in assessing how physical changes of cellular adhesion contribute to cell contact, coupling, and communication in the diabetic kidney.

Key words AFM, Cadherin, Cell adhesion, Cell-cell coupling, Membrane dynamics, Nanomedicine

1 Introduction

Effective cell-to-cell communication requires contact-dependent intercellular signaling, which relies on the interaction between cells at the adherens junction [1]. Cadherins are calcium-dependent transmembrane proteins that ligate with similar proteins on neighboring cells to form the primary point of cell-cell contact and adhesion in the tubular epithelium [2]. Cadherins have a central role in forming the multiprotein physicochemical pathway that links cell-cell contact to the actin cytoskeleton. This interaction not only increases the adhesive strength of the adherens junction, but also acts as a signaling "node" for proteins that influence adhesiveness and/or initiate intracellular signaling [3]. Since intercellular signaling requires functional cell-to-cell tethering,

Luigi Gnudi and David A. Long (eds.), *Diabetic Nephropathy: Methods and Protocols*, Methods in Molecular Biology, vol. 2067,
https://doi.org/10.1007/978-1-4939-9841-8_14,

monitoring nanoscale changes in physical adhesion can identify loss of cell function in disease. AFM-based methodologies clarify the intricate relationship between nanoscale physical changes and molecular dynamics, directly connecting biophysics with cellular function. Moreover, application of novel biophysical methods at the medical interface is pivotal in advancing early diagnostics and progressing therapeutic innovations.

Although, AFM-based force spectroscopy was primarily used as an assay to quantify molecular forces between isolated receptor-ligand binding [4], recent advancements in the separation range between cells allowed the development of single-cell force spectroscopy, which provides a description of the ligation function in situ [5–8]. The atomic force microscope (CellHesion® module, JKP Instruments, Germany) has a displacement actuator of a long traveling distance (up to 100 μm) which facilitates the measurement of complete force-displacement curves when studying the cell-to-cell separation process of large, soft cells, such as found in the tubular epithelium [9]. Retraction force-displacement curves for separating two adherent cells can be measured to determine the force and energy required to uncouple cells. The former is normally referred to as "maximum unbinding force" F_{max} and the latter the "work or energy of detachment" W_D, which can be calculated from the *F-d* separation curve. In addition, the distance of complete separation d_s and the number of tether rupture events (TREs) can be determined [9].

Here, we describe quantitative characterization of the underlying biophysical changes that accompany cell-cell adhesion in the diabetic kidney. Diabetic nephropathy currently represents the leading cause of end-stage renal disease and is characterized by a number of functional and structural disturbances [10]. Of these, tubulointerstitial fibrosis represents a key underlying pathology and is initiated in response to a loss in epithelial (E) cadherin-mediated cell-to-cell adhesion [11, 12]. While it is well documented that the pro-fibrotic cytokine, transforming growth factor-beta 1 (TGF-β1), reduces E-cadherin expression in tubular epithelial cells of the proximal nephron [13], to further understand how changes in cadherin expression, localization, and function directly affect physical adhesion requires the use of sophisticated high-resolution technologies, such as AFM-SCFS. This technique provides a reliable measurement of the minute forces involved in cell tethering and membrane dynamics. In this method, a living cell is attached on a functionalized tipless cantilever, acting this way as a probe cell, which is brought in contact with a substrate cell. A laser beam detects the vertical deflection of the cantilever, which is read on a photodetector. The total signal hitting all four quadrants of the photodetector is the sum output, which is converted in force units during calibration. Any deviation associated with the vertical deflection of the cantilever during cell separation is a measure of molecular binding. This measure of cellular adhesion can resolve subtle changes in cell-cell interactions that precede changes in function and can therefore identify underlying mechanisms linking proteomics to overt tissue complications of diabetes. These types of high-resolution, reproducible, and quantifiable measurements can be used to examine how cell adhesion and cell coupling alter in different tissue types in diabetes. The approach can resolve early physical changes that occur ahead of overt loss in function and are invaluable in understanding the basic cellular changes, which underlie many complications of the disease.

2 Materials

2.1 Tissue Culturing

1. Clonal human kidney (HK2) proximal tubule epithelial cells.
2. Tissue culture plastics.
3. Cell growth media Dulbecco's modified Eagle medium/ Ham's nutrient mixture F12 (DMEM/F12) (17.5 mM): 10% Fetal calf serum (FCS), 2 mM glutamine, 5 ng/mL epidermal growth factor (EGF), penicillin/streptomycin: 10,000 units penicillin, 10 mg streptomycin, 0.9% sodium chloride.
4. Low-glucose DMEM/F12: 50% DMEM (no glucose), 50% F-12 (10 mM).
5. Un-supplemented (serum-free) DMEM/F12.

2.2 Instrumentation

1. Integrated system for measuring cell-cell and cell-substrate interaction.
2. Inverted microscope (*see* **Note 1**).
3. BioCell temperature controller (*see* **Note 2**).
4. CCD camera.
5. Anti-vibration table.
6. Drivers and Data Processing Software.

2.3 Probes

1. Tipless cantilevers (*see* **Note 3**).
2. Glass block cantilever holder (*see* **Note 4**).
3. 2% Hellmanex solution.
4. UV treatment device.
5. Fine tweezers.
6. 25 μg/mL Poly-L-lysine.
7. 20 μg/mL Fibronectin.
8. Phosphate-buffered saline (PBS).
9. Rubber blade cell scraper, manufactured for minimum damage of cells.

3 Methods

AFM-based technology provides a powerful tool for high-resolution, broad-range single-cell force measurements. SCFS operates on the principle of molecular interaction between a probe cell and a substrate cell. A piezo actuator moves the base of a cantilever toward the surface of a sample cell in vertical direction until contact (Fig. 1). After a defined period, the cantilever is retracted while the deflection of a cantilever is continuously measured.

3.1 Cell Culture

1. HK2 cells (passages 18–30) were maintained in DMEM/F-12, which has a high basal glucose concentration of 17.5 mM to encourage cell growth and promote cell viability.
2. Cells were seeded onto 40 mm petri dishes and cultured at 37 °C in a humidified atmosphere of 5% CO_2 in air.
3. Prior to treatment, cells were cultured in DMEM/F12 low glucose (5 mM) to negate any pre-stimulatory effects of the high (17.5 mM) glucose.

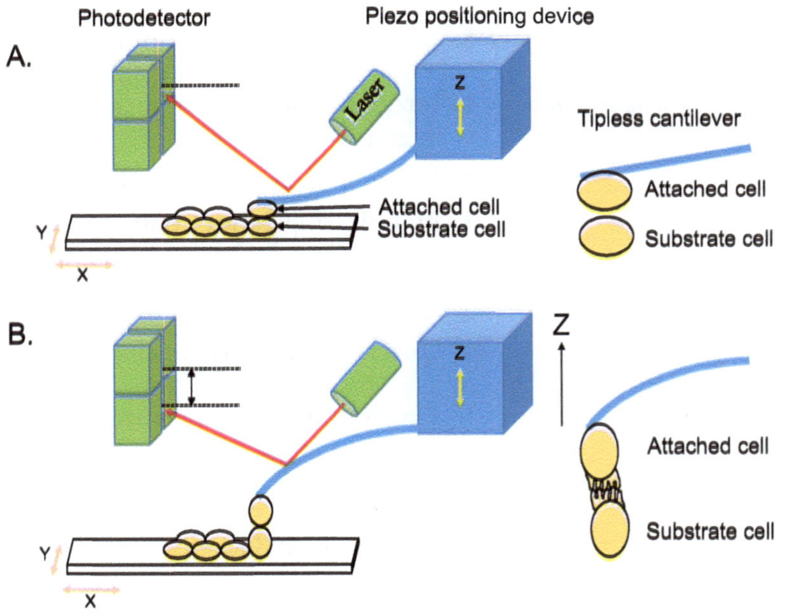

Fig. 1 A long-range piezoelectric actuator controls the position of the cantilever while any changes in deflection are detected by a quadratic photodetector. This arrangement allows high-resolution continuous measurements of force versus displacement during the separation process of two cells. In Phase A, ligation is formed when the cells are in contact and in Phase B surface molecules are unbounded during the separation process

4. Cells were cultured in low glucose containing un-supplemented (serum-free) DMEM/F12 for 48 h prior to procedure.
5. At this point cells can be treated with a designated stimulus, e.g., TGFβ1.

3.2 Sensor Preparation

AFM cantilevers for soft biological materials are very fragile and susceptible to damage. To ensure consistency between measurements, the same type and batch of the cantilevers should be used throughout an experimental project. It is suggested to test the performance of each cantilever before further use, by performing an *F-d* curve on a hard substrate.

3.2.1 Functionalization of the Cantilevers for Cell Adhesion Experiments

1. Sterilize new cantilevers using UV treatment (5 min).
2. Incubate in 25 μg/mL poly-L-lysine in PBS for 30 min at room temperature.
3. Wash cantilevers in fresh PBS.
4. Inspect surface under the optical microscope to ensure smoothness.
5. Incubate in 20 μg/mL fibronectin solution in PBS for 2 h at 37 °C.
6. Wash cantilevers in fresh PBS.
7. Repeat **steps 4** and **6** if necessary (*see* **Note 5**).
8. Store in fresh PBS solution at 4 °C and use within 3 days. Change the media daily.

3.2.2 Mounting the Cantilever on the Glass Cantilever Holder

1. Using a pair of fine tweezers, place the chip of the cantilever on the top of the glass holder.
2. Position the cantilever in the polished part making sure that it is aligned toward the middle and in parallel with the alignment marks.
3. Tighten the cantilever on the glass block to ensure that it will be secured into position during experiments.
4. Mount the glass holder into the AFM head and lock into position (*see* **Note 6**).

3.3 Instrumentation Setup

F-d curves are produced by the measurement of the cantilever deflection as a function of the piezo actuator position. Accurate detection of the cantilever's deflection is crucial as the sensitivity of this operation is directly proportional to the value of the interaction force between the probe cell and the examining cell.

3.3.1 Laser Path Alignment

Before calibrating the cantilever, we must ensure that the sum voltage output is sufficient. Whenever a new cantilever is mounted on the glass holder the laser path must be aligned, since manual

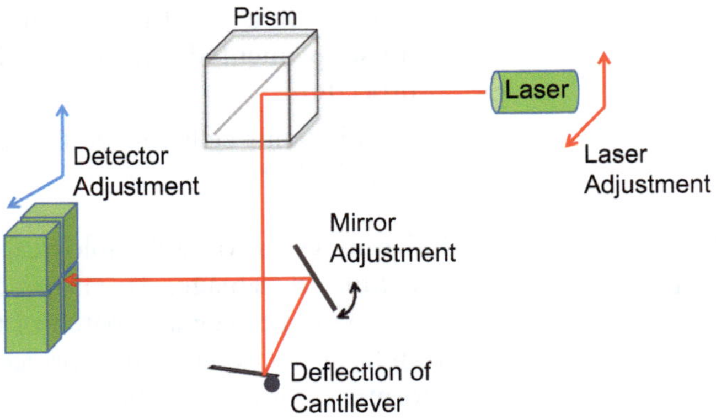

Fig. 2 Optical path of the laser. By adjusting both the mirror and the photodetector, the laser spot from the end of the cantilever can be targeted to the center of the photodetector to achieve maximum sensitivity (figure adopted from JPK's manual)

attachment results in slightly different positioning. The laser path is schematically illustrated in Fig. 2.

1. Adjust the laser spot centrally, toward the end of the cantilever (*see* **Note 7**).
2. Adjust the prism to ensure that the laser beam hits the region of the photodetector.
3. Adjust the mirror so that the maximum value of output voltage is reached.
4. Fine-tune the quadratic photodetector until the laser hits the center of it while ensuring that the lateral and vertical deflection values are close to zero.
5. The sum value should ideally be much higher than 1 V and not significantly lower than this value (*see* **Note 8**).

3.3.2 Calibration of the Cantilever

For small deflections the cantilevers approximate a Hookean spring, where the deflection is linearly correlated to the acting force. When the cantilever spring constant is known, the vertical deflection (nm) can be converted into force. Although the nominal force constant value of the cantilever is known, each cantilever must be individually calibrated (*see* **Note 9**).

1. Set the voltage at 1 V (*see* **Note 10**) and perform a *F-d* curve on a stiff, clean surface of the petri dish, as it is required to achieve a robust approach for the correct determination of the sensitivity (*see* **Note 11**).
2. Determine the sensitivity (nm/V) by the gradient of the steep linear part of the curve, close to the repulsive contact region (*see* **Note 12**).

3. Determine the spring constant of a cantilever using the thermal noise method (*see* **Note 13**).
4. Fit the function into the chosen peak.
5. Select the appropriate correction factor.

3.4 Experimental

This procedure takes place before each treatment is tested.

3.4.1 Preparation of Suspended Cells: Scrape Delivery Procedure

1. Treat the cells in a T25 flask (*see* **Note 14**).
2. Gently scrape the cells off the flask's surface using a sterile rubber blade cell scraper with low-force sweeping motion.
3. Transfer the scraped cells using a pipette in a sterile conical tube for centrifugation at 142 × *g* for 5 min at room temperature.
4. Remove the supernatant and carefully resuspend the cell pellet with fresh sterile DMEM CO_2-free media (2–3 mL depending on pellet size) (*see* **Note 15**).
5. Gently agitate the pellet using a 1000 μL pipette (3 min), to break up the cells, and ensure a uniform distribution.
6. Incubate for 5 min at 37 °C to allow recovery (*see* **Note 16**).
7. Identify a clean area on the petri dish (*see* **Note 17**) and introduce 20–30 μL of resuspended cells with gentle force to ensure that fluid movement is kept to a minimum (*see* **Note 18**).
8. Carefully place the AFM head into the stage and proceed to the next step.

3.4.2 Single-Cell Attachment Procedure

The attachment procedure (Fig. 3) must be performed rapidly (2 min); otherwise suspended cells will adhere on the substrate.

1. Set the AFM in constant force mode.
2. Set the force at 1nN, the contact time at 5 s, and the speed at 5 μm/s (*see* **Note 19**).
3. Identify a suitable cell (*see* **Note 20**) and place the arrow-shape cantilever directly above the cell.
4. Perform a *F-d* curve.
5. Once contact is established, gently position the cantilever so that the cell is attached toward the apex.
6. Inspect the attached cell and leave to recover for at least 5 min.
7. To ensure that rigid adhesion of the probe cell is achieved, move the cantilever in the medium while observing the attached cell.

3.4.3 Cell-to-Cell Adhesion

1. Set the contact force at 1 nN, contact time at 10 s, and constant speed at 5 μm/s (*see* **Note 21**).

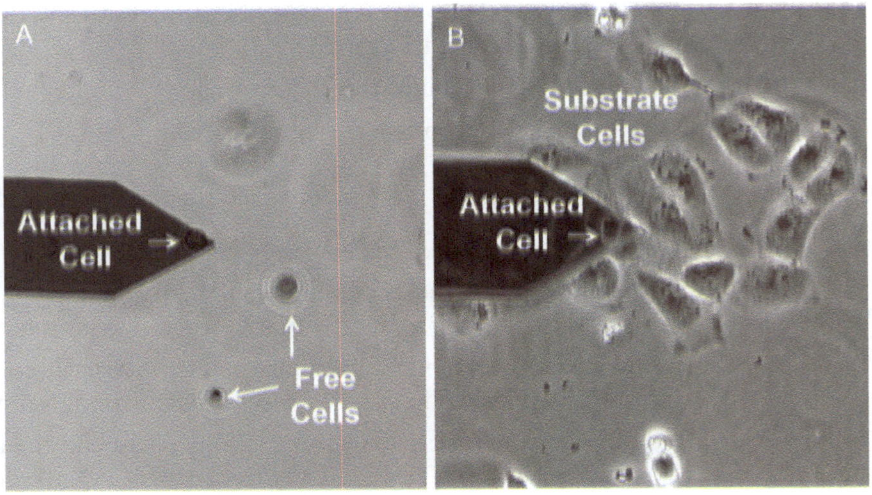

Fig. 3 (**a**) A suitable suspended (free) cell is identified and attached onto the functionalized cantilever. (**b**) The probe (attached) cell is then positioned over a substrate cell within a cell cluster before the cantilever is lowered and the attached and substrate cells are allowed to adhere under constant force (1 nN/10 s)

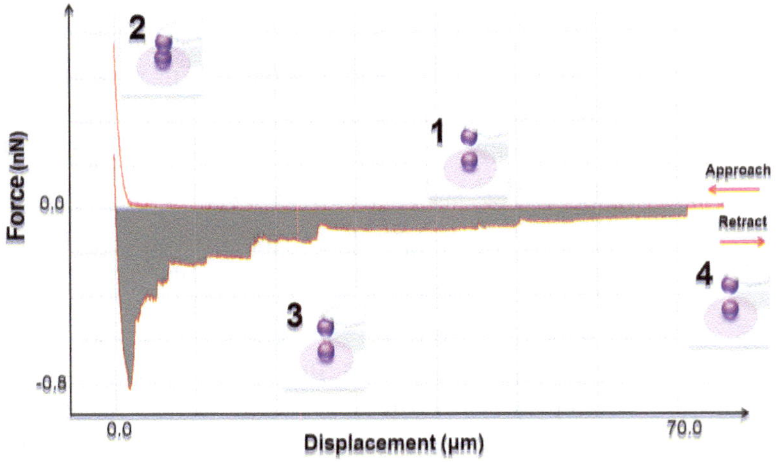

Fig. 4 A typical *F-d* curve is generated by the coupling and uncoupling of two cells. Initially the cells are bounded into a cantilever and the substrate (Phase 1). Then the cells are made to "approach" each other. After a short period of contact, the two cells adhere. During this 10-s period bonding is formed (Phase 2). Next, the cantilever is retracted and force versus displacement measured (Phase 3) until the cells are completely detached (Phase 4)

2. Identify a substrate cell and position the probe cell directly on top of nucleus (*see* **Note 22**).
3. Perform a *F-d* curve (Fig. 4).
4. Check the displacement output to ensure that the piezo is functioning in its effective range while being able to touch the cell and completely separate the cells when retracted.

5. Adjust the piezo if necessary or skip to **step 6**.
6. Allow the cells to recover for 45 s at the maximal retraction distance of the piezo.
7. Perform *F-d* ×2 on the same cells, with 45-s intervals between measurements.
8. Allow the probe cell to recover for 1 min between different cell recordings.
9. Move the cantilever gently to the next substrate cell; follow **steps 3–6** (*see* **Note 23**).
10. Perform experiments in ten cells using the same probe cell (30 *F-d* curves/dish).

3.4.4 Retraction Curve Analysis

1. Open the batch function of JPK's Data Processing.
2. Load the curves using the empty-process selection.
3. Select the function Automatically subtract the baseline.
4. Select the retract segment.
5. Select the linear part of the *F-d* curve on the *x*-axis.
6. Select the option Offset plus tilt if necessary.
7. Select the Measure Adhesion function to determine the maximum unbinding force.
8. Select the Determine the area under the curve function to calculate the work of complete detachment.
9. Select the Identify and quantify steps function (*see* **Note 24**).
10. Select Only Positive Steps (*see* **Note 25**).
11. Select the area of the retraction curve to fit the step-fitting model (*see* **Note 26**).
12. Run the automated step-fitting method to determine the tether rupture events (Fig. 5).

4 Notes

1. It is necessary to install the force spectroscopy module on an inverted microscope to maintain optical view in order to effectively manipulate the cells.
2. The temperature controller should be adjusted two degrees higher than the desired temperature to ensure that the sample is maintained at 37 °C to achieve near-physiological conditions.
3. The selection of the parameters of the cantilever depends on the type of cells and it should have a low spring constant when the sample cells are from soft tissues/organs. In addition, arrow geometry of the cantilever facilitates the manipulation and capture of the probe cell.

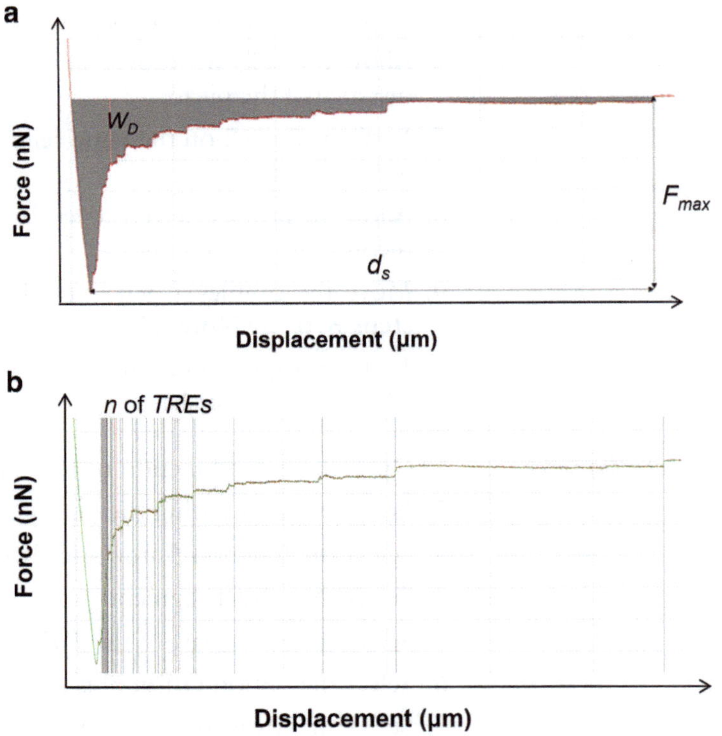

Fig. 5 Processing of *F-d* cell-to-cell adhesion curves. All processing functions are applied to the retracted part of the curve. The reference point that will be used for the determination of the adhesion parameters should be determined. Essentially this is the point of complete separation between the two cells and is specified by setting the baseline of the complete separation of the retraction curve to match the zero *x*-axis. (**a**) The detection of minimum value of force represents the maximum force required for the complete separation of the two cells. F_{max} is calculated by detecting the minimum negative value of force with respect to the *x*-axis baseline, W_D is determined by the area under the retracted part of the curve, and d_s is calculated by the difference between F_{max} and the *x*-axis point of complete separation. (**b**) The retraction curve clearly exhibits a steplike pattern as an immediate result from the rupture of surface ligations. The number of tethering rupture events can be detected by identifying sharp steps of force that occur after unbinding of ligations. TREs fall into two general areas, those in which a force ramp is preceded and those in which a mechanical deformation is preceded as the pulling distance increases

4. This specially designed cantilever holder is polished on its top and bottom surfaces, to allow transmission of light to the lenses, and therefore extra care should be taken to avoid scratching; hence they are not to be touched with hands or tweezers. The glass block can be cleaned in an ultrasonic bath using a floating rack and mild detergent.
5. Since the output sum signal depends on deflection of the laser, it is crucial to ensure that the surface of the cantilever is clean

and any residual debris should be removed from the cantilever after functionalization.

6. The way the cantilever is mounted affects the sensitivity. If the output reading is faulty, remounting the cantilever may troubleshoot.
7. The illumination of microscope can be decreased to ease the view of the laser onto the cantilever.
8. A relatively stable sum value (Volts) should be generated by the vertical and lateral deflection of the cantilever; however if the experiments are conducted in culturing media a small drift may appear. If, after the proper alignment of the laser, the sum value is significantly below 1 V or if there is high drift in the deflection of the cantilever, then a new cantilever or fresh media should be used. When using chemically modified cantilevers, it is important to use a clean region of the cantilever as the deflection site.
9. A calibrated cantilever must be recalibrated if the alignment parameters are changed or if it is loosely attached on the glass holder.
10. Higher values may compromise functionalization. Approach curves at this stage should be kept to a minimum.
11. It is crucial that this measurement is performed in the same buffer solution and temperature as in the actual experiments. Ideally, there should be space on the cultured dish, depending on the confluency; however if this is not possible a clean dish with the same experimental conditions can be used.
12. This is the distance of the cantilever vertical deflection for a given voltage difference measured by the photodetector and by calculating sensitivity deflection can then be converted into distance (nm). Typical sensitivity ranges are between 30 and 100 nm/V, as stated by the manufacturer. Sensitivity depends on the reflective characteristics of cantilever, the mounting position of the cantilever, and should be determined every time the cantilever is mounted or remounted [6].
13. For a given temperature, the amplitudes of the fluctuations depend only on the spring constant of the cantilever; hence the thermal resonance curve can be fitted to a Lorenz function to allow spring constant calculation [14]. However, the resonance of soft cantilevers in culture media is much lower and very susceptible to noise due to drifting of the cantilever, in which case a correction factor should be used to calculate the actual value of the spring constant [15]. Also, when using cantilevers for soft biological material in liquid the first resonant peak is largely affected by low-frequency noise. In that case, the second peak and a correction factor of 0.251 should be used. To increase consistency between measurements, it is suggested that cantilevers from the same batch should be used.

14. Using a flask to culture "free" cells reflects ease of accessibility when detaching cells with a scraper.
15. Experiments were performed in an instrument that is not equipped with a CO_2 chamber, hence the use of CO_2-independent media.
16. For cell attachment, please proceed with point 1 of next paragraph (section 3.4.2).
17. Perform an approach curve to adjust displacement into the piezo range prior to pipetting suspended cells. Retract the piezo (100 μm) before lifting the head.
18. Gently agitate "free" cells in the tube with a 1 mL pipette to resuspend any pelleted cells (10 s) before introducing them to the dish. To avoid fluid and particle movements, it is important to limit the amount of "free" cells entering dish.
19. Attachment force and contact time may need to be slightly adjusted between experiments; the ranges we suggest are 0.8–1.3 nN and 5–10 s.
20. Ideally a cell should have a round shape, smooth surface, and comparable diameter with the other suspended cells floating in the media. If the identified cell is relatively stable on the substrate, gently touch the head with a finger and observe whether or not the cell is affected by the fluid's motion. If not, it may be already adhered to the substrate.
21. Complete separation depends on contact time, contact force, and retraction speed. These parameters were adjusted before experiments to ensure that the maximum piezo range is sufficient for complete separation.
22. Since there is a difference in height between substrate and probe cell, fine adjustment of the lens is required to identify the exact position of contact.
23. It is advised to explore the substrate cells prior to experiments, to identify areas of potential testing cells in close proximity.
24. Unbinding of ligations can be detected by identifying sharp steps of force that occur after a main rupture of tethers and a plateau in x-axis that is dependent on cell compliance. The software is based on the work of Kerssemakers et al. [16] and works well as a step-fitting method for detecting small force jumps that correspond to bond rupture. However, the automated analysis is not fully developed and some events may not be detected. Nevertheless, differences in the molecular ligation between treatments can be observed.
25. During the retraction phase only positive steps are anticipated.
26. Zoom in the curve to determine the exact position of fitting.

Acknowledgment

This work was supported by generous support from Diabetes UK (11/0004215, 12/0004546, and 16/0005427).

References

1. Meng W, Takeichi M (2009) Adherens junction: molecular architecture and regulation. Cold Spring Harb Perspect Biol 1(6):a002899
2. Fujimoto K, Nagafuchi A, Tsukita S, Kuraoka A, Ohokuma A, Shibata Y (1997) Dynamics of connexins, E-cadherin and alpha-catenin on cell membranes during gap junction formation. J Cell Sci 110(3):311–322
3. Moreno AP, Berthoud VM, Pérez-Palacios G, Pérez-Armendariz EM (2005) Biophysical evidence that connexin-36 forms functional gap junction channels between pancreatic mouse beta-cells. Am J Physiol Endocrinol Metab 288:E948–E956
4. Benoit M, Gabriel D, Gerisch G, Gaub HE (2000) Discrete interactions in cell adhesion measured by single-molecule force spectroscopy. Nat Cell Biol 2(6):313–317
5. Franz CM, Puech P-H (2008) Atomic force microscopy: a versatile tool for studying cell morphology, adhesion and mechanics. Cell Mol Bioeng 1(4):289–300
6. Friedrichs J, Helenius J, Muller DJ (2010) Quantifying cellular adhesion to extracellular matrix components by single-cell force spectroscopy. Nat Protoc 5(7):1353–1361
7. Friedrichs J, Legate KR, Schubert R, Bharadwaj M, Werner C, Müller D, Benoit M (2013) A practical guide to quantify cell adhesion using single-cell force spectroscopy. Methods 60(2):169–178
8. Puech PH, Taubenberger A, Ulrich F, Krieg M, Muller DJ, Heisenberg CP (2005) Measuring cell adhesion forces from zebrafish using atomic force microscopy. J Cell Sci 118:4199–4206
9. Siamantouras E, Hills CE, Squires PE, Liu KK (2016) Quantifying cellular mechanics and adhesion in renal tubular injury using single cell force spectroscopy. Nanomedicine 12 (4):1013–1021
10. Wada J, Makino H (2013) Inflammation and the pathogenesis of diabetic nephropathy. Clin Sci 124:138–152
11. Zeisberg M, Neilson EG (2010) Mechanisms of tubulointerstitial fibrosis. J Am Soc Nephrol 21:1819–1834
12. Hills CE, Siamantouras E, Smith SW, Cockwell P, Liu K-K, Squires PE (2012) TGFβ modulates cell-to-cell communication in early epithelial-to-mesenchymal transition. Diabetologia 55:812–824
13. Hills CE, Squires PE (2011) The role of TGFβ and epithelial-to-mesenchymal transition in diabetic nephropathy. Cytokine Growth Factor Rev 22:131–139
14. Hutter JL, Bechhoefer J (1993) Calibration of atomic-force microscope tips. Rev Sci Instrum 64(7):1868–1873
15. Butt H-J, Jaschke M (1995) Calculation of thermal noise in atomic force microscopy. Nanotechnology 6(1):1–7
16. Kerssemakers JW, Laura ME, Laan L, Noetzel TL, Janson ME, Dogterom M (2006) Assembly dynamics of microtubules at molecular resolution. Nature 442:709–712

Part V

Transcriptome, Metabolic, and Proteomic Profiling of the Diabetic Kidney

Chapter 15

Genetic Strategies to Understand Human Diabetic Nephropathy: Wet-Lab Approaches

Laura J. Smyth, Katie Kerr, Seamus Duffy, Jill Kilner, and Amy Jayne McKnight

Abstract

Multiple genetic strategies are available to help improve understanding of diabetic nephropathy. This methods chapter provides an overview of phenotype considerations specific to diabetic nephropathy and biobank essentials, and provides detailed methodology for a common benchtop wet-lab approach (Ion Torrent semiconductor sequencing) including in silico genetic variant identification from next-generation sequencing data to identify genetic risk factors for diabetic nephropathy.

Key words Association, Diabetic nephropathy, Genome-wide, Illumina, Next-generation sequencing, Kidney, S5XL, SNP, Torrent, Trend, Variant

1 Introduction

The last decade has seen significant advances in genetic approaches to help identify common complex diseases such as diabetic nephropathy (DN) (Fig. 1). Moving beyond studies assessing small numbers of single-nucleotide polymorphisms (SNPs) by technologies such as TaqMan, Sequenom, MassARRAY iPLEX™, and Sanger sequencing [1, 2], higher throughput options such as high-density arrays and next-generation sequencing (NGS) now provide more comprehensive analysis of an individual's genome. Historically, genetic association studies for DN were plagued with lack of replication or negative reports [3]; however international collaborations are now leading to the identification of genetic risk factors that are replicated across multiple populations (Fig. 2) [4–11].

Here, we outline experimental considerations for undertaking successful genetic studies for DN. Firstly, it is critically important that the correct phenotypes are employed and clearly reported to

Luigi Gnudi and David A. Long (eds.), *Diabetic Nephropathy: Methods and Protocols*, Methods in Molecular Biology, vol. 2067, https://doi.org/10.1007/978-1-4939-9841-8_15,

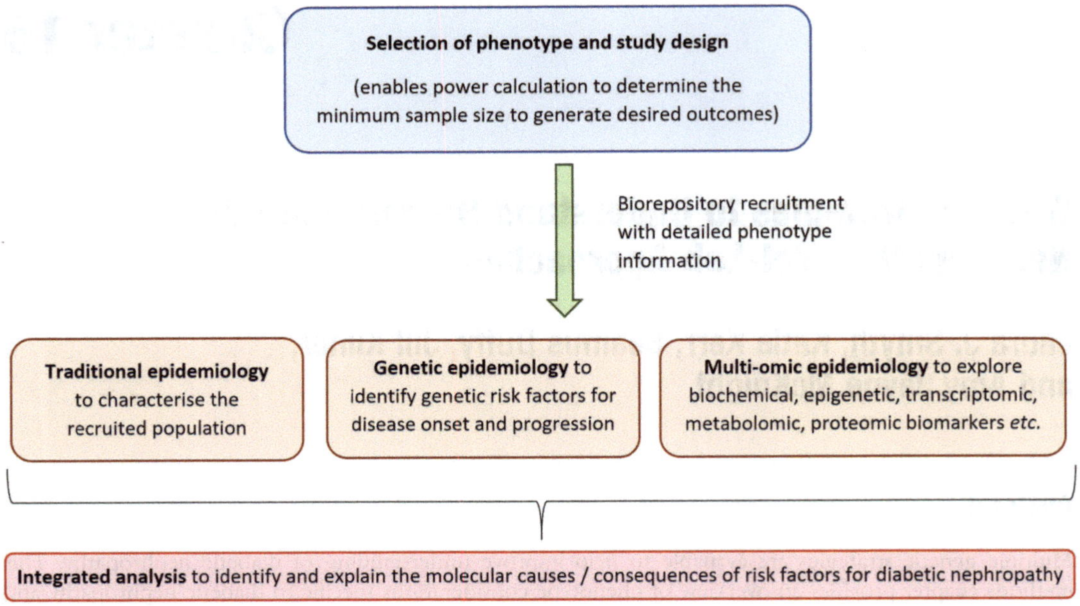

Fig. 1 Overview of strategies using human DNA to understand diabetic nephropathy

identify and replicate genetic risk factors for DN (*see* Subheading 3.1, Characterization of Participants). Standardized protocols are helpful for multicenter collections and Subheading 3.2 (Biobanking Essentials) describes a consistent approach for developing a bioresource to facilitate multiomic analysis. Sanger sequencing retains a role in validation from large-scale sequencing and fine-mapping from genome-wide association studies (GWAS), but is not described here as multiple protocols exist for this traditional technology, which include PCR amplification of targeted genetic regions, PCR cleanup, cycle sequencing, sequencing cleanup, capillary electrophoresis, and base calling [12]. Large-scale genotyping efforts such as high-density arrays and whole-genome sequencing are typically outsourced to core facilities or commercial laboratories. Instead, we outline a method for targeted next-generation semiconductor sequencing (Subheadings 2 and 3.4–3.6, Fig. 3) which is a cost-effective, benchtop approach that can be semiautomated to regularly generate high-quality sequencing data for day-to-day laboratory use. Such targeted sequencing is often used for pathway analysis, exome analysis, or validating a larger number of top-ranked SNPs from GWAS. When NGS data is generated, genetic variants must be identified based on explicitly stated parameters to allow further analysis for DN (see Chap. 16, in this volume).

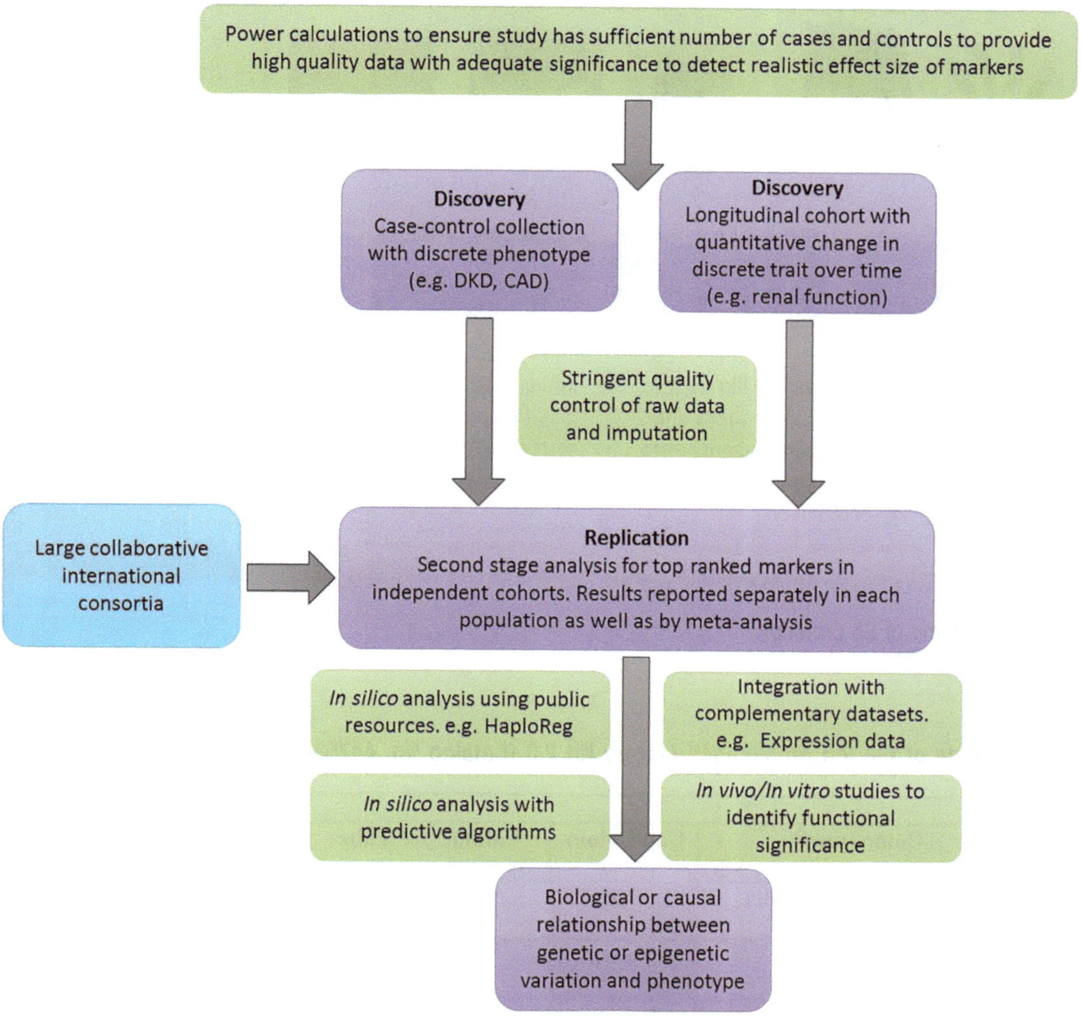

Fig. 2 Example of genome-wide association design

2 Materials for Ion S5™ Targeted Sequencing

2.1 Ion AmpliSeq™ DNA Library Preparation Materials

1. Ion AmpliSeq™ Library Kit 2.0: Each kit (Table 1) provides reagents for preparing eight libraries and contains one tube of each component. Kits are shipped on frozen gel packs and should be stored as indicated.
2. Ion AmpliSeq™ Custom and Community Panels: Typically includes one or two 2× primer pools and 384-well plates (Table 2). Order on www.ampliseq.com.
3. Complete set of Ion Xpress™ Barcode Adapters 1-96 (Catalog No. 4474517, Table 3).

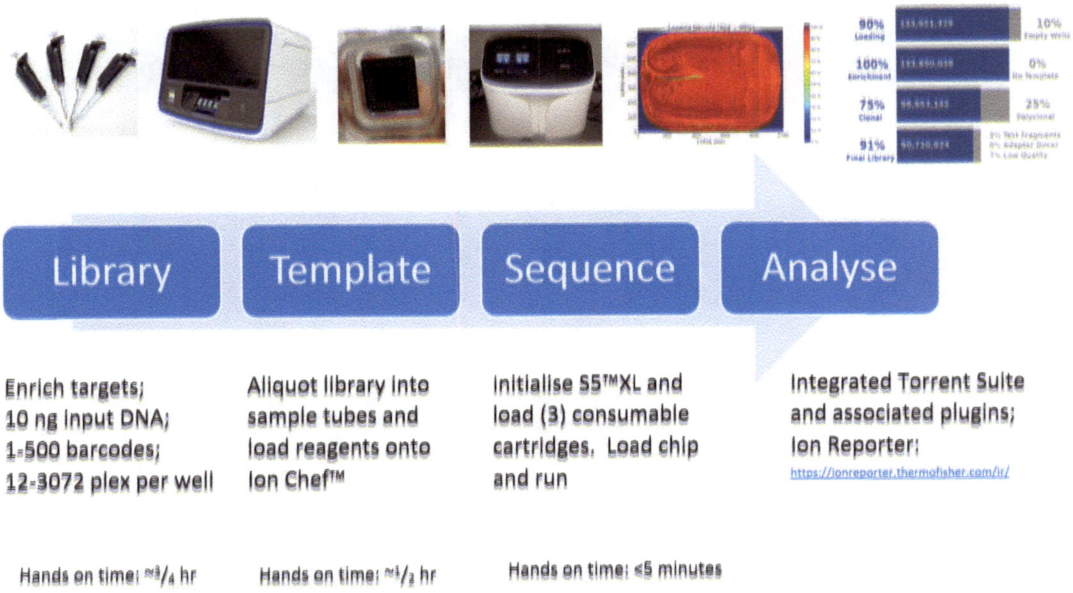

Fig. 3 Overview of S5 protocol

Table 1
Components of the Ion AmpliSeq™ Library Kit 2.0 (Catalog No. 4475345)

Component	Cap Colour	Volume per Tube	Storage
5X Ion AmpliSeq HiFi Mix	Red	40 µL	
FuPa Reagent	Brown	16 µL	
Switch Solution	Yellow	32 µL	
DNA Ligase	Blue	16 µL	
Ion AmpliSeq Adapters	Green	16 µL	
Platinum PCR Supermix HiFi	Black	400 µL	
Library Amplification Primer Mix	White	16 µL	-20 °C
Low TE	Clear	1 mL	Room temp or -20 °C

4. Thermal cycler.
5. PCR plates, 96 well.
6. Adhesive PCR film.

Table 2
Ion AmpliSeq™ custom and community panels

Average primer pairs per pool in a custom or community panel	2× Primer pools: Number of tubes per primer pool	2× Primer pools: Total tubes per box	384-Well plates: Reactions per pool	384-Well plates: Total plates per box	Storage
≤96 Primer pairs	5 Tubes (~150 reactions/ tube)	5 or 10 tubes	~1500 Reactions	Up to 6 plates	−20 °C (shipped at room temperature)
≥96 Primer pairs	20 Tubes (~150 reactions/ tube)	20 or 40 tubes	~6000 Reactions		

Table 3
Ion Xpress™ barcode adapters

Ion Xpress Barcode Adapters Kits (each kit includes 16 individually numbered barcodes)				
Component	**Cap colour**	**Quantity**	**Volume**	**Storage**
Ion Xpress P1 Adapter	Violet	1 tube	320 µL	-30 °C to -10 °C
Ion Xpress Barcode X	White	16 tubes (1 per barcode)	20 µL each	

7. Compression pads.
8. Agencourt AMPure XP beads, 450 mL.
9. Magnetic plate suitable for 96-well plate.
10. Nuclease-free water.
11. Absolute ethanol.
12. P200 pipettes.
13. Filter tips.
14. Qubit® 2.0 fluorometer.
15. Qubit® dsDNA HS Assay Kit, 500 assays (Q32854).

2.2 Materials for Using the Ion Chef™ Instrument to Prepare Template-Positive Ion Sphere Particles and Load Ion Chips

Ion 520™ and 530™ kits can be used with 200 or 400 base read libraries of any type prepared using any available library kit. A 200 and 400 base read may be loaded on the same Ion Chef™ run, but the same chip type must be used for both libraries. The Ion 540™ Kit can be used with up to 200 base read libraries of any type prepared using any available library kit.

1. Ion S5™ Ion Chef™ Supplies:
   (a) Chip adapters, x2.
   (b) Enrichment cartridge, x1.
   (c) Tip cartridge v2, x1.
   (d) PCR plate and frame seal v2, x1.
   (e) Recovery station disposable lid v2, x2.
   (f) Recovery tubes v2, x12.
2. Ion S5™ Chef solutions cartridge, x4.
3. Ion S5™ 520™, 530™, or 540™ Chef reagents cartridge, x4.
4. Ion Chef™ instrument.
5. Ion S5™XL sequencer (or another of the S5 series machines).
6. Torrent Server Life Technologies.
7. Uninterruptable power supply (UPS).
8. UltraPure 18 MΩ water system.
9. MiniFuge.
10. Microcentrifuge.
11. Vortex mixer.
12. P2, P20, P200, P1000 μL pipette set and filter tips.
13. 1.5 or 1.7 mL microcentrifuge tubes.
14. Gloves, powder free.
15. Ice bucket and ice.
16. Ion S5™ Controls, Life Technologies A27760.

2.3 Materials for Ion Torrent Sequencing Using Ion S5™ XL Materials (See Note 1)

1. Ion S5™XL Sequencing Reagents Kit containing Ion S5™XL sequencing reagents, 2 × 4 cartridges. Store in the −20 °C freezer.
2. Ion S5™XL Sequencing Solutions:
   (a) Ion S5™ Wash Solution, 2 × 4 bottles.
   (b) Ion S5™ Cleaning Solution, 1 bottle.
3. Compatible Ion Chip™ kit (Table 4).
4. Ion S5™XL Sequencer.
5. Torrent Server Life Technologies.
6. Uninterruptable power supply (UPS).

Table 4
Comparison of outputs from available S5™ platform compatible chips. The number of samples per chip depends on the number of reads required for each sample

Example panel	Ion 510 chip (3 million reads)	Ion 520 chip (6 million reads)	Ion 530 chip (30 million reads)	Ion 540 chip (90 million reads)	Ion 550 chip (130 million reads)
Ion AmpliSeq™ custom panel	Depends on the number of amplicons/genes in the panel. Smaller chips suit analyzing a smaller number of genes. Ion AmpliSeq™ Designer (https://ampliseq.com) reports primer details and the most appropriate chip for each panel for a specified number of samples				
Ion AmpliSeq™ Exome RDY panel (exome sequencing)	Insufficient reads	Insufficient reads	Not evaluated	3 Samples	6 Samples
Ion AmpliSeq™ Transcriptome Human Gene Expression (transcriptome sequencing)	Insufficient reads	Insufficient reads	2 Samples	10 Samples	16 Samples

7. Ion S5™ cartridge tool for removing CO_2 scrubber.
8. Compatible ion chip loaded with template-positive ion sphere particles.
9. Microcentrifuge.
10. Vortex mixer with a rubber platform.
11. Thermal cycler with a heated lid.
12. P2, P20, P200, P1000 μL pipette set and filter tips.
13. PCR tubes, flat cap.
14. 1.5 or 1.7 mL microcentrifuge tubes.
15. UltraPure 18 MΩ water.
16. Ice bucket and ice.
17. Isopropanol.
18. Lint-free wipes.
19. Ion S5™ Controls Kit.

3 Methods

3.1 Characterization of Participants

Historically, multiple phenotypes have been employed for cross-sectional case-control, family-based, and longitudinal studies researching genetic strategies to understand DN [13]. However, there is considerable heterogeneity in the phenotype and this leads to challenges in identifying and replicating true genetic associations. The original longitudinal progression from microalbuminuria to proteinuria with changes in glomerular filtration rate is no longer believed to be representative of DN. For example, we know that microalbuminuria may regress [14, 15], and there is little evidence of a shared genetic component between proteinuria and end-stage renal disease (ESRD) in individuals with type 1 diabetes [4]. To maximize outcomes from genetic studies for DN, large numbers of carefully phenotyped individuals, paying attention to the ethnic origin of participants, are essential and the following phenotypes should ideally be considered:

Type 1 diabetes (diagnosed less than 35 years of age and insulin dependent from diagnosis):

1. *Discrete traditional case DN versus control*: Cases developed persistent macroalbuminuria (albumin:creatine ratio >30 mg/mmol in a spot urine sample; urinary albumin excretion rate >300 mg/24 h; dipstick ++), more than 10 years after their initial diagnosis of diabetes, with concurrent retinopathy, and hypertension versus controls with at least 15-year duration of diabetes and no evidence of renal disease (albumin:creatine ratio <2.5 mg/mmol men, <3.5 mg/mmol women; urinary albumin excretion rate <30 mg/24 h) on repeat testing. Control individuals should not be taking antihypertensive medication and all individuals with microalbuminuria are excluded from both case and control groups [16, 17].
2. *Discrete extreme phenotype DN-ESRD versus long-duration control*: Cases have progressed from the DN definition in **step 1** to have ESRD requiring renal replacement therapy (dialysis or transplantation), compared to controls with more than 25 years of type 1 diabetes and no evidence of kidney disease on repeat testing.
3. *Discrete maximal inclusion microalbuminuria + DN + ESRD versus control*: All cases included in (1) + (2) combined with individuals who have microalbuminuria (albumin:creatine ratio ≥2.5–30 men, ≥3.5–30 women; urinary albumin excretion rate 20–200 mg/24 h men, 30–300 mg/24 h women) versus controls from **step 1**.
4. *Discrete microalbuminuria versus controls*: Cases with microalbuminuria versus controls from **step 1**.
5. *Discrete macroalbuminuria versus controls*: Cases with macroalbuminuria that have not progressed to ESRD versus controls from **step 1**.
6. *Discrete ESRD versus macroalbuminuria*: Cases with ESRD versus controls with macroalbuminuria.
7. *Discrete ESRD versus non-ESRD*: Cases with ESRD versus all other individuals who do not have ESRD.

8. *Discrete CKD*: Cases with CKD stages 3–5 (eGFR <45 mL/min/1.73 m^2) *versus* controls with CKD stages 1–2 (eGFR ≥45 mL/min/1.73 m^2).
9. *Discrete CKD-extreme*: Cases with CKD stage 5 (ESRD, eGFR <15 mL/min/1.73 m^2) versus controls with CKD stage 1 (eGFR ≥90 mL/min/1.73 m^2 with no overt markers of renal disease).
10. *Quantitative CKD*: Based on eGFR values for all individuals as a quantitative trait.

    Type 2 diabetes is more complex. Some individuals develop classical DN with albuminuria, hypertension, increased risk of cardiovascular disease, and premature mortality, accompanied by thickening of the glomerular basement membrane, mesangial expansion, and characteristic glomerulosclerotic nodules. Other individuals may have diabetes and kidney disease that are not associated with classical DN features, such as declining glomerular filtration rate in the absence of proteinuria. As biopsies are not routinely performed for individuals with DN in many countries, it can be challenging to clinically differentiate individuals with DN from those with chronic kidney disease (CKD) and diabetes.
11. *Discrete traditional DN versus controls*: Cases have diabetes for at least 5 years with DN diagnosed by overt proteinuria with confirmed kidney biopsy versus controls with diabetes for at least 10 years and normoalbuminuria.
12. *Discrete extreme DN versus longer duration controls*: Cases have diabetes for at least 5 years with biopsy-confirmed DN progressed to ESRD defined as a need for renal replacement therapy versus controls with diabetes for at least 15 years and no evidence of kidney disease.
13. *Discrete maximal inclusion DN + CKD + ESRD versus controls*: Cases have diabetes for at least 5 years with kidney disease that may or may not have progressed to ESRD versus controls with diabetes for at least 10 years and no evidence of kidney disease.
14. *Discrete maximal inclusion extreme DN versus controls*: Cases have diabetes for at least 5 years with kidney disease that has progressed to ESRD defined as a need for renal replacement therapy versus controls with diabetes for at least 10 years and no evidence of kidney disease.
15. *Discrete maximal inclusion microalbuminuria + DN + CKD + ESRD versus control*: All cases included in **step 13** combined with individuals who have microalbuminuria (at least two out of three measurements with albumin: creatine ratio ≥2.5 men, ≥3.5 women; urinary albumin excretion rate 20–200 mg/24 h men, 30–300 mg/24 h women) versus controls from **step 1**.

16. *Discrete ESRD versus macroalbuminuria*: Cases with ESRD versus controls with macroalbuminuria.
17. *Discrete ESRD versus non-ESRD*: Cases with ESRD versus all other individuals who do not have ESRD.
18. *Discrete CKD*: Cases with CKD stages 3–5 (eGFR <45 mL/min/1.73 m^2) versus controls with CKD stages 1–2 (eGFR ≥45 mL/min/1.73 m^2).
19. *Discrete CKD-extreme*: Cases with CKD stage 5 (ESRD, eGFR <15 mL/min/1.73 m^2) versus controls with CKD stage 1 (eGFR ≥90 mL/min/1.73 m^2 with no markers of renal disease).
20. *Quantitative CKD*: Based on eGFR values for all individuals as a quantitative trait.

3.2 Biobanking Essentials

For new cohort studies, ideally individuals would be recruited with diabetes and followed up every 2 years with detailed phenotype information and biological samples collected for as long as possible to evaluate changes over time. Examples of acquired genetic changes over time may be mitochondrial mutations or telomere length, while complementary changes to SNPs and structural DNA variation may involve differential methylation, changing gene expression levels, or changes to biochemical biomarkers (*see* **Notes 2** and **3**). Biorepositories should aim to collect at least whole blood in EDTA tubes, PAXgene (https://www.preanalytix.com/products/blood/rna-/-mirna/paxgene-blood-rna-tube-ivd/NL?cHash=7a86399709f1fc95ac588e891b36c6f0), serum, glucose, and plasma, alongside urine for analysis (Fig. 4). Ideally

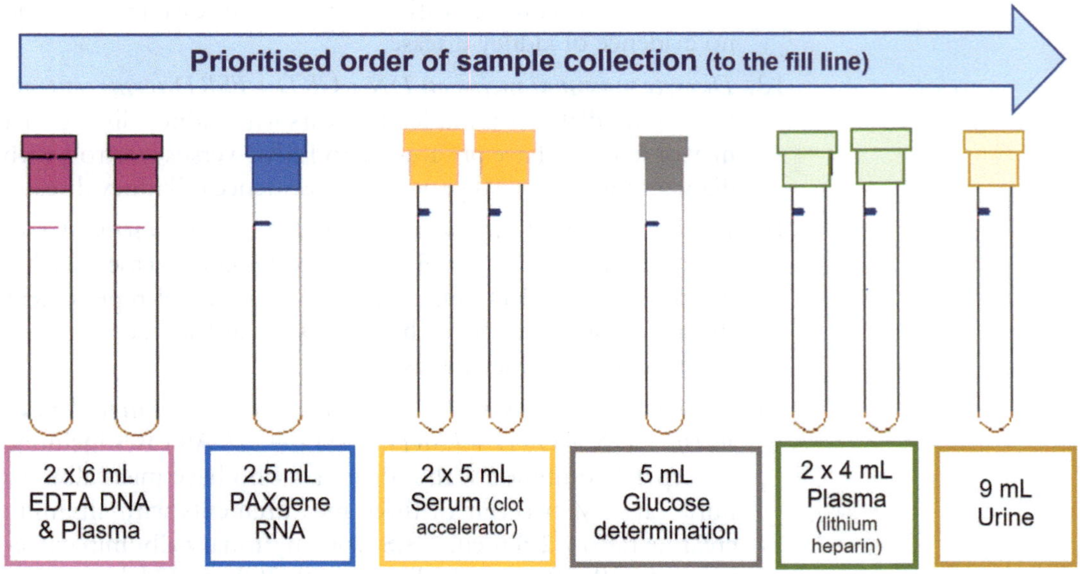

Fig. 4 Specimen tubes for sample collection

fasting samples would be collected with timed urine samples alongside details regarding diet, infections, and exercise, but pragmatically this may not be feasible for large-scale collections. Prolonged or timed urine collections are challenging, with spot urine samples (where albumin is expressed as urinary albumin concentration, albeit influenced by [urine], or a urinary albumin:creatine ratio) proving cost effective [18]. The quality of any laboratory test relies on provision of a high-quality sample. Several steps are required to obtain the best possible samples and it is essential that samples are correctly processed, ideally by a limited number of people following the same protocol, using the same equipment, in a single testing center with limited transportation occurring quickly under standard environmental conditions to preserve the integrity of samples. The method described here facilitates collection and storage of samples using approaches that create a flexible future-proofed resource as much as possible. It is recommended that rigorous quality control (QC) is integrated at all stages with centralized standardized processing that is audit tracked at every stage. Note that individual precautions will exist for safe sample handling of potentially infectious material, which indicates that samples must be handled following relevant legal requirements onsite. Any area contaminated with blood or serum must be disinfected immediately with 10% bleach (hypochlorite at 0.5% final concentration) or another approved disinfectant that meets the health and safety guidelines on your site. Specimens must be handled in a safe manner and according to applicable legal guidance or requirements.

1. Create a sample collection record sheet such as the template in Table 5 and ensure that it is completed in full at each stage.
2. Generate relevant barcodes for tubes (*see* **Note 4**) that enables storage of anonymized samples that can be tracked to relevant phenotype information. Label each tube with the relevant unique sample identifiers and place in a dark racked polystyrene box in preparation for sample collection.
3. Using a single-injection blood draw kit, collect blood samples in the order shown in Fig. 4. Gently invert 180° EDTA, PAXgene, and glucose tubes eight times immediately following collection. Urine should be collected in any approved collection tube and transferred to the urine vial.
4. Process each tube as required, remembering to complete the sample processing record. Relevant microtubes suitable for cryostorage should be individually labeled in preparation for sample processing and final sample storage.
   (a) EDTA tubes for DNA and plasma: Ensure that centrifuge buckets are balanced and spin both tubes at 1680 × *g* for 10 min in a refrigerated centrifuge at 4 °C. This removes

Table 5
Example of a sample collection record sheet

Unique barcode identifier	Biological sample tube identifier	Date, time, and initials of collection	Date, time, and initials of sample lab arrival	Date, time, and initials of process step 1	Date, time, and initials of process step 2	Storage location	Comments (any protocol deviation)
A123456B	A123456B_EDTA1	01/01/18_AJM	01/01/18_AJM	02/01/18_JK	02/01/18_JK	Slots 1–4, box 1, shelf 1; −80 °C freezer 1	
	A123456B_EDTA2	01/01/18_AJM	01/01/18_AJM	02/01/18_JK	02/01/18_JK	Slots 5–7, box 1, shelf 1; −80 °C freezer 1	
	A123456B_PAX	01/01/18_AJM	01/01/18_AJM	02/01/18_JK	02/01/18_JK	Slot 1, box 2, shelf 1; −80 °C freezer 1	
	A123456B_serum1	01/01/18_AJM	01/01/18_AJM	02/01/18_JK	02/01/18_JK	Slots 1–3, box 3, shelf 1; −80 °C freezer 1	
	A123456B_serum2	01/01/18_AJM	01/01/18_AJM	02/01/18_JK	02/01/18_JK	Slots 3–6, box 3, shelf 1; −80 °C freezer 1	
	A123456B_glucose	01/01/18_AJM	01/01/18_AJM	02/01/18_JK	02/01/18_JK		
	A123456B_plasma1	01/01/18_AJM	01/01/18_AJM	02/01/18_JK	02/01/18_JK	Slots 1–3, box 4, shelf 1; −80 °C freezer 1	
	A123456B_plasma2	01/01/18_AJM	01/01/18_AJM	02/01/18_JK	02/01/18_JK	Slots 3–6, box 4, shelf 1; −80 °C freezer 1	
	A123456B_urine	01/01/18_AJM	01/01/18_AJM	02/01/18_JK	02/01/18_JK	Slots 1–9, box 5, shelf 1; −80 °C freezer 1	

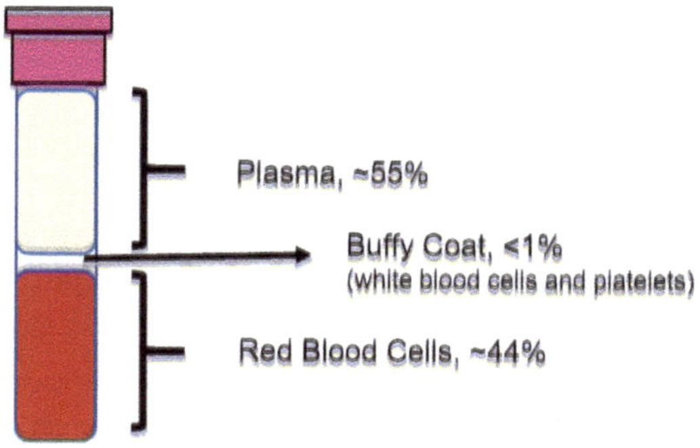

Fig. 5 Buffy Coat

cells with the resulting supernatant (~55% of the total sample, Fig. 5) being plasma that should be extracted into as many sterile 1 mL cryotubes that can be filled using clean Pasteur pipettes taking care not to disturb the buffy coat. Carefully collect the buffy coat (~1% of the total sample) from each EDTA tube and aliquot this into two 1 mL microtubes. Discard the red blood cells (~44% of the total sample) using the appropriate safety regulations for your laboratories. Keep tube lids closed as much as possible throughout this procedure and store samples at least at −20 °C or ideally −80 °C. It is critically important to minimize freeze-thaw cycles for these samples to preserve sample integrity.

(b) PAXgene tube: Leave for at least 2 h at room temperature (15–25 °C); samples can be stored at room temperature for 3 days. Freeze upright at −20 °C for at least 24 h before transferring to −80 °C freezer.

(c) Serum and plasma tubes: These should be left on the bench at room temperature for 30 min before centrifuging at 1680 × *g* for 10 min at 4 °C. The supernatant should be aliquoted into respective plasma and serum tubes in as many 1 mL aliquots as possible in cryostorage microtubes and store at −80 °C.

(d) Glucose tube: This tube contains potassium oxalate and sodium fluoride representing a cost-effective approach to preserve glucose in whole blood (*see* **Note 5**). Centrifuge at 1680 × *g* for 10 min at 4 °C. In a similar manner to that above, use a clean Pasteur pipette to transfer two 1 mL aliquots into storage cryomicrotubules, taking care not to disturb underlying cells, and store at −80 °C.

(e) Urine vial: Gently invert the urine five times to mix. Using a clean Pasteur pipette take 9 × 1 mL aliquots into cryostorage microtubes and store at −80 °C.

Other samples that may be collected if resources permit include the following:

- Feces: expensive to handle and store with challenges for collection.
- Hair and fingernails: provide limited information, challenges to collect consistently, complicated by external products such as cosmetics, soaps, and shampoo.
- Saliva: can be used for nucleic acid analysis, but blood-derived DNA and RNA are preferred to generate high-molecular-weight DNA suitable for whole-genome projects and immortalized beta cell lines. Complications from periodontal disease and oral microbiome.

3.3 Study Design

Once the phenotype(s) has been defined, the study design must be carefully considered; there is no statistical test or molecular technique that can compensate for a poorly designed study. Ideally collections should be as large as possible, but pragmatism typically dictates sample size for any study based on recruitment pool, bioresource costs, and molecular capacity for laboratory tests. Common study designs include the following (Fig. 6):

- *Multigenerational pedigrees*: excellent for identifying rare disease genes with large effect sizes in families; this design is of more limited use for common, complex diseases. It is challenging to recruit sufficient multigenerational individuals in a family for later onset conditions when older generations may not be able to participate due to geographical distance, disability, or death.
- *Case-control collections*: relatively inexpensive, represent the easiest approach to recruit large numbers of unrelated participants who have diabetes with/without DN, and provide more statistical power than similarly sized, family-based collections [19, 20]. Case-control collections may be subject to population stratification and substructure effects that influence false conclusions drawn from the data, but these can be limited by strict inclusion criteria or adjusted in the analysis model downstream.
- *Sib-pair cohort*: difficult to collect for later onset conditions and small numbers available, particularly of twins concordant or discordant for DN.
- *Parent-offspring cohort:* family-based collections overcome many population stratification effects and allow for assessment of parent-of-origin effects. They are an expensive approach to generate genotyping data and are similarly challenged by collecting biological samples from parents of adults with DN.

It is important to harmonize phenotypes and study designs where possible for multicenter studies. Typically for NGS projects there are more samples available for sequencing than the funding

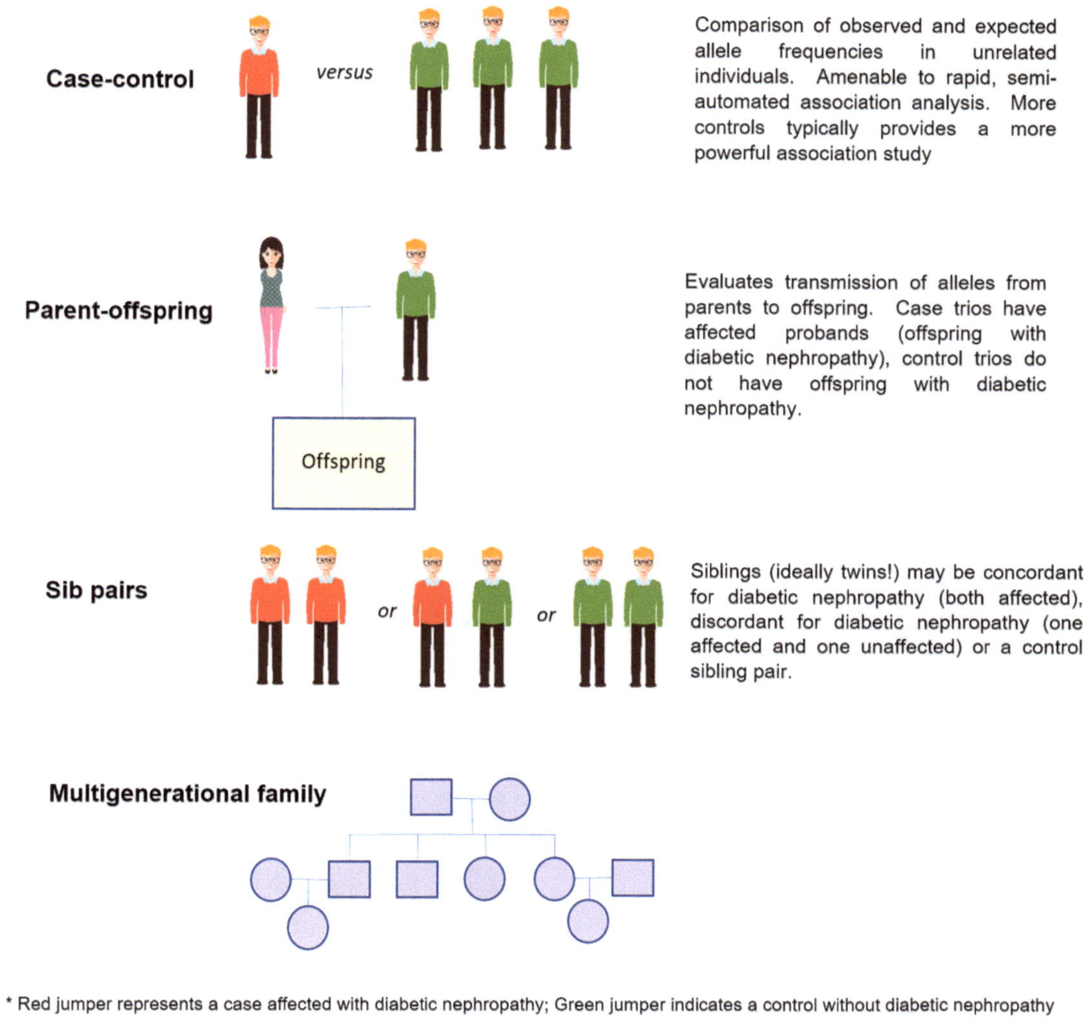

Fig. 6 Common study designs

budget will facilitate. There are software tools such as G-STRATEGY [21] that help to prioritize sample selection for efficient sequencing in common complex disease studies to maximize a study's power to identify genetic risk factors in association studies.

3.4 Ion AmpliSeq™ DNA Library Preparation Method (Figs. 3, 7, and 8, See Notes 6–9)

Amplify target regions from 10 ng of genomic DNA (gDNA) with the Ion AmpliSeq™ ready-to-use custom or commercial primer pools. The AmpliSeq™ library preparation approach is suitable for Torrent or Illumina sequencing. For panels that contain multiple primer pools, prepare a separate target amplification reaction for each primer pool. The resulting amplicons are treated with FuPa reagent, which contains enzymes to partially digest the primers and phosphorylate the amplicons. The amplicons are then ligated to ion

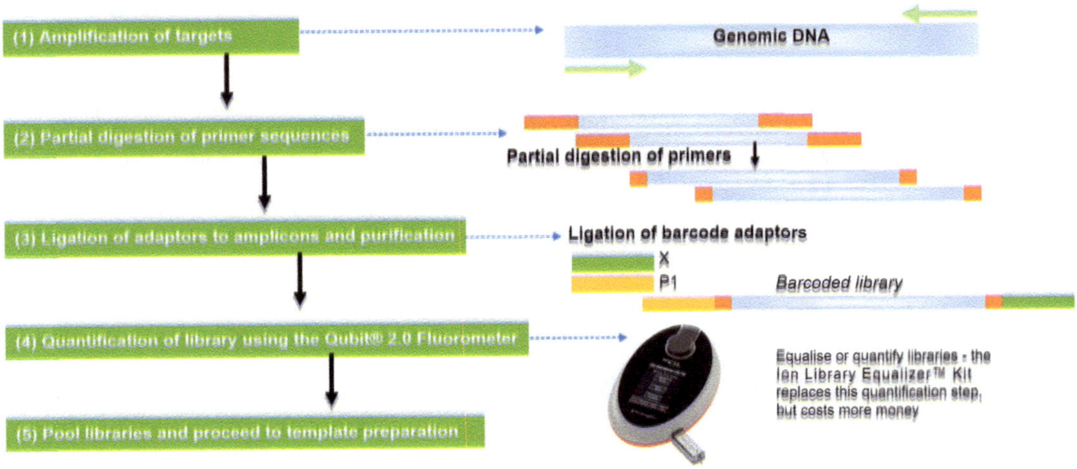

Fig. 7 Ion AmpliSeq™ DNA library workflow

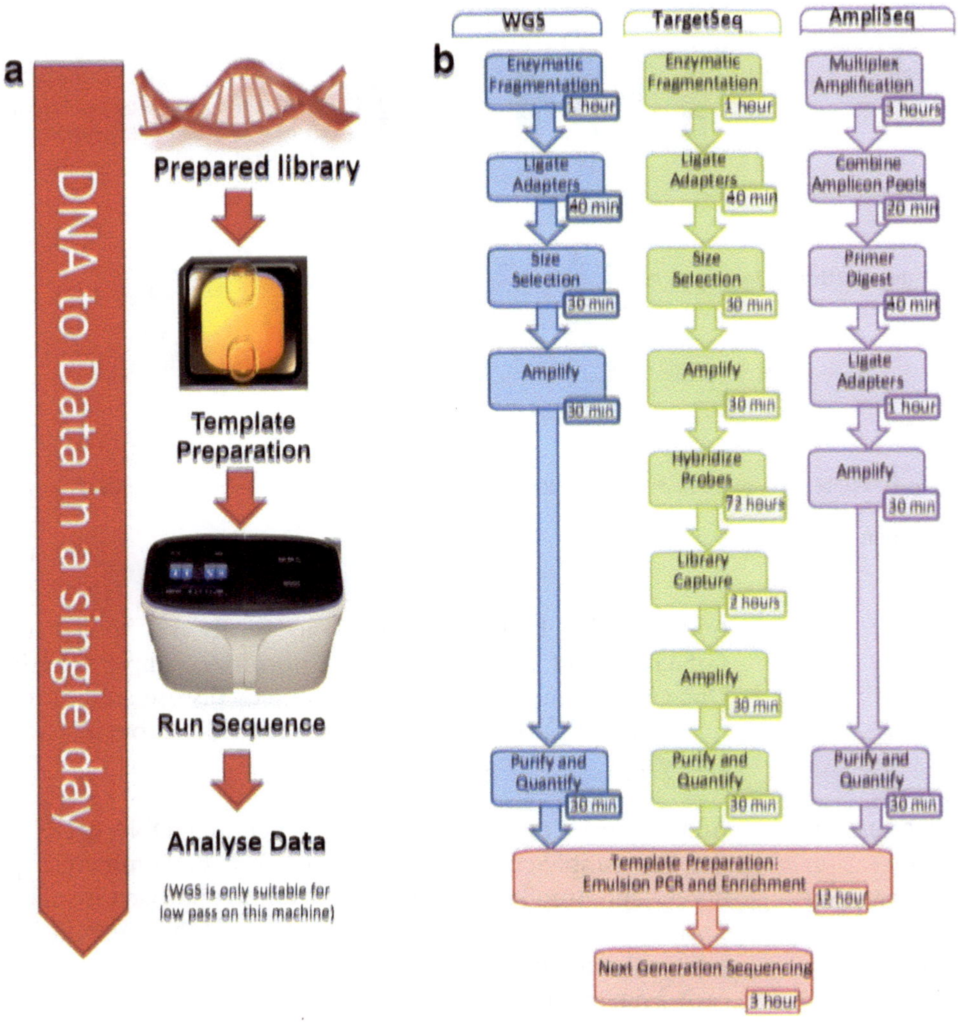

Fig. 8 Comparison of targeted sequencing approaches. This figure provides the rationale for using AmpliSeq™ to provide more targeted information than whole-genome sequencing (WGS) and compared to the timeframes and complexity of using a hybridization approach such as TargetSeq™ to analyze the same targets for the same samples

adapters with barcodes and purified. Libraries are amplified, purified, and then quantified using the Qubit® 2.0 Fluorometer (*see* **Note 10**). Combining libraries with the use of barcode adapters maximizes chip use while minimizing cost and labor.

3.4.1 DNA Input Requirements

For each target amplification reaction, use 10 ng of gDNA. The maximum volume of DNA per reaction depends on the concentration of the Ion AmpliSeq™ Primer Pool employed.

3.4.2 Library Preparation

Amplify Targets

1. For each DNA/primer pool combination, add the components in Table 6 to a single well of a 96-well PCR plate. Prepare a master mix for multiple reactions (*see* **Note 11**).
2. Seal the plate with MicroAmp adhesive film and ensure a tight seal by applying pressure with an applicator to prevent evaporation. Spin the plate to collect droplets if necessary.
3. Place a MicroAmp Compression Pad on the plate, load the plate in the thermal cycler, and run the program in Table 7 to amplify target genomic regions. PCR products can be stored at 10 °C overnight or for longer periods, at −20 °C.

Table 6
Components required to amplify target genomic regions

Component	Volume	Master mix (×8)
5× AmpliSeq™ HiFi Mix (Red Cap)	4 μL	32 μL
2× Ion AmpliSeq™ Primer Pool	10 μL	80 μL
gDNA (10 ng)	γ μL (<6 μL)	–
Nuclease-free water	(6–γ)	8×(6–γ), e.g., 8 × 4 = 32 μL
Total	20 μL	e.g., 144 μL

For example, for DNA stock at 5 ng/μL: gDNA volume = 2 μL nuclease-free water = (6 − 2) = 4 μL (master mix 4 × 8 = 32 μL)

Table 7
Thermal cycler program to amplify target genomic regions

Stage	Step	Temperature	Time
Time ~1.5 h			
Hold	Activate the enzyme	99 °C	2 min
17 Cycles	Denature Anneal and extend	99 °C 60 °C	15 s 4 min
Hold	–	10 °C	Hold (may be held at 10 °C overnight)

Partially Digest Primer Sequences

1. Carefully remove the plate seal.
2. Add 2 μL of FuPa Reagent (brown cap, *see* **Note 12**) to each amplified sample to a total volume of 22 μL.
3. Seal the plate with MicroAmp adhesive film, vortex thoroughly, and spin down to collect droplets.
4. Place the MicroAmp Compression Pad on the plate, load the plate in the thermal cycler, and run the program in Table 8.

Ligate Adapters to the Amplicons and Purify

1. Combine and dilute adapters. For each barcode X chosen, prepare a mix (Table 9) of Ion P2 Adapter and Ion Xpress™ Barcode X at a final dilution of 1:4 for each adapter. Diluted adapters should be stored at −20 °C. (The mix below will be sufficient for three 96-well plates; after the first plate, store the mix at −20 °C until needed for the second plate. The volumes may however be scaled as necessary.)
2. Next, set up and run the ligation reaction. If there is visible precipitate in the Switch Solution, vortex or pipette up and down at room temperature to resuspend.
3. Carefully remove the plate seal and add the components in Table 10 to each well containing digested sample. (Switch Solution and adapters can be combined before addition.)

Table 8
Thermal cycler program to partially digest primer sequences

Temperature (°C)	Time
Time ~40 min	
50	10 min
55	10 min
60	20 min
10	Hold (for up to 1 h)

Table 9
Mix for the combination and dilution of adaptors

Component	Volume (μL)
Ion P1 Adapter	2
Ion Xpress™ Barcode X	2
Nuclease-free water	4
Total	8

Table 10
Components of the ligation reaction

Component	Volume (μL)
Switch Solution (yellow cap)	4
Diluted barcode adapter mix	2
Total volume (including 22 μL digested amplicons)	28

Table 11
Program of the ligation reaction

Temperature (°C)	Time
Program name: amplig (~40 min)	
22	30 min
72	10 min
10	Hold (up to 1 h)

4. Add 2 μL of DNA ligase to each well.
5. Seal the plate with MicroAmp adhesive film, vortex thoroughly, and spin down to collect droplets.
6. Place a MicroAmp Compression Pad on the plate, load in the thermal cycler, and run the program in Table 11 (*see* **Note 13**).
7. The unamplified library is then purified. Carefully remove the plate seal and add 45 μL (1.5× sample volume) of Agencourt AMPure XP Reagent to each library and pipette up and down five times to thoroughly mix the bead suspension with the DNA.
8. Incubate the mixture for 5 min at room temperature.
9. Place the plate in a magnetic rack (DynaMag-96 Side Magnet) and incubate for 2 min or until solution clears.
10. Carefully remove and discard the supernatant without disturbing the pellet.
11. Add 150 μL of freshly prepared 70% ethanol and move the plate side to side in the two positions of the magnet to wash the beads.
12. Remove and discard the supernatant without disturbing the pellet.
13. Repeat **steps 11** and **12** for a second wash.

14. Ensure that all ethanol droplets are removed from the wells. Keeping the plate in the magnet, air-dry the beads at room temperature for 5 min. Do not overdry or allow the beads to crack. Proceed immediately to Qubit® 2.0 Fluorometer.

Quantify the Amplified Library with the Qubit® 2.0 Fluorometer

Ion AmpliSeq™ libraries must be amplified prior to quantification to enrich amplifiable material and obtain sufficient material for accurate quantification. Amplify the library using Platinum PCR Supermix High Fidelity and then purify each library. Quantify using the Qubit® 2.0 Fluorometer. After quantification, determine the dilution factor that results in a concentration of ~100 pM.

1. Remove the plate containing the Ion AmpliSeq™ library from the magnet and add 50 μL of Platinum PCR Supermix High Fidelity and 2 μL of Library Amplification Primer Mix to each bead pellet (the Supermix and Primer Mix may be combined before addition).
2. Seal the plate with MicroAmp adhesive film, vortex thoroughly, and spin down to collect droplets.
3. Place the plate back on the magnet for at least 2 min, and then carefully transfer ~50 μL of supernatant from each well to a clean plate without disturbing the pellet.
4. Place a MicroAmp Compression Pad on the plate, load in the thermal cycler, and run the program in Table 12. Samples may be stored at −20 °C at this point.
5. The amplified library is then purified using a two-round purification process with Agencourt AMPure XP Reagent. Add 25 μL (0.5× sample volume) of Agencourt AMPure XP Reagent to each plate well containing ~50 μL of sample. Pipette up and down five times to thoroughly mix the bead suspension with the DNA.
6. Seal the plate with MicroAmp adhesive film.
7. Incubate the mixture for 5 min at room temperature.

Table 12
Thermal cycling program to amplify the library

Stage	Temperature (°C)	Time
Time ~10 min		
Hold	98	2 min
5 Cycles	98 64	15 s 1 min
Hold	10	Hold

8. Place the plate in the magnet for 3 min or until the solution is clear.
9. Carefully transfer the supernatant from each well to a single well of a new 96-well PCR plate, without disturbing the pellet. *Do NOT discard supernatant as it contains the desired amplicons.*
10. To the supernatant from **step 9**, add 60 μL (1.2× original sample volume) of Agencourt AMPure XP Reagent. Pipette up and down five times to thoroughly mix the bead suspension with the DNA.
11. Seal the plate with MicroAmp adhesive film.
12. Incubate the mixture for 5 min at room temperature.
13. Place the plate in the magnet for 3 min or until the solution is clear.
14. Carefully remove and discard the supernatant without disturbing the pellet. *Save the bead pellet as the amplicons are bound to the pellet.*
15. Add 150 μL of freshly prepared 70% ethanol to each well and move the plate side to side in the magnet to wash the beads.
16. Remove and discard the supernatant without disturbing the pellet.
17. Repeat **steps 15** and **16** for a second wash.
18. Ensure that all ethanol droplets are removed from the wells. Keeping the plate in the magnet, air-dry the beads at room temperature for 5 min. *Do not overdry.*
19. Remove plate from magnet and add 50 μL of low TE to the pellet to disperse the beads.
20. Seal the plate with MicroAmp adhesive film, vortex thoroughly, and spin down to collect droplets.
21. Place the plate in the magnet for at least 2 min and analyze 1 μL of each amplified library using the Qubit® 2.0 Fluorometer. Amplified libraries typically have concentrations of 300–1500 ng/mL.
22. To determine the amplified library concentration firstly make a 1:200 working dilution of Qubit® dsDNA HS reagent using the Qubit® dsDNA HS Buffer.
23. Combine 1 μL of the amplified Ion AmpliSeq™ library with 199 μL of dye reagent, mix well, and incubate for at least 2 min.
24. Prepare Qubit® standards as per user guide.
25. Measure the concentration on the Qubit® 2.0 Fluorometer.
26. Calculate the concentration of the undiluted library using the "Calculate Stock Concentration" button on the Qubit® 2.0 Fluorometer.

(a) Based on the calculated library concentration, determine the dilution that results in a concentration of ~26 pM (see example calculation below). This is based on 22 ng/mL for amplicons up to 275 bp.

Sample Calculation:	
Qubit® results: concentration	=2.52 ng/mL
Stock concentration	=504 ng/mL
	=0.504 ng/μL
	=504 pg/μL
Molar concentration	=2760.3 pM (from Molar calculator)
Dilution factor	=Library concentration (pM) = 2760.3 = 106.17
	26 pM
	1 μL Library + 105.17 μL water yields 26 pM

27. The undiluted library can be stored at 4–8 °C for up to 1 month or for longer term storage at −20 °C. *Do NOT dilute before storing.*

Combining Ion AmpliSeq™ Libraries

Combined amplicon libraries are generated from multiple DNA samples using barcoded adapters for sequencing on the same ion chip. *Remember to dilute the DNA as calculated above before commencing.*

Barcoded libraries from different samples are prepared using Ion Xpress™ Barcode Adapters 1–96 Kits. The number of combined libraries that can be accommodated in a single sequencing run depends on:

1. The size of the chip
2. The ability to reliably quantify and combine barcoded libraries
3. The coverage required

Note: The total volume of library required for the Ion Chef™ is 70 μL.

3.5 Using the Ion Chef™ Instrument to Prepare Template-Positive Ion Sphere Particles and Load Ion Chips Ready for Semiconductor Sequencing on the Ion S5™ XL

The Ion Chef™ System allows for simple, high-throughput, template preparation, and ion chip loading. The instrument consists of a deck area, LED lighting bars, Microscan Vision sample tracking system with camera and barcode reader, and a 15 W UVC germicidal lamp. The deck contains separate tip racks for clean and used tips, as well as a mixing station where reagents, solutions, and samples are loaded. The mixing station is used to prepare for the emulsion PCR, which is then set up and run in the thermal cycler. Following PCR, the two tube centrifuges are used to break the emulsion, releasing, and pelleting the ISPs. The ISPs are recovered, washed, and transferred to the enrichment module. The enrichment module houses a linear magnet and enrichment for template-positive ion sphere particles is performed with paramagnetic beads. The enriched library is prepared for loading during which the sequencing primer is annealed and sequencing polymerase bound. Once ready, this is transferred to the chip centrifuge and loaded onto the chips.

The Ion Chef™ run takes approximately 10 h to complete and is normally performed overnight. The run should be timed to finish around 9.30 a.m. the following morning, allowing adequate time to get the Ion S5™XL Sequencer initialized. The chips must be removed from the Ion Chef™ as soon as the run stops and either sequenced or stored straight away. After use, it is essential that the Ion Chef™ deck is cleared and the UV clean completed.

3.5.1 Preparation for the Ion Chef™ Run

1. Prepare and dilute the libraries. Libraries must be prepared in advance. They should be quantified using the Qubit® 2.0 Fluorometer and then stored in the freezer until required. The dilution factors should be calculated using the library calculator with the kit (*see* **Note 14**).
2. Prepare the planned runs. Create a *Planned Run* on the *Torrent Server* that is connected to the Ion Chef™ (*see* **Note 15**).
3. Handling ion chips: It is important to note that the chip *can be damaged by electrostatic discharge*. To avoid damage:
   (a) Do not wear gloves when transferring chips on and off the instrument.
   (b) Ground yourself before touching any chips.
   (c) Always hold ion chips gently by their side edges.
   (d) Only place the chip into the chip centrifuge bucket or designated storage box.
   (e) Never place the chip directly on the bench or other surface.
4. Prepare the consumables:
   (a) Remove the specific *Ion Chef™ reagent cartridge* (according to the kit being used) from the freezer and leave on the bench to equilibrate to room temperature for at least 45 min before use.
   (b) Collect the specific *Ion Chef™ solution cartridge* (according to the kit being used).
   (c) Collect one box of *Ion Chef™ supplies* containing 1× enrichment cartridge v2, 2× chip adapters, 1× tip cartridge v2, 1× PCR plate and frame seal v2, 12× recovery tubes v2, and 2× recovery station lids v2.

3.5.2 Setting Up the Ion Chef™

1. Turn on the Ion Chef™ instrument by pressing the button on the front panel.
2. Ensure that the instrument was cleaned following the previous run. If in doubt, then perform the UV clean *before* loading the deck with consumables.
3. Open the door by pressing 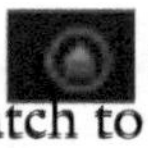 at top right-hand side of the touchscreen. Wait for the latch to open. Using both hands, lift the instrument door to the top until it clicks.
4. Ensure that the empty tip cartridge from the previous run is in the Used Tip Rack position. Check that the rack does not contain any tips.
5. Place the new tip rack into the new tip rack position. To do this:
   (a) Pull the lock latch forward to allow the locking bracket to move upwards.
   (b) Slot the new tip rack in place.
   (c) Close the bracket.
6. Place the PCR plate in the thermal cycler position.
7. Place the PCR lid seal under the thermal cycler heated lid.
8. Ensure that the specific Ion Chef™ reagent cartridge has been at room temperature for 45 min. Tap the reagent cartridge on the bench to ensure that all reagents are at the bottom of the tubes.
9. Using a P200 pipette, transfer 70 μL of sample 1 to the respective tube in the reagent cartridge. Replace the tube cap loosely. Carefully record the sample tube barcode and corresponding sample number; it is vital to know which library is in which sample tube. Do the same with the second sample.
10. Loosen the caps of the NaOH tube and the empty tube in the reagent cartridge.
11. Insert the reagent cartridge into the back slot of the mixing station (the chilled block), as shown in the deck layout. Ensure that the cartridge clicks into place and it is flush with the deck.
12. Remove the four loosely attached lids from the reagent cartridge.
13. Tap the Ion Chef™ solution cartridge on the bench and slot into the front block of the mixing station. Ensure that it clicks into place and is flush with the deck.
14. Load the 12 recovery tubes into the two recovery centrifuges on the right-hand side of the deck. Ensure that they are all correctly inserted into the centrifuge buckets and that the buckets are secure.
15. Place a *recovery centrifuge lid v2* over each centrifuge, in the correct orientation. Make certain that the lids snap completely

into place by applying firm downward pressure along the lid perimeter. Close the main lid.

16. Load the *enrichment cartridge v2*, pressing down to ensure that it is flush with the deck of the chef.
17. Load the *chip-loading centrifuge*:
    (a) Remove a bucket from the chip-loading centrifuge. Place a new chip into the bucket. Align the chip adapter to the chip ensuring that the barcode is visible. Slot the tabs at the reservoir end into the slots in the bucket. Squeeze the flexible tabs at the opposite end into the bucket slots locking the adapter into place. Repeat for the second chip (*see* **Note 16**).
    (b) Place the adapter/bucket assemblies into the chip-loading centrifuge.
    (c) Check that the metal strip on top of the chip-loading centrifuge can open and close with ease. When the strip is closed, the marker holes on top indicate chip A and chip B. The chip in Position A will be loaded with the library sample that was pipetted into Position A of the reagent cartridge. Similarly, Position B will be the second library (*see* **Note 17**). Record the chip barcodes and their position in the rotor. *IMPORTANT! Ensure that the metal strip is left open.*
    (d) Ensure that the centrifuge buckets are securely seated. Check that the rotor is balanced and can turn freely.
    (e) Close the chip-loading centrifuge lid.
18. *Confirm that the deck has been loaded correctly.* Ensure that all components are flush with the deck, reagent caps have been removed, centrifuge lids are closed, and there are no objects that could crash with the robotic arm during operation.

3.5.3 Starting the Ion Chef™ Run

1. On the Ion Chef™ screen, press *Set up run*.
2. From the *Set up run* menu, select either *step-by-step* assistance or *quick start* run. *Normally select step by step and follow the on-screen instructions to check that all of the components are present and in the correct place.*
3. When prompted, close the door by lifting gently upwards using both hands, and then supporting to bring it down before clicking into place (there should be a click from each side as the door engages).
4. When prompted, touch *Start Check*. The vision system will scan the deck ensuring that everything is compatible, in the correct place, and all barcodes can be read.
5. This takes approximately 4 min.

6. If any problems are detected, these will be displayed on the screen. For example:
   (a) If the precautionary message "Check that the new tip rack is full, and the waste one is empty" is displayed, then check that this is so. Then click *Yes* to start the run.
   (b) If the sample tube barcodes cannot be read or the machine detects that the lids are still on these tubes (even though they have been removed) then click *No* to go back. Try moving the barcode slightly, or move the tubes, before allowing the Ion Chef™ to check everything again (*see* **Note 18**).
   (c) If there is an error relating to the breaking centrifuge, be very careful to check that all recovery tubes have been correctly inserted and that all buckets are securely seated in the rotor before allowing the Ion Chef™ to check everything again (*see* **Note 19**).
7. When the *Deck scan* is complete, touch Next to display the *Data Destination* screen.
8. Confirm that the correct Ion S5™XL Kit and Chip type are displayed. Ensure that the chip barcode, sample ID (that you noted down earlier), and planned run name match up. If not, use the drop-down menu to select the correct run plan for your sample.
   (a) *IMPORTANT:* Ensure that the chip position, chip barcode (this is vital as the Ion Chef™ and S5™XL sequencer uses this to track the sample), sample name, and planned run name have been recorded for each sample.
   (b) Click *Next.*
9. On the *Run Options* screen, select *Time* and set the Ion Chef™ to complete the run at a suitable time, which must coordinate with initialization of the Ion S5™XL completing at, e.g., 9.30 a.m. You can select up to 24 h, but to maintain DNA quality you should keep this within 20 h. Click *Next* to start the run.

3.5.4 Quality Control

QC samples may be used to assess templating efficiency. Under *Run Options*, the *Time* option allows QC samples to be collected after the Ion Chef™ run finishes. If QC is required:

- *Collect unenriched samples from the reagent cartridge.*
  - Library A can be sampled in Library Sample Tube A.
  - Library B can be sampled in Library Sample Tube B.
- *Collect enriched samples from the enrichment cartridge v2 (ES).*
  - Library A can be sampled in Position E of the ES.
  - Library B can be sampled in Position A of the ES.

Alternatively, under *Run Options* the *Pause* option may be used to collect these samples when the instrument pauses prior to chip loading (~11 h into the run). The run must be restarted as soon as the door is closed.

3.5.5 After the Run Has Finished

Remove the chips immediately and proceed to sequencing the first chip on the Ion S5™XL. Store the second chip in the chip storage box and place into the fridge until later.

Remember to clear the deck of the Ion Chef™. Store reagents and solutions until good sequencing has been confirmed. Dispose of all other waste according to site guidelines and perform the integrated Ion Chef™ UV clean.

3.6 Ion Torrent Sequencing Using the Ion S5™XL (See Note 20)

Before starting this protocol, the planned runs must be created and the Ion Chef™ set up to run overnight using the specific Ion Chef™ Kit and chips (*see* **Note 21**). The first stage of this protocol is to clean and initialize the Ion S5™XL ready for use in this massively parallel sequencing protocol. Then, the Ion Chips™ (loaded with template-positive ion sphere particles, annealed sequencing primer, and bound sequencing polymerase) are removed from the Ion Chef™ Instrument. Finally, using the Ion S5™XL, the post-light, semiconductor sequencing run is performed. During sequencing, dNTPs (A, G, C, T) "flow" across the chip one at a time, in a particular pattern (*see* **Note 22**). When a dNTP becomes incorporated, a hydrogen ion is released which is detected as a pH change. This signal pattern is directly translated into digital form to produce an ionogram. Data is transferred to the server as an SFF file which converts the raw signal into base calls. The quality data for the run must be checked and the base calls are downloaded (quality info and nucleotide info are contained in the .bam file).

3.6.1 Preparations for the Run

1. The S5™ system uses RFID technology to verify that the proper reagents are loaded and have not expired. An error message will be displayed if a problem is detected (*see* **Note 23**).
2. Remove the Ion S5™ Sequencing reagent cartridge from the freezer and equilibrate to room temperature for 15–45 min before use. Keep in the foil packaging until immediately before use—the unopened cartridge may be returned to storage if sequencing is delayed for any reason.
3. Holding the bottle of Ion S5™ wash solution, invert five times and then swirl at an angle to thoroughly mix the milky solution. Remove the screw-cap lid and check that the sipper and filter are attached properly. If detached, then reattach them and securely close the lid.
4. Dry ice (solid CO_2) should be kept away from areas where wash solutions or sources of molecular biology-grade water for the Ion S5™XL System are used. High air concentrations of

subliming CO_2 may influence the pH of such solutions. The stability of the pH of these solutions is a critical factor in the performance of the Ion S5™XL System (*see* **Note 24**).

3.6.2 Clean and Initialize the Ion S5™XL System

1. Ensure that the Ion S5™XL sequencer is switched on by pressing the on/off button (*see* **Note 25**).
2. The sequencer must be cleaned before each initialization. This required cleaning is normally performed automatically after the sequencing run has finished. However, if the sequencing run has not completed properly (e.g., there was a power cut) a clean must be performed (*see* **Note 26**).

3.6.3 Initializing the Ion S5™XL System (Takes ~40 min, See Note 27)

1. Ensure that the reagent cartridge has equilibrated to room temperature for 15–45 min.
2. On the touch screen *Main Menu*, press *Initialize*. The instrument door, chip, and reagent cartridge clamps will unlock.
3. When prompted, remove the Ion S5™ wash solution bottle to access the waste reservoir. Then remove and empty the waste reservoir to drain with copious volumes of water.
4. Reinstall the empty waste reservoir. Note: The waste container sits on a balance that detects when the container is NOT empty. The waste needs emptied between chips.
5. Remove the used Ion S5™ sequencing reagent cartridge and replace with the new cartridge which has been equilibrated to room temperature.
6. Remove the red cap from a new Ion S5™ wash solution bottle that has been thoroughly mixed and install:
   (a) Attach the bottle.
   (b) Swing the base of the bottle toward the machine.
   (c) Press firmly inward to secure the bottle into position.
7. Pull the chip clamp out and ensure that the used chip from the previous sequencing run is properly seated in the chip clamp. Then push the clamp fully into the locking position (*see* **Notes 28** and **29**).
8. If necessary, install a new Ion S5™ cleaning solution bottle (each bottle will complete four cleans). Tighten the cap securely before installing (sometimes the cap can be a bit loose).
9. Close the door and touch *Next* on the screen.

3.6.4 Remove Chips from the Ion Chef™ (See Note 30)

1. Once the Ion Chef™ has stopped, open the instrument door by pressing 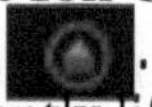. Wait until the latch opens, and then using both hands gently lift the door until the latch mechanism at the top engages.

2. Open the lid of the chip-loading centrifuge.
3. Gently remove the chip/bucket assemblies from the centrifuge.
4. Remove and discard the chip adapter from each chip by applying pressure to both ends.
5. Handling chips only by their side edges:
   (a) Keep the first chip to be sequenced in the centrifuge bucket, ready for safe transport to the sequencer.
   (b) Place the other into a chip storage box and store it in the fridge until required (6–8 h maximum).
6. Return empty buckets to the Ion Chef™.
7. Close the door of the Ion Chef™ using both hands to lift slightly, then gently close, and push to lock (*see* **Notes 31** and **32**).

3.6.5 Sequencing the Chip on the Ion S5™XL Sequencer

1. Select *Run* on the *Main Menu*. The door and chip clamp will be unlocked.
2. Remove the used sequencing chip.
3. Secure the chip loaded with template-positive ion sphere particles into the chip clamp.
4. Push the chip clamp fully into engage.
5. Close the instrument door and press *Next*.
6. Confirm that the correct *Planned Run* has auto-populated, and then press *Next*.
7. Confirm that the run details are correct for your run, or make changes using the buttons and drop-down menus if necessary. IMPORTANT!! *Post-Run Clean is automatically selected for each chip*. If running two chips per initialization:
   (a) *Deselect Post-Run Clean for the first chip*. If you forget to do this, cleaning will be performed automatically after the first chip has been sequenced, reagents are wasted, and the machine needs to be reinitialized for the second chip.
   (b) *Select Post-Run Clean for the second chip* to perform automatic cleaning after the sequencing run has finished.
8. Confirm that the instrument door is closed. Then press *Next* and the run will begin (*see* **Note 33**).
9. The run varies in length depending on the chip type.
10. A thumbnail report is available to view shortly after the sequencing run is started. The main data takes a few hours to transfer to the server before it can be downloaded and ultimately analyzed. User-friendly applications are available and are directly linked to the sequencing data to align sequences

to a reference genome and call variants with customized parameters.

11. Set up the second chip in the same way (*see* **Notes 34** and **35**).

4 Notes

1. It is critically important that only full kits with the same version numbers are employed for Ion Torrent™ runs. Mixing and matching components from different versions of kits may result in a failed or suboptimal run.
2. Peripheral venous blood should be collected after participants are seated quietly for 5 min. There are multiple options to collect saliva samples for downstream DNA studies, but blood-derived DNA is more flexible for downstream uses where available. Be aware that preservatives/anticoagulants in collection tubes can influence results; for example anticoagulants may result in artificially increased cytokine levels.
3. Many tests performed on serum or plasma get better results from a fasting specimen; however this is challenging for individuals with diabetes in particular so fasting samples are rarely obtainable. Early-morning sample collection is best for fasting samples in people with diabetes. Fasting is defined as no consumption of food or beverage, other than water, for 9–12 h before testing.
4. Other manufacturers of appropriate tubes are available; we routinely use BD vacutainers for consistency, https://www.bd.com/en-uk/products/blood-and-urine-collection/blood-collection-tubes. Pediatric color-coded Vacutainer® tubes are useful for smaller volumes and to differentiate pediatric from adult samples where necessary. It helps laboratory logistics to have microtube lids to match the color of lids of primary sample collection tubes.
5. For the glucose tube, the protocol suggests a cost-effective option. However, a Glucomedics tube is the most suitable for minimizing glycolysis if there is budget for that [22].
6. Thaw components that contain enzymes on ice and keep them on ice during procedure(s). All other components including primer pools may be thawed at room temperature. Best results are obtained if these are briefly vortexed and spun down before use. Pipette viscous solutions slowly and ensure complete mixing by vigorous vortexing.
7. If there is visible precipitate in the Switch Solution or the tube cap after thawing, vortex at room temperature to resuspend.

8. Allow AMPure™ beads at least 40 min to reach room temperature before use.
9. Minimize freeze thawing of Ion AmpliSeq™ Primer Pools by aliquoting as needed.
10. Using the optional Ion Library Equalizer™ Kit (catalog number: 4482298, Thermo Fisher Scientific, or equivalent) simplifies the library preparation by removing the need to quantify and dilute libraries prior to sequencing. This kit has a relatively long shelf life (typically 18 months) but represents an additional financial cost in the protocol.
11. Primer pool and 5× Ion AmpliSeq™ HiFi Mix are viscous. Pipette slowly and mix thoroughly. PCR setup should be on ice.
12. Ensure that the lid of this FuPa reagent is securely closed after use. We found it advantageous to wrap the tube in parafilm prior to refreezing to minimize evaporation.
13. At this point, take out the Platinum PCR Supermix High Fidelity and Library Amplification Primer and put on ice to defrost. Also take out the AMPure Beads and allow them to come to room temperature. This takes at least 40 min.
14. To maximize high-quality results, the library should not be diluted until <4 h before starting the Ion Chef™ run; otherwise the quality of the data will deteriorate. Libraries should ideally be diluted in nuclease-free water. Diluted libraries may be stored in the fridge for later use (max 48 h).
15. Remember that a separate planned run is required for each chip, so if two chips are being prepared then two planned runs must be entered.
16. Loading can fail if the adapter is incorrectly fitted. Also note that the top of the chip may be labeled but do not obstruct the barcode or the reader may object.
17. In exceptional circumstances, if only one chip is to be loaded, the Ion S5™ series chip balance must be used in Position B, but remember that it is not cost effective to run one chip on the Ion Chef™.
18. Do not proceed with the run until these error messages are cleared; it is possible, but is not recommended as a run with uncleared errors frequently crashes. It may take numerous checking and moving attempts before these error messages clear, but it is essential to ensure that they do.
19. Do not proceed with the run until this error message is cleared. It may be necessary to swap the recovery tubes from one centrifuge to the other, and/or swap the recovery station lids

before these error messages clear, but it is essential to ensure that they do.

20. The Ion GeneStudio S5™ platform is a series of next-generation sequencing instruments that support different sequencing chips depending on the output required—note that the sequencing kits cost the same, but the chip price is different.
21. To maximize lab efficiency assuming a standard working day, the Ion Chef™ run should be timed to finish at around 9.30 a.m. The chips, loaded with template-positive ion sphere particles, must be removed immediately when the run is completed and either sequenced or stored. Initialization of the Ion S5XL™ should be started at 8 a.m., which allows 1.5 h to ensure that the Ion S5XL™ is ready to sequence the first chip as soon as the Ion Chef™ stops.
22. The maximum number of flows is 1100; therefore for example, it is possible to run 400 base read and a small RNA run from the same bottle of W2.
23. To avoid error messages, check the compatibility and expiry date of all reagents before loading onto the sequencer. RFID regulatory info may be found under Options → Regulatory Information.
24. Ensure that the software is running an updated version at least 2 days before a planned run—it can take >24 h for software updating to complete.
25. When the sequencer door is opened, the chip moves out of the clamp. Work quickly and accurately to prepare the instrument for initialization so that the chip is only briefly out of the clamp; otherwise there may be backflow of air into the lines.
26. If it is necessary to perform a manual clean follow the steps below:
    (a) On the touchscreen *Main Menu*, press *Clean*. The instrument door will unlock.
    (b) Remove the Ion S5™ wash solution bottle to access the waste reservoir. Then remove and empty the waste reservoir to drain with copious volumes of water.
    (c) Carefully reinstall both the empty waste reservoir and the used Ion S5 wash solution bottle.
    (d) Keep the used reagent cartridge in position.

    Note: The cleaning routine pumps cleaning solution into the wash solution bottle and the reagent cartridge making them unsuitable for sequencing.

    (e) Ensure that a used chip is in the chip clamp. Then push the clamp fully into engage.

(f) Close the instrument door and press *Next*. Cleaning takes approximately 35 min to complete. Upon completion the door opens and the chip and cartridge clamps disengage.

(g) Without delay, proceed to initialization.

27. Following initialization, the first run must be started as soon as possible and the second run within 24 h to get the maximum Gb output of sequencing data.
28. Moving the chip clamp out and in ensures that the instrument will recognize the chip and minimizes the errors.
29. The chip can be damaged by electrostatic discharge. To avoid damage, never place the chip directly on the bench or other surface; only place the chip onto a grounding plate or into the custom ion centrifuge adapter/rotor bucket or designated storage box. Do not wear gloves when transferring chips on and off the instrument.
30. As soon as the Ion Chef™ run stops, the chips must be removed straight away and either sequenced or stored to preserve quality.
31. Remember to clean the Ion Chef™ immediately after the sequencing run has been started.
32. Remember to lift the stored chip out of the fridge 30 min prior to sequencing. Keeping it in the chip storage box, store in the dark to equilibrate to room temperature with minimal degradation before use.
33. During a run, do not touch the Ion S5XL™ as this could reduce the quality of the measurements. Do not open the instrument door as this will spoil the consumables.
34. If sequencing has failed, empty the nucleotide cartridge into a suitable container and check whether the liquid is clear or cloudy. If cloudy, then the filter may either be faulty or detached during the run.
35. Having used the Ion Chef™ we would not go back to the more manually intensive One Touch™ + Enrichment System™ preparation method; the Ion Chef™ generates more consistent results across multiple users, is amenable to easy training, and is cost effective for staff time. From our evaluated S5XL™ (in 2016) we would not return to PGM™ or Proton™ for these analyses. The Ion S5™ has no gas or 18.2 mΩ water requirement for initialization. It has a faster initialization time compared to the other machines, meaning more chips can be run per week, generating more data. The S5™ minimizes user error with less hands-on steps in the protocol and only four containers of RFID-tagged consumables, which typically have a longer shelf life than PGM™ or Proton™ kits. There is an embedded clean in the run plan for the S5™, which means runs

can be set up on a Friday evening without someone needing to be present to clean within 24 h of a complete run. A smaller quantity of chemical waste is produced during the S5™ sequencing run; the machine itself requires less bench space and there are fewer bottles. Overall this means that less storage space is required than had been for the earlier Ion Torrent™ NGS machines. The reagent cartridges are bulky and require considerable storage space at −20 °C if preparing for high-throughput use.

References

1. McKnight AJ, Currie D, Patterson CC, Maxwell AP, Fogarty DG, Warren UKGSG (2009) Targeted genome-wide investigation identifies novel SNPs associated with diabetic nephropathy. HUGO J 3(1-4):77–82. https://doi.org/10.1007/s11568-010-9133-2
2. McKnight AJ, Woodman AM, Parkkonen M, Patterson CC, Savage DA, Forsblom C, Pettigrew KA, Sadlier D, Groop PH, Maxwell AP, Warren UKGSG (2009) Investigation of DNA polymorphisms in SMAD genes for genetic predisposition to diabetic nephropathy in patients with type 1 diabetes mellitus. Diabetologia 52(5):844–849. https://doi.org/10.1007/s00125-009-1281-3
3. McKnight AJ, Duffy S, Maxwell AP (2015) Genetics of diabetic nephropathy: a long road of discovery. Curr Diab Rep 15(7):41. https://doi.org/10.1007/s11892-015-0610-9
4. Chan Y, Lim ET, Sandholm N, Wang SR, McKnight AJ, Ripke S, Consortium D, Consortium G, Consortium G, Consortium I, Consortium PGC, Daly MJ, Neale BM, Salem RM, Hirschhorn JN (2014) An excess of risk-increasing low-frequency variants can be a signal of polygenic inheritance in complex diseases. Am J Hum Genet 94(3):437–452. https://doi.org/10.1016/j.ajhg.2014.02.006
5. Germain M, Pezzolesi MG, Sandholm N, McKnight AJ, Susztak K, Lajer M, Forsblom C, Marre M, Parving HH, Rossing P, Toppila I, Skupien J, Roussel R, Ko YA, Ledo N, Folkersen L, Civelek M, Maxwell AP, Tregouet DA, Groop PH, Tarnow L, Hadjadj S (2015) SORBS1 gene, a new candidate for diabetic nephropathy: results from a multi-stage genome-wide association study in patients with type 1 diabetes. Diabetologia 58(3):543–548. https://doi.org/10.1007/s00125-014-3459-6
6. Sandholm N, Forsblom C, Makinen VP, McKnight AJ, Osterholm AM, He B, Harjutsalo V, Lithovius R, Gordin D, Parkkonen M, Saraheimo M, Thorn LM, Tolonen N, Waden J, Tuomilehto J, Lajer M, Ahlqvist E, Mollsten A, Marcovecchio ML, Cooper J, Dunger D, Paterson AD, Zerbini G, Groop L, Consortium S, Tarnow L, Maxwell AP, Tryggvason K, Groop PH, FinnDiane Study G (2014) Genome-wide association study of urinary albumin excretion rate in patients with type 1 diabetes. Diabetologia 57(6):1143–1153. https://doi.org/10.1007/s00125-014-3202-3
7. Sandholm N, McKnight AJ, Salem RM, Brennan EP, Forsblom C, Harjutsalo V, Makinen VP, McKay GJ, Sadlier DM, Williams WW, Martin F, Panduru NM, Tarnow L, Tuomilehto J, Tryggvason K, Zerbini G, Comeau ME, Langefeld CD, Consortium F, Godson C, Hirschhorn JN, Maxwell AP, Florez JC, Groop PH, FinnDiane Study G, the GC (2013) Chromosome 2q31.1 associates with ESRD in women with type 1 diabetes. J Am Soc Nephrol 24(10):1537–1543. https://doi.org/10.1681/ASN.2012111122
8. Sandholm N, Salem RM, McKnight AJ, Brennan EP, Forsblom C, Isakova T, McKay GJ, Williams WW, Sadlier DM, Makinen VP, Swan EJ, Palmer C, Boright AP, Ahlqvist E, Deshmukh HA, Keller BJ, Huang H, Ahola AJ, Fagerholm E, Gordin D, Harjutsalo V, He B, Heikkila O, Hietala K, Kyto J, Lahermo P, Lehto M, Lithovius R, Osterholm AM, Parkkonen M, Pitkaniemi J, Rosengard-Barlund M, Saraheimo M, Sarti C, Soderlund J, Soro-Paavonen A, Syreeni A, Thorn LM, Tikkanen H, Tolonen N, Tryggvason K, Tuomilehto J, Waden J, Gill GV, Prior S, Guiducci C, Mirel DB, Taylor A, Hosseini SM, Group DER, Parving HH, Rossing P, Tarnow L, Ladenvall C, Alhenc-Gelas F, Lefebvre P, Rigalleau V, Roussel R, Tregouet DA, Maestroni A, Maestroni S, Falhammar H, Gu T, Mollsten A, Cimponeriu D, Ioana M, Mota M, Mota E, Serafinceanu C, Stavarachi M, Hanson RL,

Nelson RG, Kretzler M, Colhoun HM, Panduru NM, Gu HF, Brismar K, Zerbini G, Hadjadj S, Marre M, Groop L, Lajer M, Bull SB, Waggott D, Paterson AD, Savage DA, Bain SC, Martin F, Hirschhorn JN, Godson C, Florez JC, Groop PH, Maxwell AP (2012) New susceptibility loci associated with kidney disease in type 1 diabetes. PLoS Genet 8(9): e1002921. https://doi.org/10.1371/journal.pgen.1002921

9. Sandholm N, Van Zuydam N, Ahlqvist E, Juliusdottir T, Deshmukh HA, Rayner NW, Di Camillo B, Forsblom C, Fadista J, Ziemek D, Salem RM, Hiraki LT, Pezzolesi M, Tregouet D, Dahlstrom E, Valo E, Oskolkov N, Ladenvall C, Marcovecchio ML, Cooper J, Sambo F, Malovini A, Manfrini M, McKnight AJ, Lajer M, Harjutsalo V, Gordin D, Parkkonen M, Finn-Diane Study Group JT, Lyssenko V, McKeigue PM, Rich SS, Brosnan MJ, Fauman E, Bellazzi R, Rossing P, Hadjadj S, Krolewski A, Paterson AD, Dcct/Edic Study Group JCF, Hirschhorn JN, Maxwell AP, Genie Consortium DD, Cobelli C, Colhoun HM, Groop L, McCarthy MI, Groop PH, Consortium S (2017) The genetic landscape of renal complications in type 1 diabetes. J Am Soc Nephrol 28(2):557–574. https://doi.org/10.1681/ASN.2016020231
10. Todd JN, Dahlstrom EH, Salem RM, Sandholm N, Forsblom C, FinnDiane Study G, McKnight AJ, Maxwell AP, Brennan E, Sadlier D, Godson C, Groop PH, Hirschhorn JN, Florez JC (2015) Genetic evidence for a causal role of obesity in diabetic kidney disease. Diabetes 64(12):4238–4246. https://doi.org/10.2337/db15-0254
11. van Zuydam NR, Ahlqvist E, Sandholm N, Deshmukh H, Rayner NW, Abdalla M, Ladenvall C, Ziemek D, Fauman E, Robertson NR, McKeigue PM, Valo E, Forsblom C, Harjutsalo V, Finnish Diabetic Nephropathy S, Perna A, Rurali E, Marcovecchio ML, Igo RP Jr, Salem RM, Perico N, Lajer M, Karajamaki A, Imamura M, Kubo M, Takahashi A, Sim X, Liu J, van Dam RM, Jiang G, Tam CHT, Luk AOY, Lee HM, Lim CKP, Szeto CC, So WY, Chan JCN, Hong Kong Diabetes Registry Theme-based Research Scheme Project G, Ang SF, Dorajoo R, Wang L, Clara TSH, McKnight AJ, Duffy S, Warren, Genetics of Kidneys in Diabetes Study G, Pezzolesi MG, Consortium G, Marre M, Gyorgy B, Hadjadj S, Hiraki LT, Diabetes C, Complications Trial /Epidemiology of Diabetes I, Complications Research G, Ahluwalia TS, Almgren P, Schulz CA, Orho-Melander M, Linneberg A, Christensen C, Witte DR, Grarup N, Brandslund I, Melander O, Paterson AD, Tregouet D, Maxwell AP, Lim SC, Ma RCW, Tai ES, Maeda S, Lyssenko V, Tuomi T, Krolewski AS, Rich SS, Hirschhorn JN, Florez JC, Dunger D, Pedersen O, Hansen T, Rossing P, Remuzzi G, Micro SUmf, Macrovascular hard endpoints for Innovative diabetes Tools C, Brosnan MJ, Palmer CNA, Groop PH, Colhoun HM, Groop LC, McCarthy MI (2018) A genome-wide association study of diabetic kidney disease in subjects with type 2 diabetes. Diabetes 67(7):1414–1427. https://doi.org/10.2337/db17-0914
12. Graham CA, Hill AJM (2001) DNA sequencing protocols. In: Methods in molecular biology, vol 167. Humana Press/Springer, New York/Berlin
13. Ho K, McKnight AJ (2014) The changing landscape of diabetic kidney disease: new reflections on phenotype, classification, and disease progression to influence future investigative studies and therapeutic trials. Adv Chronic Kidney Dis 21(3):256–259. https://doi.org/10.1053/j.ackd.2014.03.002
14. Perkins BA, Ficociello LH, Silva KH, Finkelstein DM, Warram JH, Krolewski AS (2003) Regression of microalbuminuria in type 1 diabetes. N Engl J Med 348(23):2285–2293. https://doi.org/10.1056/NEJMoa021835
15. Chida S, Fujita Y, Ogawa A, Hayashi A, Ichikawa R, Kamata Y, Takeuchi A, Takano K, Shichiri M (2016) Levels of albuminuria and risk of developing macroalbuminuria in type 2 diabetes: historical cohort study. Sci Rep 6:26380. https://doi.org/10.1038/srep26380
16. McKnight AJ, Patterson CC, Pettigrew KA, Savage DA, Kilner J, Murphy M, Sadlier D, Maxwell AP, Warren UKGoKiDSG (2010) A GREM1 gene variant associates with diabetic nephropathy. J Am Soc Nephrol 21(5):773–781. https://doi.org/10.1681/ASN.2009070773
17. Marshall SM (2004) Recent advances in diabetic nephropathy. Postgrad Med J 80(949):624–633. https://doi.org/10.1136/pgmj.2004.021287
18. Gross JL, de Azevedo MJ, Silveiro SP, Canani LH, Caramori ML, Zelmanovitz T (2005) Diabetic nephropathy: diagnosis, prevention, and treatment. Diabetes Care 28(1):164–176
19. Risch NJ (2000) Searching for genetic determinants in the new millennium. Nature 405(6788):847–856. https://doi.org/10.1038/35015718
20. McGinnis R (2000) General equations for Pt, Ps, and the power of the TDT and the affected-

sib-pair test. Am J Hum Genet 67 (5):1340–1347. https://doi.org/10.1016/S0002-9297(07)62965-6

21. Wang M, Jakobsdottir J, Smith AV, McPeek MS (2016) G-STRATEGY: optimal selection of individuals for sequencing in genetic association studies. Genet Epidemiol 40 (6):446–460. https://doi.org/10.1002/gepi.21982

22. Dimeski G, Yow KS, Brown NN (2015) What is the most suitable blood collection tube for glucose estimation? Ann Clin Biochem 52 (Pt 2):270–275. https://doi.org/10.1177/0004563214544708

Chapter 16

Genetic Strategies to Understand Human Diabetic Nephropathy: In Silico Strategies for Molecular Data—Association Studies

Marisa Canadas-Garre, Laura J. Smyth, Kerry Anderson, Katie Kerr, and Amy Jayne McKnight

Abstract

Multiple genetic strategies are available to help improve understanding of diabetic nephropathy. This chapter provides detailed methodology for a single-nucleotide polymorphism association study and meta-analysis, using a protocol suitable for targeted SNP or genome-wide association studies, to identify genetic risk factors for diabetic nephropathy.

Key words Association, Diabetic nephropathy, Genome-wide, Imputation, Meta-analysis, Plink, RAREMETAL, Rvtests, SNP, Trend

1 Introduction

The last decade has seen significant advances in computational approaches to help identify common complex diseases such as diabetic nephropathy. Moving beyond studies using an individual single-nucleotide polymorphism (SNP) to more comprehensive genotype data from high-density arrays imputed to an appropriate reference genome, and whole-genome sequencing approaches, requires significantly more computing power and customized software. Historically, genetic association studies for diabetic nephropathy were plagued with lack of replication or negative reports [1]; however international collaborations are now leading to the identification of genetic risk factors that are independently replicated across multiple populations with harmonized phenotypes [2–9].

There is typically heterogeneity evident in phenotypes and/or variables reported across publications so it is critically important that the correct phenotypes are consistently employed for association studies investigating diabetic nephropathy (*see* Chap. 15 in this volume). Conducting robust in silico analyses that are transparent

Luigi Gnudi and David A. Long (eds.), *Diabetic Nephropathy: Methods and Protocols*, Methods in Molecular Biology, vol. 2067, https://doi.org/10.1007/978-1-4939-9841-8_16,

and follow clear guidelines is essential. Meta-analysis is now a typical component of genetic association studies to improve power, place results in context, and provide evidence that genetic risk factors are observed across multiple populations [7, 10, 11].

Here, we describe detailed methodology for the analysis of a SNP association study and meta-analysis, using a protocol suitable for targeted SNP or genome-wide association studies, to identify genetic risk factors for diabetic nephropathy.

2 Materials

2.1 Hardware Requirements for Larger Scale Studies

Computer workstation with Windows and Unix or Linux operating system. Ideally a computer with multiple cores and access to a minimum of 100 Tb of storage and 192 Gb RAM.

2.2 Software for Large-Scale Association Studies and Meta-analysis

Multiple tools exist for these analyses, but this protocol focuses on two commonly used tools that can be downloaded to individual computers, facilitate in-house analysis, and enable integration of summative data to meta-consortia.

1. **Plink 1.9**: **PLINK** is a free, open-source whole-genome association analysis toolset, designed to perform a range of basic, large-scale analyses in a computationally efficient manner [12, 13]. Plink can work both in Windows and Linux operative systems.
2. **Rvtests**: Rare Variant Tests, or **RVTESTS**, is a flexible Linux software package for genetic association studies [14]. Although it was designed specifically for the analysis of rare variants, it can also be used for common variants and supports the analysis of autosomal and X-linked variants for both unrelated and related (family-based) individuals. Both quantitative trait and binary trait are supported.
3. **Perl**: Perl is a programming language. In this procedure, we will use the Perl script **run-IBD-QC.pl**.
4. **RAREMETAL**: **RAREMETAL** is a computationally efficient tool for meta-analysis of rare variants genotyped using sequencing or arrays [15]. RAREMETAL can be used with a variety of input file formats, supports association analysis in related and unrelated individuals, and performs conditional association analyses.

2.3 Software for SNP-Based Meta-analysis

There are multiple software packages available for meta-analysis from open source to commercial resources; these differ substantially in ease of use, analysis features, and cost. The protocol described here uses RevMan version 5.3 [16], which is freely available for academic research and was developed by the Cochrane community evaluating evidence in systematic reviews.

3 Methods

3.1 Methods for Primary Association Analysis

The aim of this protocol is to detect SNP associations using individual genome-wide association (GWA) analysis to identify the SNPs and then a GWA meta-analysis to increase the power of the study. The first step starts with the quality control of the genotype data, followed by the individual GWA for chromosomes 1–22 in each study, and finally the meta-analysis of the summary statistics (Fig. 1). The present procedure focuses on more common variants (minor allele frequency, MAF >1%), although the software tools used also provide options for specific tests for rare variants (MAF <1%). This procedure assumes that the user is familiar in basic Windows and Unix/Linux operative systems.

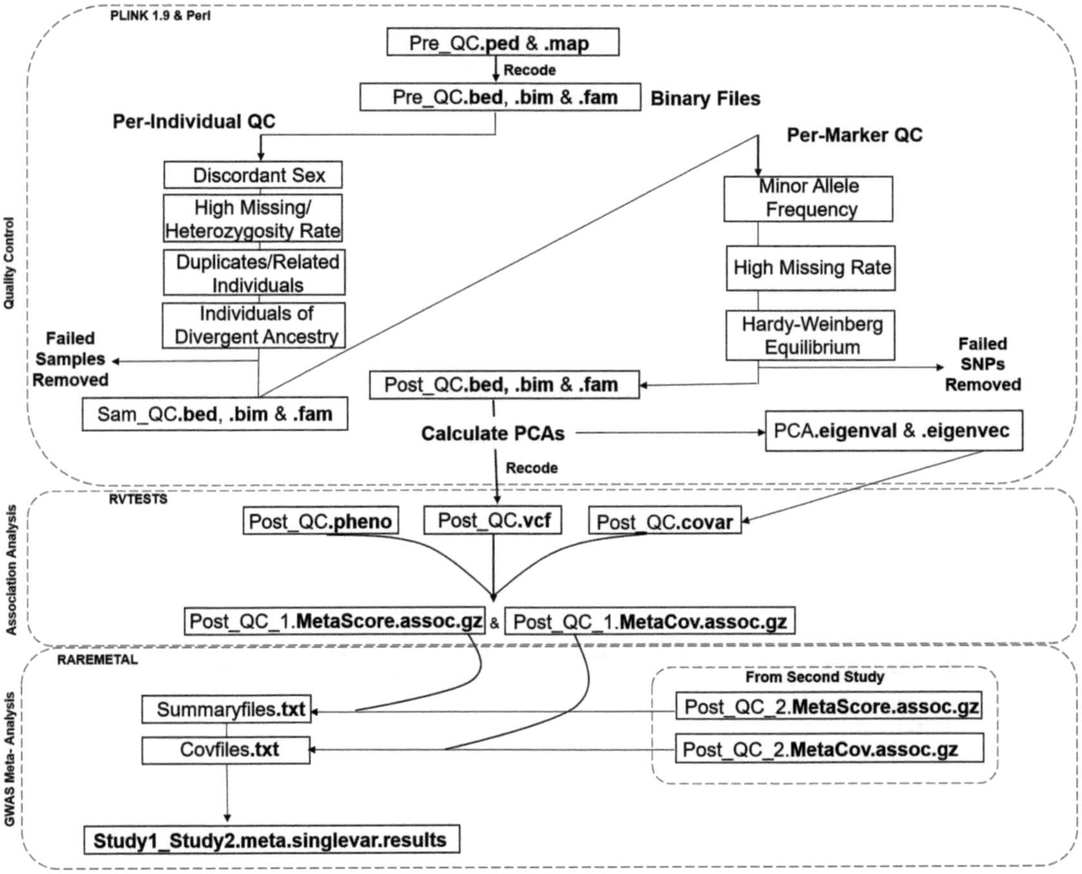

Fig. 1 Outline of GWAS quality control, association, and GWAS meta-analysis

3.1.1 Creating the Computer Environment and Essential Files

Step 1: Set the Working Directory

Create a new folder and copy the .ped and .map files. This is also the folder where all output files will be saved after each command.

This protocol assumes that you are working with Pre_QC.ped and Pre_QC.map files, containing the genotype data for analysis before standard quality control has been performed.

Step 2: Download the Software Tools

Subheading 2.2 includes hyperlinks to each of the software documentation websites, where the programs can be found. Compile the software or download the executables in the same folder where the .ped and .map files are located.

3.1.2 GWAS Quality Control with PLINK (See Notes 1–4)

This step can be performed in Windows or Linux.

Data Files

Most platforms and software used to directly genotype SNPs will output data in the standard PED and MAP file formats for PLINK. Both the .map and the .ped files must have consistent filenames so plink recognizes them as part of the same study (e.g., myfile.ped and myfile.map).

PED File

The PED file is a non-header white-space (space or tab) delimited file composed of the following (Fig. 2):

The first six columns include general information and are mandatory:

First column: Family ID (FID): it should be alphanumeric.

Second column: Individual ID (IID): it should be alphanumeric.

The combination of family and individual ID should uniquely identify a person.

Third column: Paternal ID (FATID).

Fourth column: Maternal ID (MATID).

FID	IID	FATID	MATID	SEX	PHENO	rs1		rs2		rs3		rs4		rs5	
FAM1	1	0	0	1	1	G	G	A	A	A	A	C	C	G	G
FAM1	2	0	0	1	2	G	G	A	A	A	A	C	C	G	G
FAM1	3	0	0	1	2	G	G	A	A	A	A	C	C	G	G
FAM2	1	0	0	1	2	G	G	A	A	A	A	C	C	G	G
FAM2	2	0	0	1	2	G	G	A	A	A	A	C	C	G	G
FAM2	3	0	0	1	2	G	G	A	A	A	A	C	C	G	G
FAM3	1	0	0	1	2	G	G	A	A	A	A	C	C	G	G
FAM3	2	0	0	1	2	G	G	A	A	A	A	C	C	G	G
FAM3	3	0	0	1	2	A	A	G	G	G	G	C	C	G	G

Fig. 2 Example of a PED file. Headers indicating the content of each column are shown for educational purposes only

Fifth column: Sex, coded as 1 for males, 2 for females, and any other for unknown or missing data.

Sixth column: Phenotype of Affection Status, coded as 1 for unaffected individuals (controls), 2 for affected individuals (cases), and 0 or −9 for missing values. The phenotype can also be a quantitative trait instead of affection status, as long as the decimal point is coded with a period/full stop character and not a comma. Only one phenotype in the sixth column can be included in the PED file. If more phenotypes are required, they can be incorporated into the analysis with additional commands in PLINK using additional files.

The seventh and subsequent columns indicate the genotypes for the different SNPs, in the order given by the MAP file. They can be coded by any character (e.g., 1, 2, 3, 4, or A, C, G, T). Missing genotypes are coded with 0. Each SNP must have two alleles (i.e., both alleles are either present or absent).

MAP File

The MAP file is a non-header white-space (space or tab) delimited file which provides the order of the SNPs in the PED file. By default, each line of the MAP file describes a single marker and must contain exactly four columns (Fig. 3):

First column: chromosome (1–22, X, Y, or 0 if unplaced).

Second column: rs# or SNP identifier.

Third column: Genetic distance (morgans): can be fixed to 0.

Fourth column: Base-pair position (bp units).

Step 1: Creation of BED Files

Timing: ≈5–20 min, depending on the size of the PED and MAP files.

The first step consists of the conversion of PED and MAP files (Pre_QC.ped and Pre_QC.map files) into binary BED files, designed to be more computationally efficient and optimize time and resources for the analysis of large-scale data sets [13].

CHROMOSOME	SNP IDENTIFIER	GENETIC DISTANCE	BASE PAIR POSITION
24	rs2534636	0	2657176
24	rs2058276	0	2668456
24	rs2075640	0	2722506
24	rs35284970	0	2734854
24	rs9786209	0	2739468
24	rs9786748	0	2743754

Fig. 3 Example of a MAP file. Headers indicating the content of each column are shown for educational purposes only

In Windows: open the Command Prompt window. There are several ways to do this:

- Type "Command Prompt" in the search window in the taskbar and click on the Command Prompt Desktop Application.
- Press the Windows key and +R from the keyboard to open the Run command, type *cmd*, and press enter.

For simplicity, the commands in this section will be referred to Windows.

In Linux: open a Terminal. The commands will be the same, but preceded by ./.

Change the directory to the folder you created, containing the PED and MAP files and the software:

In Windows: **cd path\to\your\folder**.

In Unix/Linux: **cd path/to/your/folder**.

Type the following command in the Command Prompt:

```
plink --file Pre_QC --make-bed --out Pre_QC
```

PLINK creates a .log file (Pre_QC.log) that details (among other information):

- The implemented commands.
- The number of cases and controls in the input files.
- Any excluded data and the genotyping rate in the remaining data.

The log file is very useful for checking whether the software is successfully completing commands and tracking all changes that have been made in the files.

Step 2: Per-Individual QC

Step 2.1: Identification of Individuals with Discordant Sex Information

Timing: ≈5 min.

Use **PLINK** to calculate the mean homozygosity rate across X-chromosome markers for each individual in the study.

The command in the Command Prompt would be:

```
plink --bfile Pre_QC --check-sex --out checksex
```

This operation produces the **checksex.sexcheck** file, which can be imported into an Excel file as text (Fig. 4).

Produce a list of individuals with discordant sex data by exporting to Excel and filtering by **STATUS=PROBLEM**. Add the family ID (FID) and individual ID (IID) of the samples to a file named "**Fail_sexcheck.txt**" (one individual per line, tab delimited).

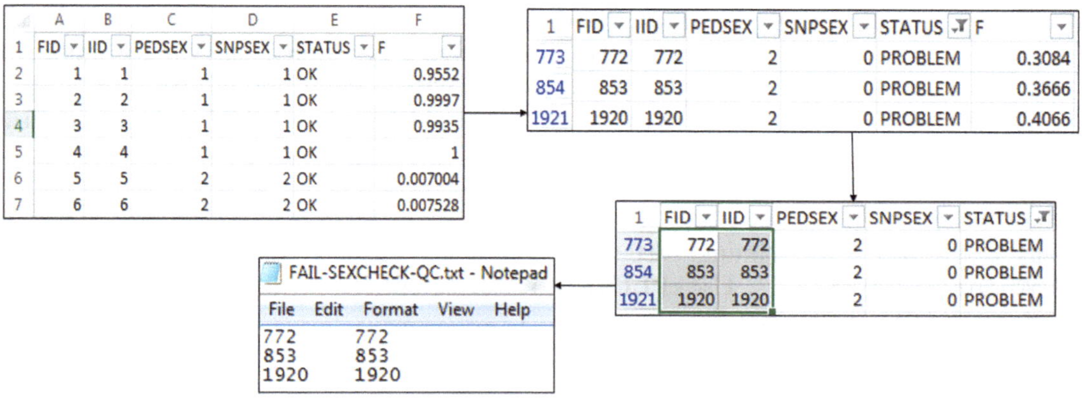

Fig. 4 Identification of individuals with discordant sex information using Excel

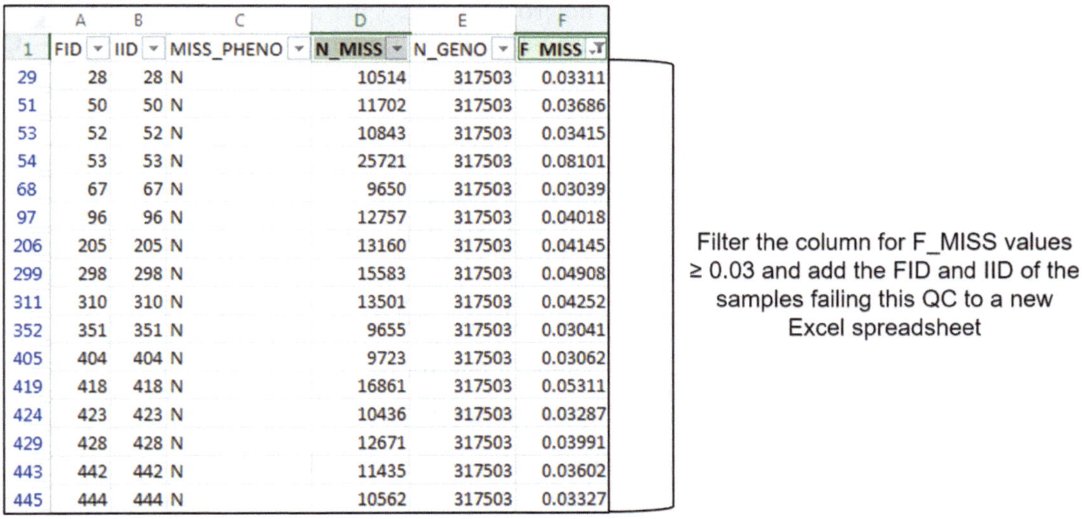

Fig. 5 Identification of individuals with elevated missing data rates using Excel

Step 2.2: Identification of Individuals with Elevated Missing Data Rates

Timing: ≈10 min.

Use **PLINK** to calculate missing data rates, by creating the files **.imiss** and **.lmiss**.

The command in the Command Prompt would be:

```
plink --bfile Pre_QC --missing --out missingness
```

This operation produces two files (**missingness.imiss and missingness.lmiss**), which can be imported into an Excel file as text (Fig. 5).

Import the **missingness.imiss** file:

- The fourth column in the **.imiss** file (N_MISS) indicates the number of missing SNPs.

- The sixth column in the **.imiss** file (F_MISS) indicates the proportion of missing SNPs per individual. We are going to **exclude all individuals with a genotype failure rate ≥0.03,** so filter the column for F_MISS values ≥0.03 and add the FID and IID of the samples failing this QC to a new Excel spreadsheet.

Step 2.3: Identification of Individuals with Outlying Heterozygosity Rate

Timing: ≈10 min.

Use **PLINK** to calculate heterozygosity by creating the **.het** file.

The command in the Command Prompt would be:

```
plink --bfile Pre_QC --het --out heterozygosity
```

This operation produces a file (**heterozygosity.het**), which can be imported into an Excel file as text.

Import the heterozygosity.het file and calculate the Observed heterozygosity rate per individual with the formula (N(NM) − O (Hom))/N(NM). The values can be found in the heterozygosity. het file:

- The third column indicates the observed number of homozygous genotypes [O(Hom)].
- The fifth column indicates the number of nonmissing genotypes [N(NM)] per individual.

Calculate mean and standard deviation, and the values:

- Mean + **3** × standard deviation.
- Mean − **3** × standard deviation.

The individuals with a heterozygosity rate ± **3** standard deviation from the mean will be excluded from the analyses. To do so, filter the column with the **observed heterozygosity rate per individual** by the calculated values (individuals with heterozygosity rate > (mean + **3** × standard deviation) **OR** individuals with heterozygosity rate < (mean − **3** × standard deviation)) (Fig. 6). Add the FID and IID of the samples failing this QC to the Excel spreadsheet created in the previous step (missingness). Export the Excel spreadsheet into a tab-delimited text file with the name **Fail_miss_het.txt**.

Step 2.4: Identification of Duplicated or Related Individuals

Step 2.4.1: Creation of the Pruned Input File

Timing: ≈10 min.

Duplicated or related individuals will be identified using only a subset of SNPs to calculate the values in the identity by state, IBS matrix. These SNPs are selected so that no pair of SNPs (within a given number of base pairs) has an r^2 value greater than a given threshold (typically, 0.2).

Create a tab-delimited text file named HLA.txt containing the HLA region, to be excluded.

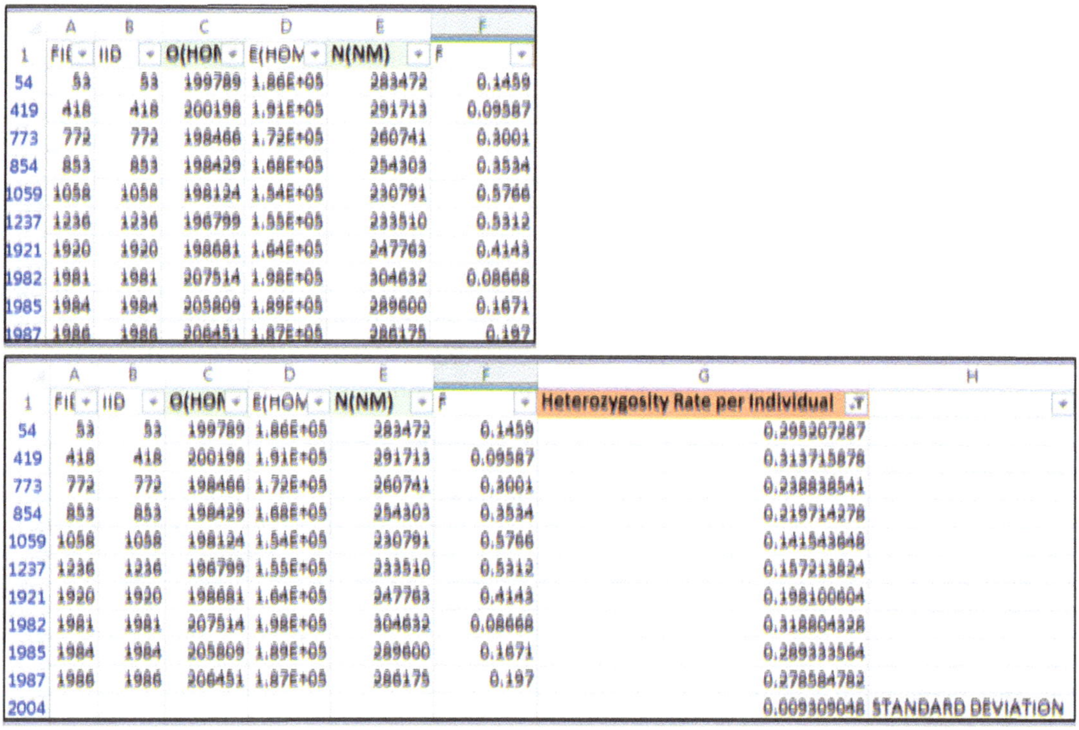

	A	B	C	D	E	F
1	FI(	IID	O(HON	E(HON	N(NM)	F
54	53	53	199789	1.86E+05	283472	0.1459
419	418	418	200198	1.91E+05	291713	0.09587
773	772	772	198466	1.72E+05	260741	0.3001
854	853	853	198429	1.68E+05	254303	0.3534
1059	1058	1058	198124	1.54E+05	230791	0.5766
1237	1236	1236	196799	1.55E+05	233510	0.5312
1921	1920	1920	198681	1.64E+05	247763	0.4143
1982	1981	1981	207514	1.98E+05	304632	0.08668
1985	1984	1984	205809	1.89E+05	289600	0.1671
1987	1986	1986	206451	1.87E+05	286175	0.197

	A	B	C	D	E	F	G	H
1	FI(	IID	O(HON	E(HON	N(NM)	F	Heterozygosity Rate per Individual	
54	53	53	199789	1.86E+05	283472	0.1459	0.295207287	
419	418	418	200198	1.91E+05	291713	0.09587	0.313715878	
773	772	772	198466	1.72E+05	260741	0.3001	0.238838541	
854	853	853	198429	1.68E+05	254303	0.3534	0.219714278	
1059	1058	1058	198124	1.54E+05	230791	0.5766	0.141543648	
1237	1236	1236	196799	1.55E+05	233510	0.5312	0.157213824	
1921	1920	1920	198681	1.64E+05	247763	0.4143	0.198100604	
1982	1981	1981	207514	1.98E+05	304632	0.08668	0.318804328	
1985	1984	1984	205809	1.89E+05	289600	0.1671	0.289333564	
1987	1986	1986	206451	1.87E+05	286175	0.197	0.278584782	
2004							0.009309048	STANDARD DEVIATION

Fig. 6 Identification of individuals with outlying heterozygosity rate using Excel

The content of the file should be (tab delimited) 6 25500000 33500000 8 HLA.

```
plink --file Pre_QC --exclude HLA.txt --range --indep-pairwise
50 5 0.2 --out Pre_QC
```

The file **Pre_QC.prune.in** is created, including the list of SNPs to be kept for the IBS matrix generation.

Step 2.4.2: Identification of Duplicated or Related Individuals

Use **PLINK** to generate pairwise IBS for all pairs of individuals in the study based on the new file with the SNP subset.

The command in the Command Prompt would be:

```
plink --bfile Pre_QC --extract Pre_QC.prune.in --genome --out
Pre_QC
```

This operation produces a file (**ibs.genome**), which cannot be imported into Excel due to its size.

To identify all pairs of individuals with an IBD >0.185, a perl script (**run-IBD-QC.pl**) is used. The code in this program uses the **.genome** and **.imiss** files, identifies the individual call rates stored in the **.imiss** file, and outputs the IDs of the individuals with the lowest call rate to a "**Fail_ibd.txt**" file for subsequent removal (Fig. 7).

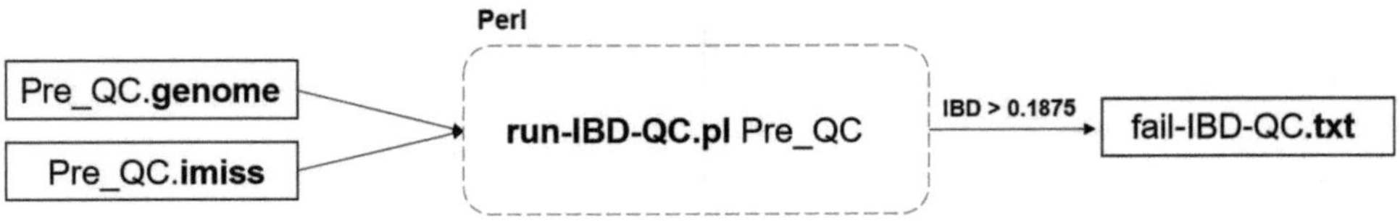

Fig. 7 Identification of duplicated or related individuals using Perl

Step 2.5: Identification of Individuals of Divergent Ancestry

Timing: ≈10 min.

Use **PLINK** to generate an IBS matrix for all pairs of individuals in the study based on the reduced marker set.

First, use **PLINK** to create the Z-scores with the following command in the Command Prompt:

```
plink --bfile Pre_QC --cluster --neighbour 1 5
```

This operation produces a file (**neighbour.nearest**), which can be imported into an Excel file as text (Fig. 8). Import the data in this file to an Excel file and identify the individuals with a Z score <4 standard deviation units. Add the FID and IID of the samples failing this QC to a file named "**Fail_neigh.txt**."

Step 2.6: Removal of All Individuals Failing QC

Timing: ≈5 min.

Make a Fail_indiv.txt file merging all the individuals failing the previous QC steps (merge Fail_sexcheck.txt, Fail_miss_het.txt, Fail_ibd.txt, Fail_neigh.txt). You can do this in Excel.

Use PLINK to remove all individuals failing QC from the original Pre_QC file set and create a new **Sam_QC** file set:

```
plink --bfile Pre_QC --remove Fail_indiv.txt --make-bed --out
Sam_QC
```

Step 3: Per-Marker QC

Timing: ≈5 min.

Variants failing the following thresholds will be excluded:

- Minor allele frequency: 0.01.

  Filters out variants with MAF >1%.
- SNP missingness: 0.05.

  Filters out variants with missing calls >5%.
- Hardy-Weinberg equilibrium: 0.00005.

  Filters out variants failing a Hardy-Weinberg equilibrium (HWE) exact test ($p < 1 \times 10^{-5}$).

Use PLINK with the following command in the Command Prompt:

```
plink --bfile Sam_QC --maf 0.01 --geno 0.05 --hwe 1e-5 --make-
bed --out Post_QC
```

This operation generates a **Post_QC** binary file ready to be used in the association analysis.

	A	B	C	D	E	F	G
1	FII	IID	N	MIN_D	Z	FII	IID
9878	1976	1976	2	0.7176	-6.6	Z:	
9879	1976	1976	3	0.7175	-6.6	Less than "-4"	
9880	1976	1976	4	0.7164	-6.622	1951	1951
9881	1976	1976	5	0.7163	-9.449	1955	1955
9883	1977	1977	2	0.7178	-6.608	1952	1952
9884	1977	1977	3	0.7177	-6.604	1954	1954
9885	1977	1977	4	0.7165	-6.591	1955	1955
9886	1977	1977	5	0.7161	-9.51	1951	1951
9888	1978	1978	2	0.718	-6.546	1954	1954
9889	1978	1978	3	0.7179	-6.546	1953	1953
9890	1978	1978	4	0.7166	-6.577	1951	1951
9891	1978	1978	5	0.7163	-9.436	1955	1955
9893	1979	1979	2	0.7183	-6.474	1952	1952
9894	1979	1979	3	0.7181	-6.507	1953	1953
9895	1979	1979	4	0.7171	-6.455	1951	1951

Fig. 8 Identification of individuals of divergent ancestry using Plink

3.1.3 Association Analysis (See Notes 5-6)

The software for the association analysis will be Rvtests, run under Unix/Linux environment.

This procedure is designed for genotyped SNPs from autosomes in unrelated individuals from homogenous ancestry. If the dataset contains individuals of several ancestral groups, they should be analyzed separately (*see* **Note 7**).

As this procedure is designed to perform meta-analysis with the summary statistics of several individual GWAS, for each study, components of single-variant association score statistics and a variance covariance matrix for score statistics will be calculated.

We will assume that there is no sample overlap and therefore the analysis can be done separately for each study.

Data Files

Timing: $\approx$10 min.

Dataset

The dataset used for this step will be the Post_QC file generated after quality control. Rvtests does not support BED input files, so this file will be converted into a VCF (variant call format) file. Files in both plain text format and gzipped format are supported.

To convert the BED file into VCF format, use PLINK with the following command in the Command Prompt:

```
plink --bfile Post_QC --recode vcf-iid --out Post_QC
```

This will generate a VCF file named **Post_QC.vcf** to be used in the association analysis.

fid	iid	fatid	matid	sex	age	DKD	mAlb	pheno3
FAM1	1	0	0	2	30	2	2	1
FAM1	2	0	0	1	31	1	1	1
FAM1	3	0	0	1	32	1	2	1
FAM2	1	0	0	1	33	1	2	1
FAM2	2	0	0	1	34	2	1	2
FAM2	3	0	0	1	35	2	1	2
FAM3	1	0	0	2	36	2	2	1
FAM3	2	0	0	1	37	2	2	2

Fig. 9 Example of a phenotype file for Rvtests. Headers indicating the content of each column are mandatory (DKD: diabetic kidney disease, mAlb: microalbuminuria)

Phenotype File

This is a tab-delimited text file with headers that contains at least six columns indicating the phenotypes (clinical data on each study subject) for association analysis, one row per individual (Fig. 9). For the purpose of this procedure, we will assume that the phenotype file is named Post_QC.pheno and includes columns for two phenotypes, one binary, diabetic kidney disease (DKD), and one quantitative trait, microalbuminuria (mAlb):

First column	fid	Family ID
Second column	iid	Individual ID
Third column	fatid	Phenotype 1
Fourth column	matid	Phenotype 2
Fifth column	sex	Gender
Sixth column	Phenotype 1 (e.g., DKD)	
Seventh column	Phenotype 2 (e.g., mAlb)	

Missing values should be indicated as *NA*.

The flag *--mpheno* (followed by the column number) or *--pheno-name* (followed by the phenotype name as indicated in the header) is used to specify a given phenotype.

Covariate File

Timing: ≈10 min.

The covariate file has the same format than the phenotype file, but the variables included are covariates (Fig. 10). The flags *--covar* and *--covar-name* are used to specify covariates for single-variant association analysis; this parameter is optional.

First column	fid	Family ID
Second column	iid	Individual ID
Third column	fatid	Phenotype 1
Fourth column	matid	Phenotype 2
Fifth column	sex	Gender
Sixth column	Covariate 1 (e.g., age)	
Seventh column	Covariate 2 (e.g., pca1)	

fid	iid	fatid	matid	sex	age	pheno	pca1	pca2	pca3	pca4	pca5
FAM1	1	0	0	2	30	2	0.005346	-0.005	0.001356	-0.00838	-0.00931
FAM1	2	0	0	1	31	1	0.000414	-0.00728	-0.0056	-0.00381	-0.00838
FAM1	3	0	0	1	32	1	-0.00931	-0.00998	-0.00735	0.010219	-0.00381
FAM2	1	0	0	1	33	1	-0.00838	0.019179	-0.00431	0.004114	0.010219
FAM2	2	0	0	1	34	2	-0.00381	0.009888	0.007359	-0.01019	0.004114
FAM2	3	0	0	1	35	2	0.010219	-0.0033	-0.00133	-0.00998	-0.01019
FAM3	1	0	0	2	36	2	0.004114	-0.00313	-0.00377	0.019179	-0.00381
FAM3	2	0	0	1	37	2	-0.01019	-0.00321	0.003825	0.009888	0.010219

Fig. 10 Example of a covariate file for Rvtests. Headers indicating the content of each column are mandatory (PCA: principal component analysis)

Missing values should be indicated as *NA*.

For the purpose of this procedure, we will assume that the covariate file is named Post_QC.covar and includes columns for the covariates age and sex.

The covariate file may also contain the eigenvec values of the principal component analysis (PCA) to use as covariates in the association analysis and adjust for population substructure (Fig. 1). For the purpose of this procedure, we will assume that the names of the columns containing the PCA values are pca1, pca2 ... pca20.

To calculate these values, use PLINK with the following command in the Command Prompt:

```
plink --bfile Post_QC --cluster --pca --read-genome Pre_QC.
genome --out PCA
```

This generates a text file with 20 PCA values that can be added to the .covar file.

Step 1: Association Test for Binary Traits

Timing: ≈10 min.

For the purpose of this procedure, we will assume that we are evaluating the development of DKD and that we are considering as potential confounders the variables sex, age, and five PCA.

Open the terminal in the Unix/Linux environment and type the following command:

```
./rvtest --inVcf Post_QC.vcf \
--pheno Post_QC.pheno \
--pheno-name DKD \
--covar Post_QC.covar \
--meta score,cov[windowSize=500000] \
--covar-name age,sex,pca1,pca2,pca3,pca4,pca5 \
--out Post_QC_1
```

This will generate four files to be used in the meta-analysis:

- Two of them contain the summary statistics and covariance matrix:

  - Summary score statistics files: Post_QC_1.MetaScore.assoc.gz.
  - Covariance files: Post_QC_1.MetaCov.assoc.gz.
- This also generates tabix-indexed .tbi files of those two files.

Repeat for each individual study.

Step 2: Association Test for Quantitative Traits

Timing: ≈10 min.

(*See* **Note 8**) For the purpose of this procedure, we will assume that we are evaluating the development of mAlb in DKD patients and that we are considering as potential confounders the variables sex, age, and five PCA. To specify that the phenotype is continuously distributed, the --qtl\flag can be added to the command.

Open the terminal in the Unix/Linux environment and type the following command:

```
./rvtest --inVcf Post_QC.vcf \
--pheno Post_QC.pheno \
--pheno-name mAlb \
--covar Post_QC.covar \
--meta score,cov[windowSize=500000]\(see Note 9)
--covar-name age,sex,pca1,pca2,pca3,pca4,pca5 \
--qtl \
--out Post_QC_1
```

3.1.4 GWAS Meta-analysis

In this procedure, we will use RAREMETAL to perform single-variant meta-analysis using summary statistics of two studies on DKD (*see* **Notes 10** and **11**).

Data Files

Input Files

The four files generated by Rvtests will be used to provide the summary statistics, but two additional files listing the names of those files must be created.

Summary Files

These are plain-text files listing the names of the MetaScore.assoc.gz files. In this example, the included files should be:

Post_QC_1.MetaScore.assoc.gz

Post_QC_2.MetaScore.assoc.gz

Covariance Files

These are plain-text files listing the names of the MetaScore.assoc.gz files. In this example, the included files should be:

Post_QC_1.MetaCov.assoc.gz

Post_QC_2.MetaCov.assoc.gz

Step 1: Meta-analysis Test

Timing: ≈10 min.

To perform single-variant meta-analysis of the two GWAS studies, use the following command:

```
./raremetal --summaryFiles Summaryfiles \
--covFiles Covfiles \
--prefix Study1_Study2 \
--hwe 1.0e-05 \
--callRate 0.95
```

This command filters summary statistics based on HWE *p*-value and variant call rate, generates single-variant meta-analysis results, and produces summary results in .pdf format.

- The following output will be generated:
  - Study1_Study2.meta.plots.pdf (QQ plots and Manhattan plots)
  - Study1_Study2.meta.singlevar.results
  - Study1_Study2.raremetal.log

3.2 Methods for SNP-Based Meta-analysis

Where top-ranked SNPs are identified from GWAS and meta-GWAS or mega-GWAS studies, often independent replication is performed in new cohorts and smaller scale meta-analysis is then essential to show the significance and direction of effect across all cohorts (*see* Fig. 11, **Note 12**).

3.2.1 Search Parameters

Initially, the phenotype must be explicitly determined and target SNPs (typically SNPs that are top-ranked from previous association testing) identified for meta-analysis. Remember to include alternate names for each SNP and all SNPs in linkage disequilibrium with the target SNP(s). Meta-analysis of GWAS is now often undertaken and it is important that association results from these high-density SNP screens and whole-genome sequencing data are included in meta-analysis where possible (*see* **Notes 13** and **14**). At this stage clear inclusion and exclusion criteria should be identified; for example:

Inclusion criteria	Exclusion criteria
• English language publication • Human study • Case-control/cohort study • Defined kidney disease • Genotype counts/frequencies available	• Pharmacological based study • No genotypic data available for the correct gene • Nonhuman study • Duplicate research

3.2.2 Electronic Database Search

Online resources should be systematically searched including Cochrane library, EMBASE, MEDLINE, PubMed, Web of Science, conference abstracts, Grey Lit, and OpenGrey resources for specific SNPs and/or genes of interest. Each search must be independently performed by two trained investigators within a specific timeframe (typically from inception of each database until the latest realistic date before the meta-analysis commences); this date should be recorded carefully. All search terms should be explicitly retained

Identify clear inclusion and exclusion criteria

Select keywords and filter parameters for searches

Electronic database search

Cochrane library, EMBASE, MEDLINE, PubMed, Web of Science, conference abstracts, Grey Lit and OpenGrey resources should be searched for specific SNPs or genes of interest; remember to include SNPs in linkage disequilibrium with the target SNP

Record the number of results returned and remove duplicates

Be careful to remove research presented in abstract & paper form, which may be slightly different

Abstract screening

Remove articles who do not meet the inclusion criteria based on title, keywords and abstract

Full text screening

Be careful to note reasons why research is excluded at this stage

Additional relevant papers may be identified from bibliographies during full-text screening

Final study selection for data extraction

Record all unique research that meets inclusion criteria and create a standard template for relevant data extraction, including recording covariates and quality control steps employed in the original publication. For example:

Unique reference identifying study	Unique SNP identifier (noting LD for target SNP)	Case phenotype	Control phenotype	Number of cases: controls	Case genotype counts (11/12/22)	Control genotype counts (11/12/22)	Reported Hardy-Weinberg equilibrium	Reported p value	Reported odds ratio (95% CI)	Calculated p value	Calculated odds ratio (95% CI)	Calculated Hardy-Weinberg equilibrium	Comments
1 (Muggin *et al.*, 2011; PMID 1234567)	Rs12345	Persistent macroalbuminuria, retinopathy and hypertension in type 1 diabetes	>20 years type 1 diabetes with no renal disease	48:197	34/10/04	104/82/11	none	0.03	OR=2.15; 95% CI=0.88–5.27,	0.12	OR=1.55; 95% CI=0.89, 2.72	0.0285	

Final study selection for quantitative analysis

The completed data extraction template is reviewed to identify SNPs with at least three populations (including your study) with the same ethnicity to enable meta-analyses

Quantitative meta-analysis

Using a relevant statistical program (e.g. RevMan5) perform meta-analyses; generate Forest plots, evaluate bias (funnel plot), and report results.

Fig. 11 Overview of targeted, SNP-based meta-analysis

for future use, with the results of each search (total number of results returned) recorded with the date each study was conducted.

3.2.3 Screening Results

Primary screening of results should be performed independently by at least two trained reviewers, with a third reviewer consulted where disagreements are noted.

Stage 1 Screening

The title, keywords, and abstract of each article returned from each search are read to ensure that each article meets the stated inclusion criteria. Where articles clearly meet the exclusion criteria, mark them as excluded (e.g., duplicates, not written in English, no data for SNP of interest) and transfer them to a separate file, carefully noting why each study was excluded so that it can be reported later. Be cautious at this point and keep in the results any study that may meet the inclusion criteria. Where a study may contain slightly different participant numbers, but clearly reports results on a particular SNP in the same population, use the study with the larger sample size to provide the greatest power assuming that the phenotype is appropriate.

Stage 2 Screening

Studies that still meet the inclusion criteria are then screened more comprehensively with the entire full text of articles being read independently by the two reviewers. Paying careful attention, select studies that still meet the inclusion criteria and note reasons for excluding studies; studies excluded at this stage should be transferred to a new file as they may be requested by external reviewers. At this stage, the bibliographies of each article should be read and additional relevant papers are identified and added to the file of included studies; please carefully record which studies were identified using this approach. Forward citation screening using tools such as the Web of Science or Google Scholar may identify more recent articles that cite shortlisted papers after publication. Again, any discrepancies in results should be resolved with a third independent reviewer.

3.2.4 Data Extraction

By this stage a file should exist listing all unique studies that meet the inclusion criteria; this is the final studies selected for data extraction. Using a template similar to that provided in Fig. 11, record all relevant data, including details on covariates used in each study, ethnicity of participants, and quality control steps described in the original publication; a new row should be taken for each relevant SNP to facilitate downstream analysis. At a minimum, extracted data for each row of each study in this file (i.e., each relevant unique variant per publication) should include explicit phenotype definitions, total number of individuals in each group for a study, ethnicity (consistently coded using the IGSR: The International Genome Sample Resource), unique SNP identifiers, genotype counts/frequencies/allele counts, and reported significance values. Once data extraction is complete, studies should be reviewed and those SNPs where three or more studies report genotype data for the same SNP (or a SNP in strong linkage disequilibrium r^2 >0.8 with the target SNP) using similar phenotype criteria are selected for meta-analysis.

3.2.5 Meta-analysis

For studies that meet the final review of inclusion criteria, Hardy-Weinberg equilibrium should be calculated in case and control groups separately and compared to that reported (if any) in the original publication. Allele frequencies should be calculated from genotype counts or, suboptimally, estimated from genotype frequencies if necessary. P values and odds ratios with 95% confidence intervals should be calculated and compared to those reported in the original publication. Meta-analysis should be conducted using RevMan (see steps below for RevMan version 5.3). Forest plots should be generated and heterogeneity levels (I^2) [17] calculated for each SNP analysis. Either a fixed or a random effects model should be selected to pool study estimates. Where little or no heterogeneity is found (I^2 of less than 25%), a fixed effects model is the more powerful approach. However if there is found to be a significant variation between studies (I^2 of more than 25%), a random effects model may be more appropriate to minimize the risk of type 1 error as a result of not considering between study heterogeneity. Sex-specific and ancestry-specific analysis should be performed where sufficient data is available to minimize heterogeneity across studies. All study methodology should conform to international guidelines such as STrengthening the REporting of Genetic Association studies (STREGA) [18, 19] and Meta-analysis Of Observational Studies in Epidemiology (MOOSE) criteria [20].

Step 1: Open Review Manager 5.3 and select Create a new review (Fig. 12).

Step 2: The New Review Wizard opens. Click Next to continue (Fig. 13).

Step 3: Next, select the Type of Review that you wish to create. The best option here is *Flexible review*; subtype *Qualitative*. Click *Next* to continue (Fig. 14).

Step 4: Following this, enter a *Title* for your review. Click *Next* to continue (Fig. 15).

Step 5: Select the *Full review* option. Click *Finish* to exit the wizard (Fig. 16).

Step 6: You are then presented with the following screen from which you are able to enter the data for analysis (Fig. 17).

Step 7: Initially, click on *Studies and references* from the left-hand-side menu. Select *Add Study* from under the *Included studies* heading in the main panel. The *New Study Wizard* opens. Enter

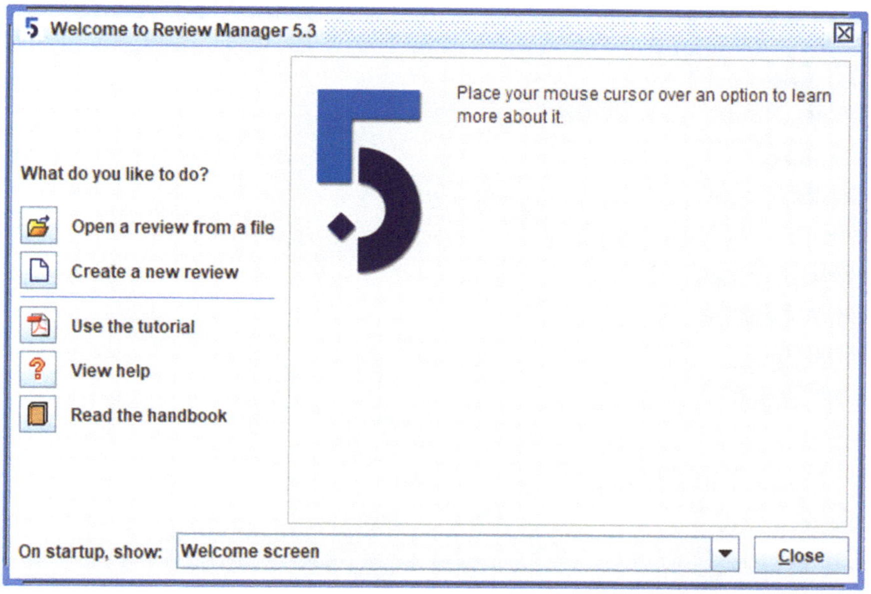

Fig. 12 Screenshots illustrating the RevMan step-by-step protocol

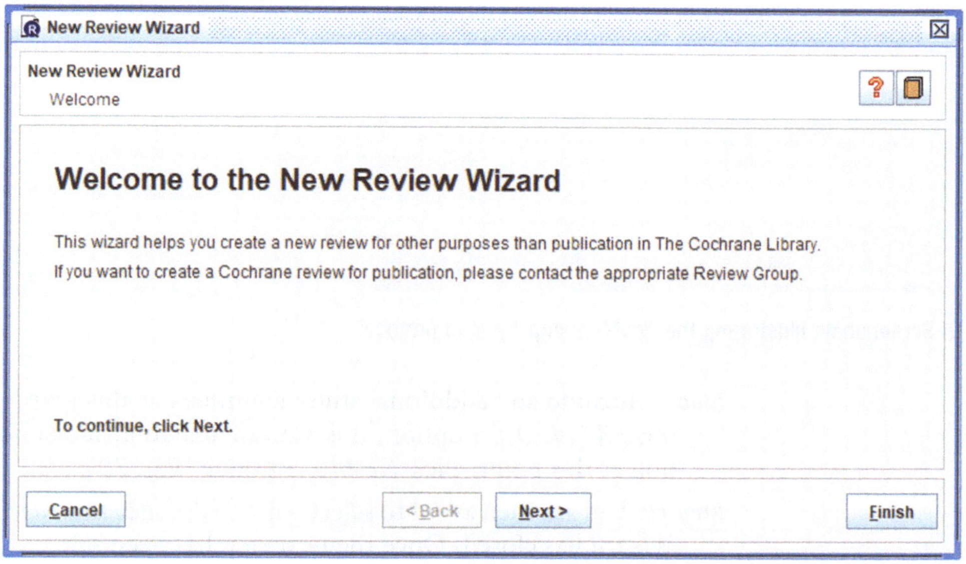

Fig. 13 Screenshots illustrating the RevMan step-by-step protocol

a *Study ID* into the menu which opens; the first author and year of publication are useful to include here. Click *Next* to continue (Fig. 18).

Step 8: Following this, you select your *Data source* from the drop-down menu. *Published data only (unpublished not sought)* selected for this study. Click *Next* to continue (Fig. 19).

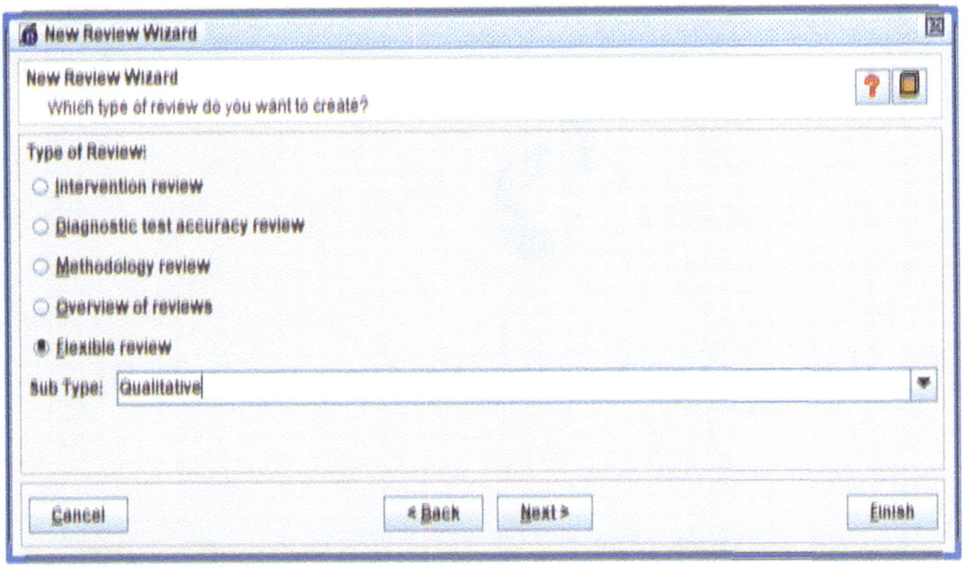

Fig. 14 Screenshots illustrating the RevMan step-by-step protocol

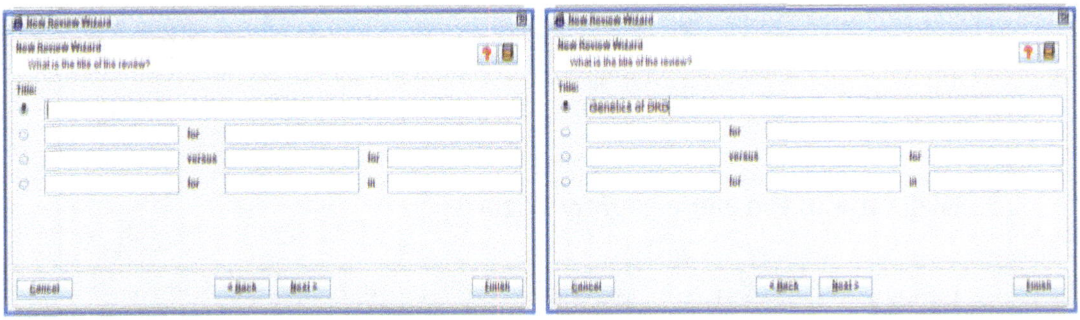

Fig. 15 Screenshots illustrating the RevMan step-by-step protocol

Step 9: Include any additional study identifiers at this point using the *Add identifier* option. It is not essential to include information at this point; click *Next* to continue (Fig. 20).

Step 10: You are then asked to select what to do once the *New Study Wizard* has closed. Once the next step has been selected, click *Finish* to exit the wizard (Fig. 21).

Step 11: Once you return to the main Review Manager 5.3 screen, the study that you have entered the data for will be included under *Included studies* (Fig. 22).

Step 12: Next, select the *Data and analyses* option from the left-hand screen to enable you to add data. Select *Add comparison* from under the *Data and analyses* heading in the main screen (Fig. 23).

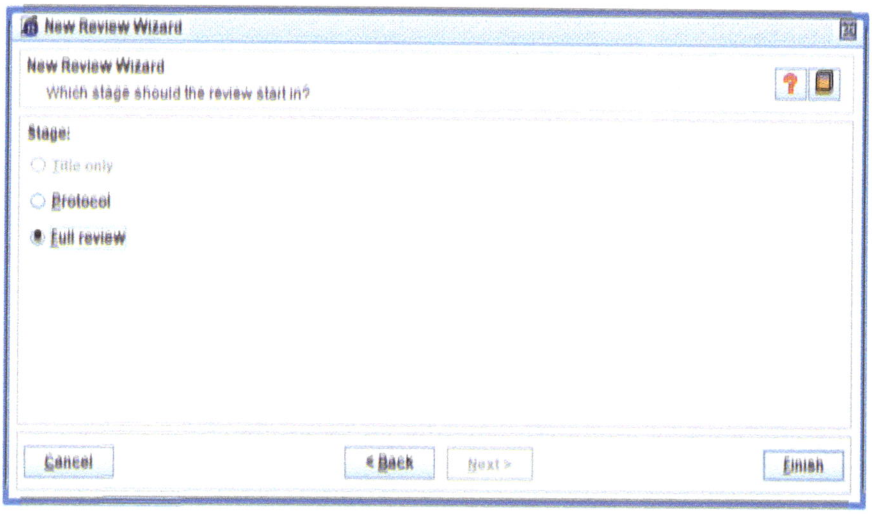

Fig. 16 Screenshots illustrating the RevMan step-by-step protocol

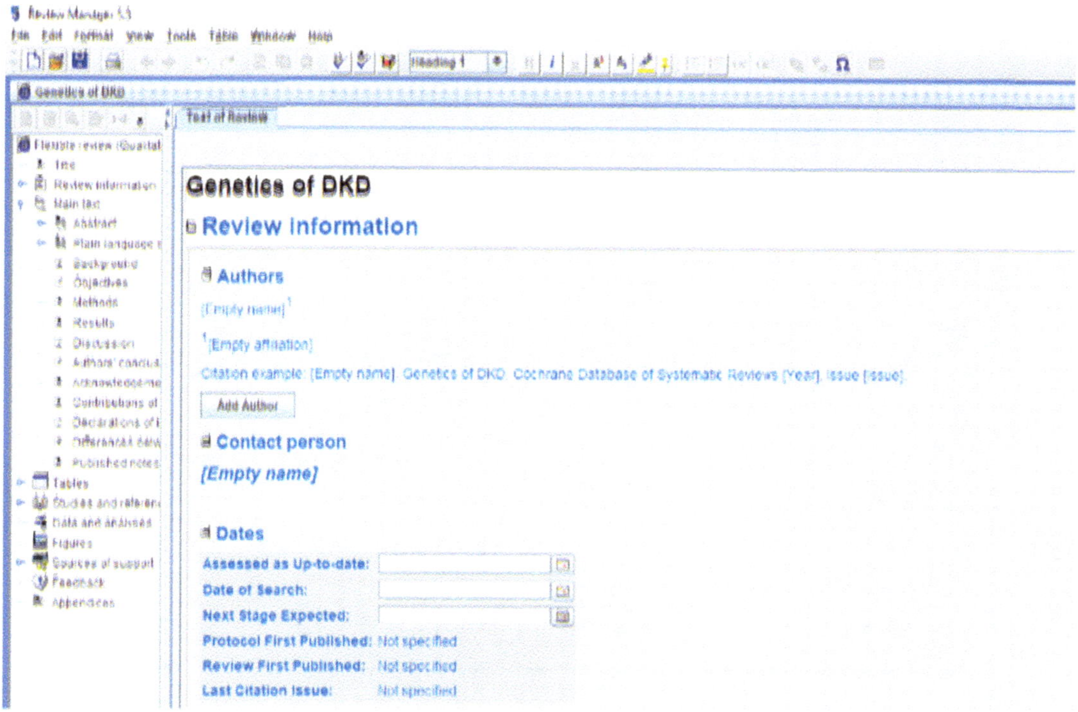

Fig. 17 Screenshots illustrating the RevMan step-by-step protocol

Step 13: The *New Comparison* Wizard opens. Enter a *Name* before clicking *Next*. In order to track your SNP analyses, enter the phenotype of interest to be analyzed here (Fig. 24).

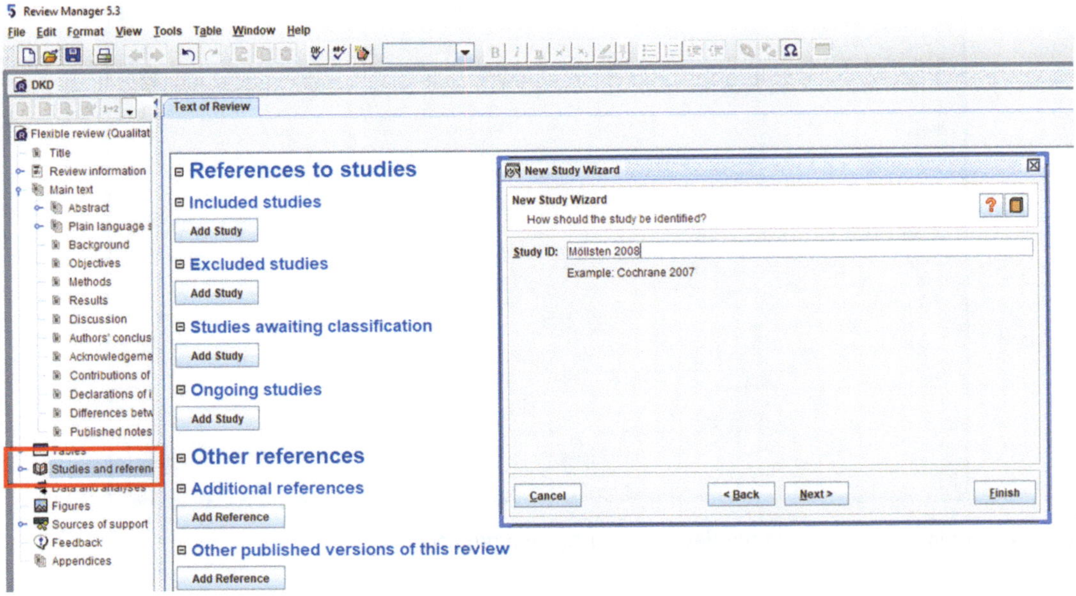

Fig. 18 Screenshots illustrating the RevMan step-by-step protocol

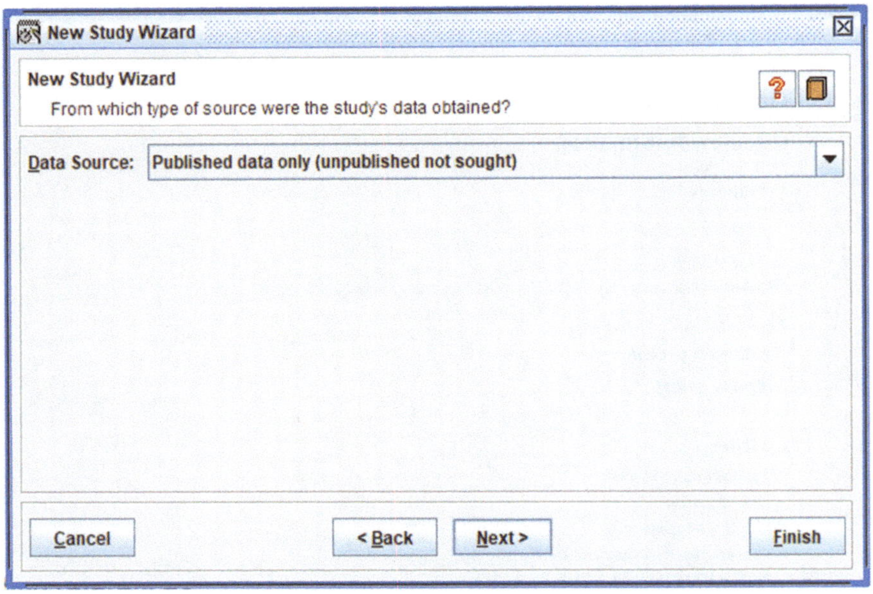

Fig. 19 Screenshots illustrating the RevMan step-by-step protocol

Step 14: You are then asked to select what to do once the *New Comparison wizard* has closed. Once the next step has been selected, click *Continue* (Fig. 25).

Step 15: Select from the list of options the *Data Type* that you will enter. A description of each is provided. *Dichotomous* is selected here. Click *Next* (Fig. 26).

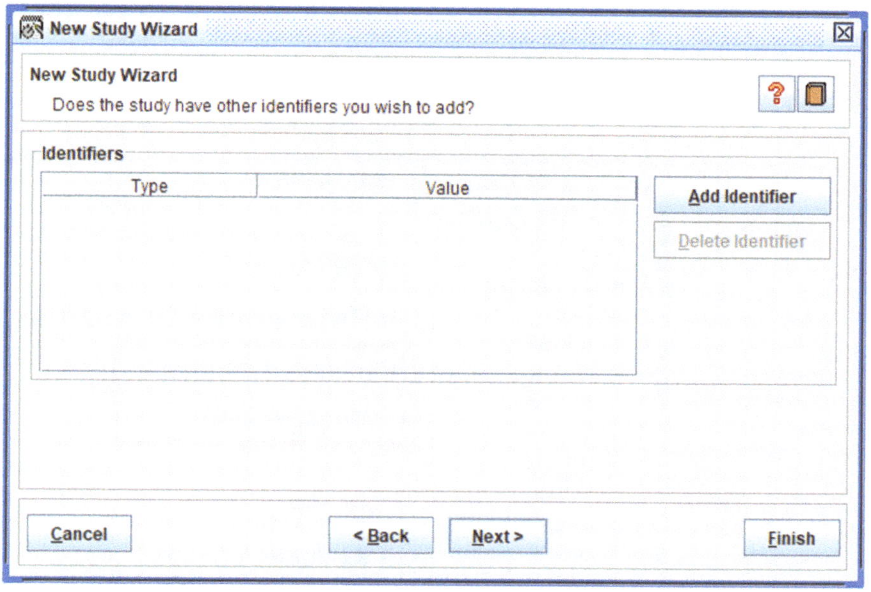

Fig. 20 Screenshots illustrating the RevMan step-by-step protocol

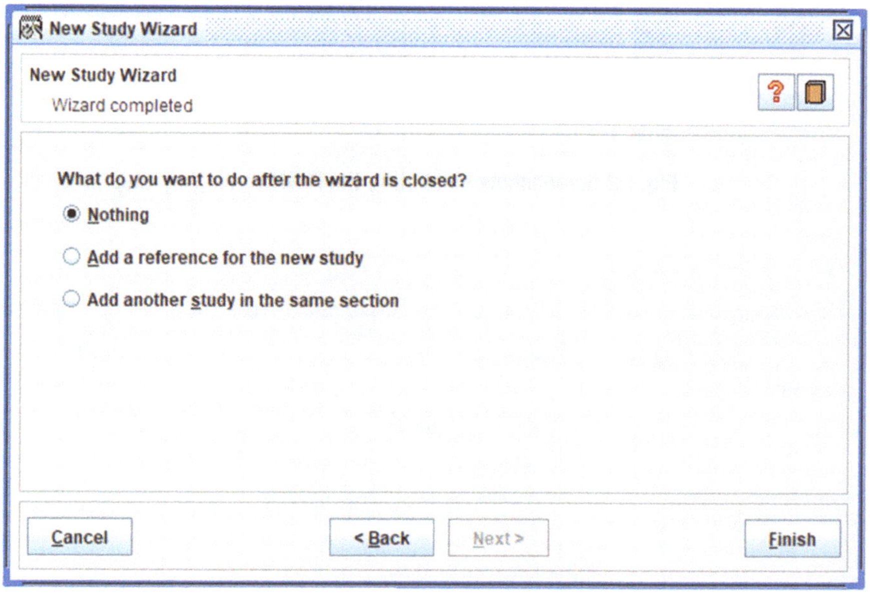

Fig. 21 Screenshots illustrating the RevMan step-by-step protocol

Step 16: Enter the *Name* of your comparison (or SNP in this example) and the *Group labels*, i.e., Case and Control. Click *Next* (Fig. 27).

Step 17: Next you select the *Statistical Method*, *Analysis Model*, and *Effect Measure* for this comparison. For SNP comparisons, select *Mantel-Haenszel* (*Statistical Method*), *Random Effects*

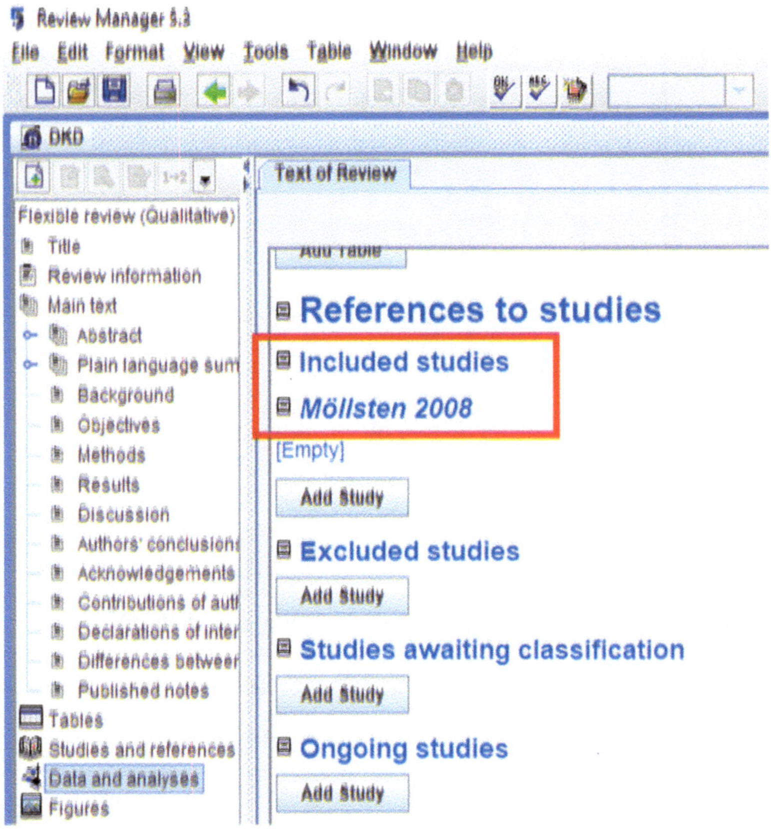

Fig. 22 Screenshots illustrating the RevMan step-by-step protocol

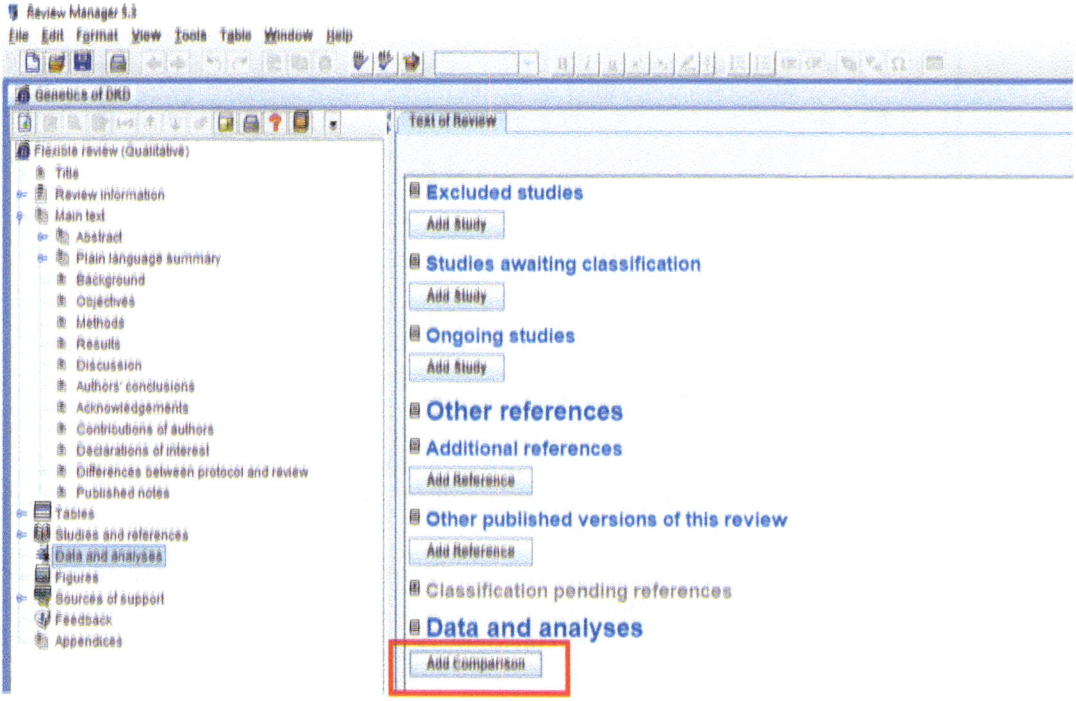

Fig. 23 Screenshots illustrating the RevMan step-by-step protocol

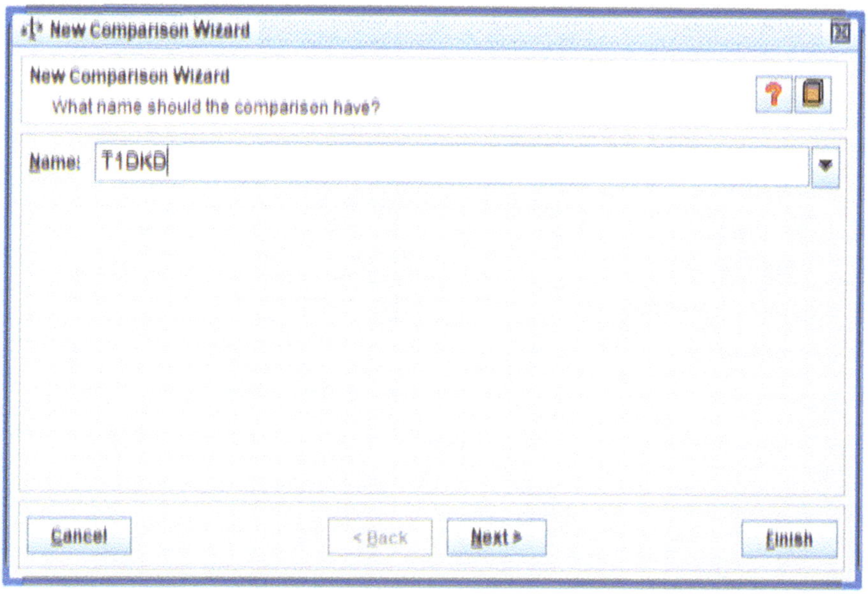

Fig. 24 Screenshots illustrating the RevMan step-by-step protocol

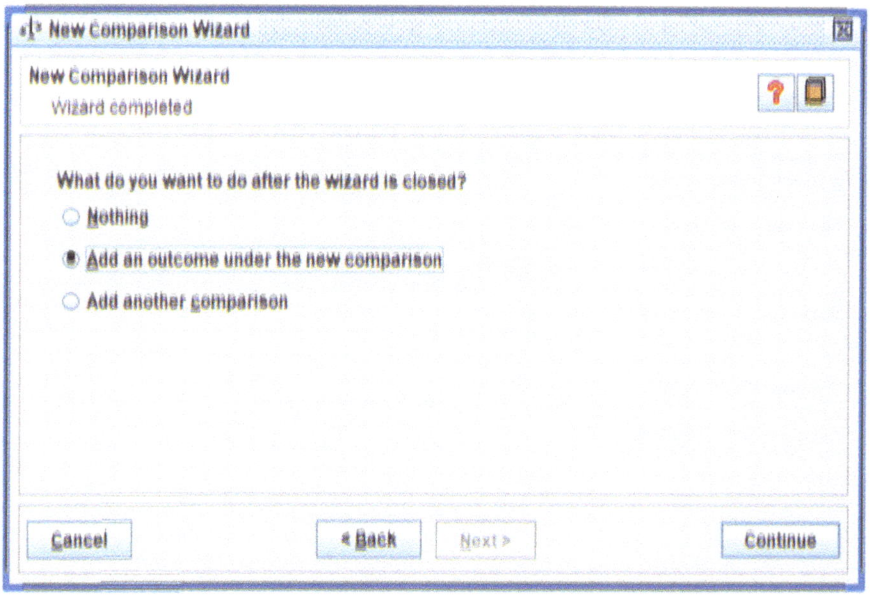

Fig. 25 Screenshots illustrating the RevMan step-by-step protocol

(*Analysis Model*), and *Odds Ratio* (*Effects Measure*). Click *Next* (Fig. 28).

Step 18: Following this, you must indicate the ***analysis details***. The preset options are ***Totals and subtotals*** and ***95% Confidence intervals*** for both the ***studies*** and the ***total***. Click *Next* (Fig. 29).

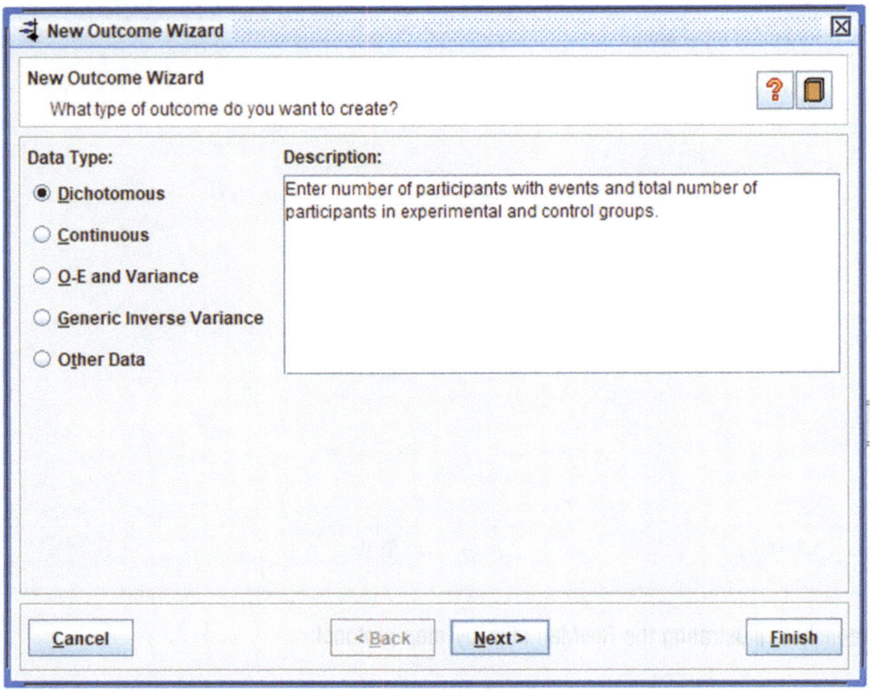

Fig. 26 Screenshots illustrating the RevMan step-by-step protocol

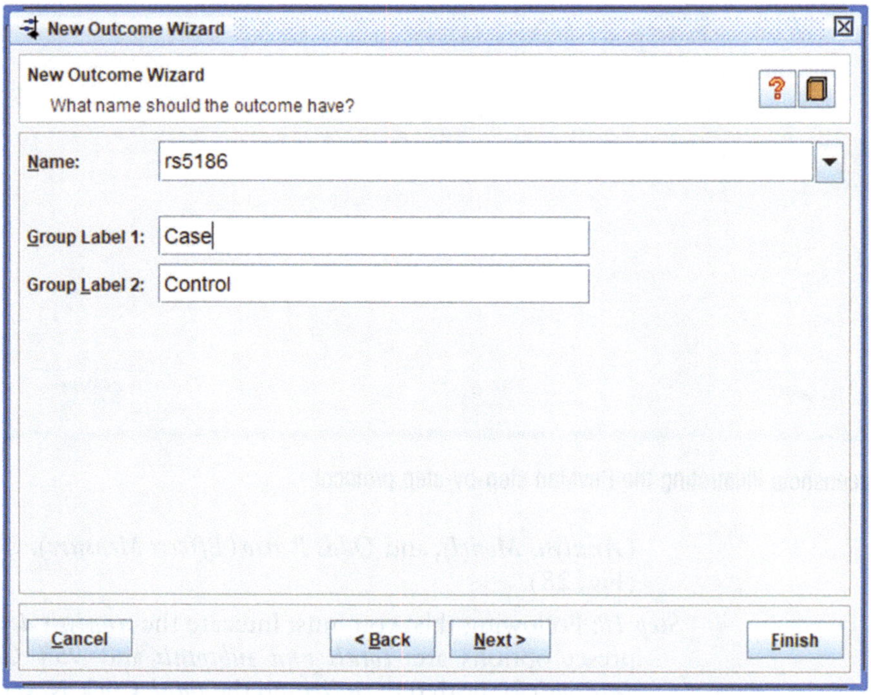

Fig. 27 Screenshots illustrating the RevMan step-by-step protocol

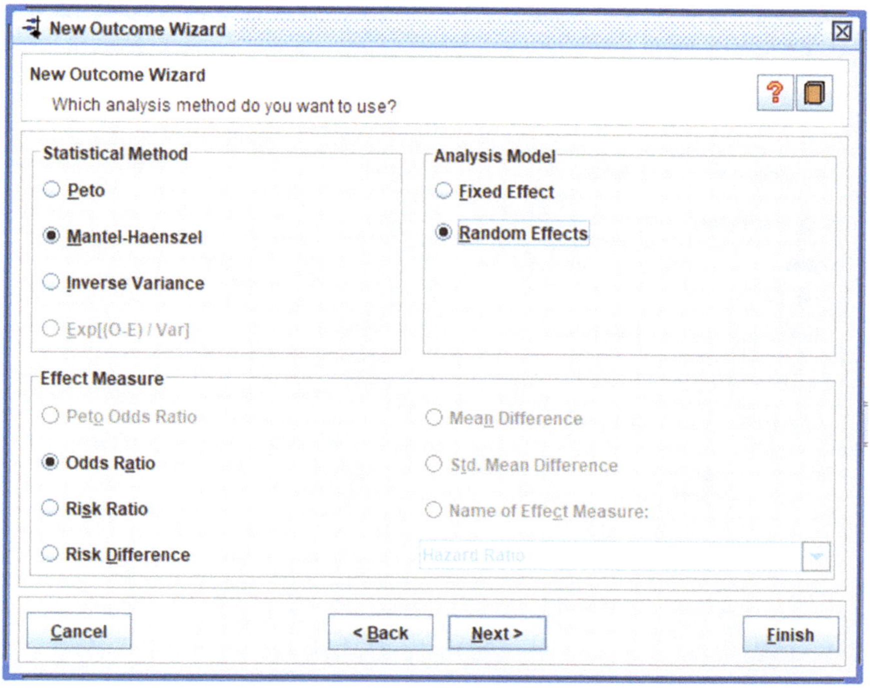

Fig. 28 Screenshots illustrating the RevMan step-by-step protocol

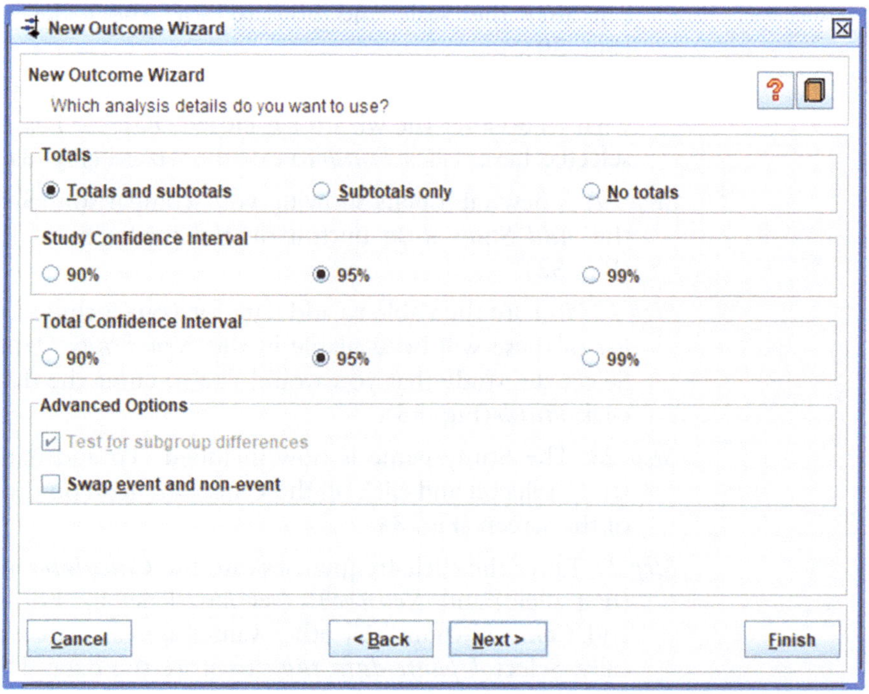

Fig. 29 Screenshots illustrating the RevMan step-by-step protocol

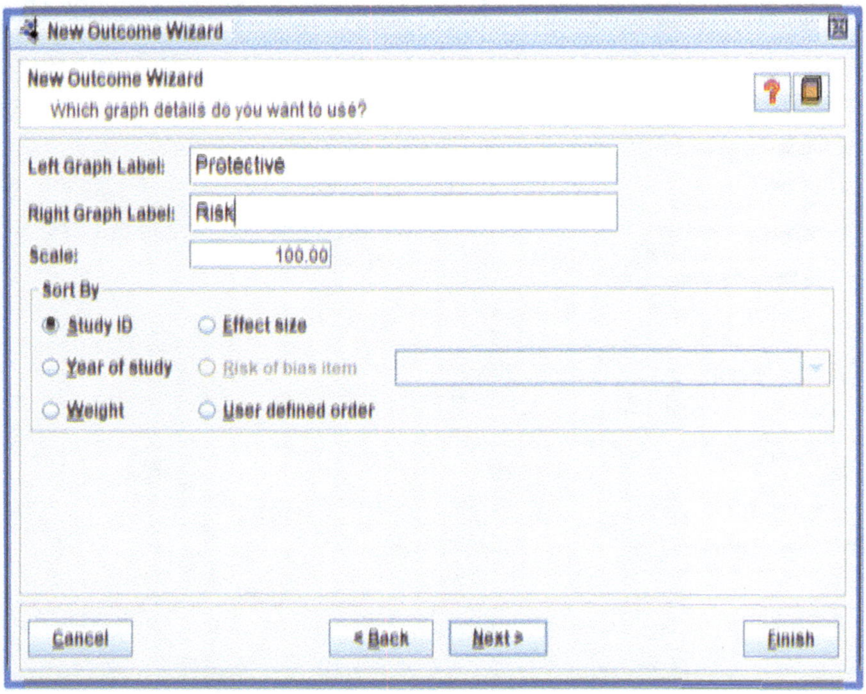

Fig. 30 Screenshots illustrating the RevMan step-by-step protocol

Step 19: Next, you must indicate the graph details. Label the *Left Graph Label*, Protective, and the *Right Graph Label*, Risk. You can alter the Scale and how to Sort the order of studies (Fig. 30).

Step 20: The wizard has now been completed and you must select what to do after the wizard has closed. *Edit the new outcome* is selected here. Click *Finish* to exit the wizard (Fig. 31).

Step 21: A new tab opens showing your comparison (SNP). Click the *Add Study data* button on the top right of the screen (Fig. 32).

Step 22: You are then able to add data for your included studies. A list of these will be available in the *New Study Data Wizard*. Select the study that you would like to enter the data for and click *Finish* (Fig. 33).

Step 23: The Study name is now included. To add data for this study, select it and click on the *Calculator* icon on the top right of the screen (Fig. 34).

Step 24: Enter the allele frequencies into the *Calculator* into *Events* (first allele) and *Non-events* (second allele) for both the *Case* and *Control* groups. All other values are calculated automatically. Select *Update data table* to store the data. This can be edited if required *via* the same means (Fig. 35).

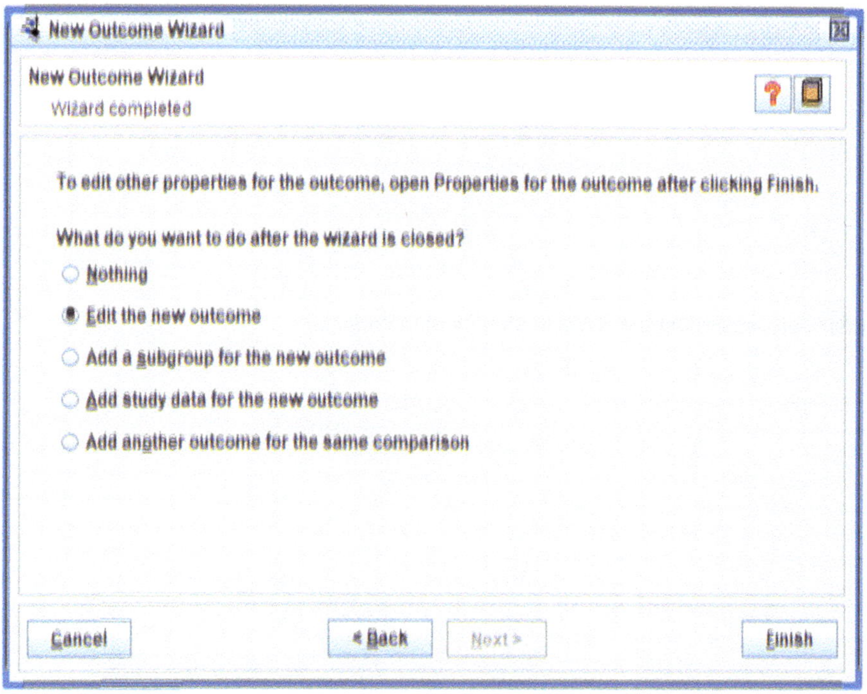

Fig. 31 Screenshots illustrating the RevMan step-by-step protocol

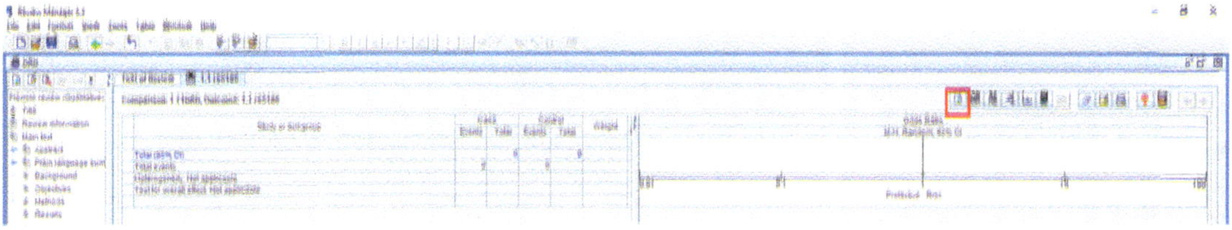

Fig. 32 Screenshots illustrating the RevMan step-by-step protocol

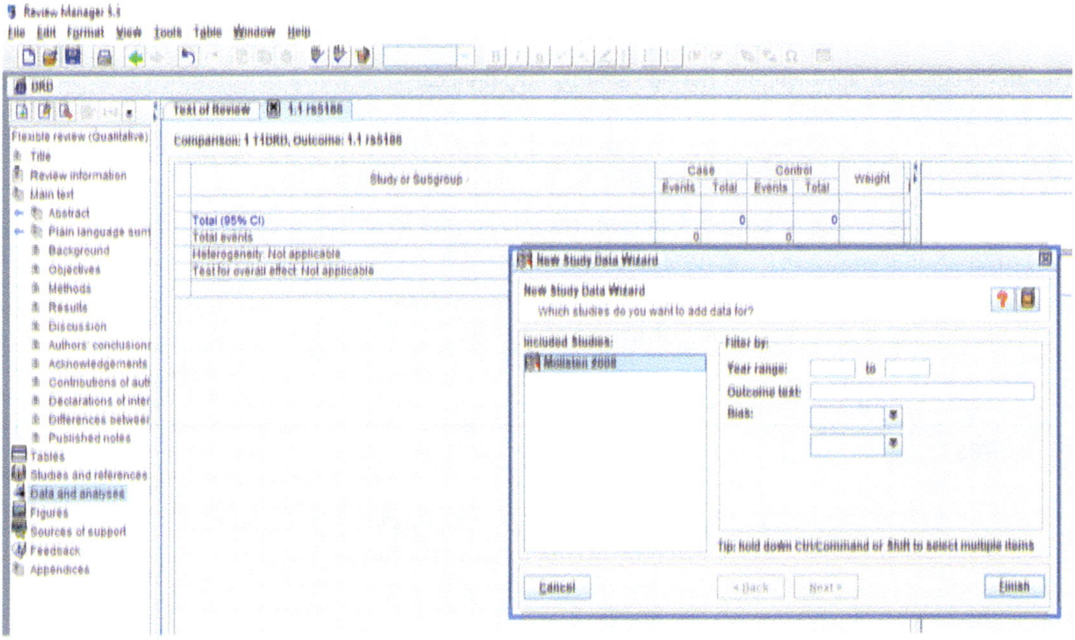

Fig. 33 Screenshots illustrating the RevMan step-by-step protocol

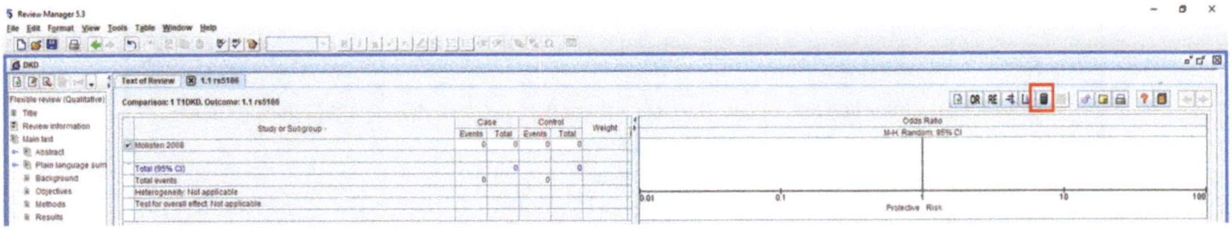

Fig. 34 Screenshots illustrating the RevMan step-by-step protocol

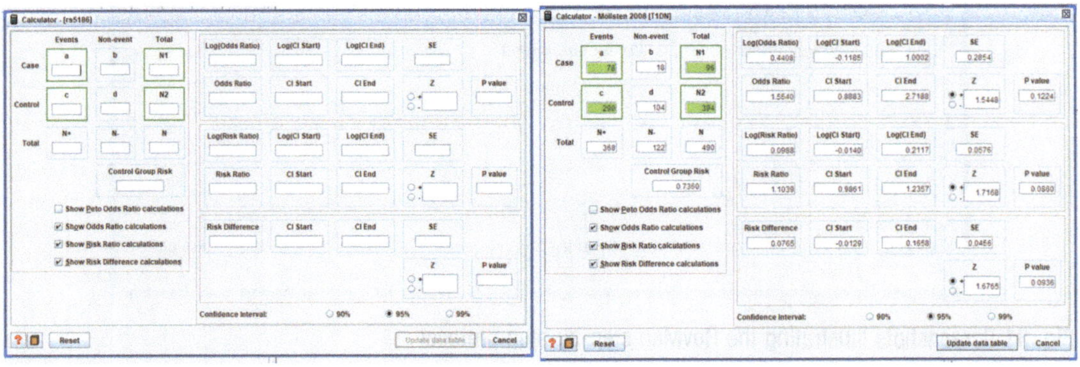

Fig. 35 Screenshots illustrating the RevMan step-by-step protocol

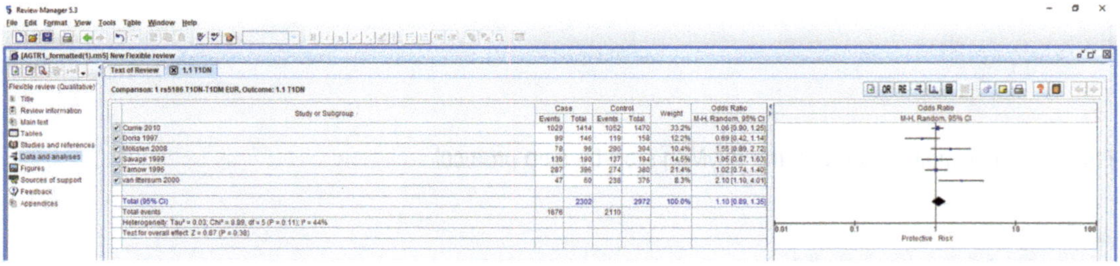

Fig. 36 Screenshots illustrating the RevMan step-by-step protocol

Step 25: This method is completed for all studies. A sample completed table is included below (Fig. 36).

Step 26: Click on the *Forest plot* icon to generate the following style of image (Fig. 37).

Step 27: Click on the *Funnel plot* icon to generate the following style of image (Fig. 38).

4 Notes

1. Quality control (QC) in targeted SNP studies should be less restricted by quality control filters:

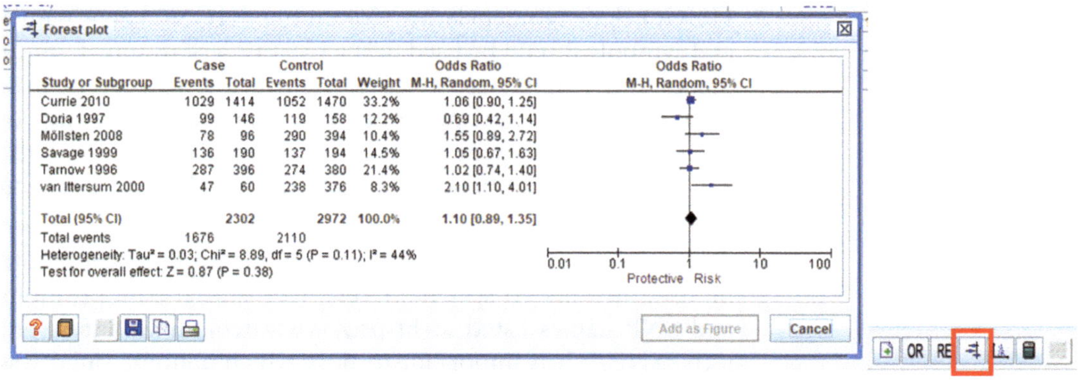

Fig. 37 Screenshots illustrating the RevMan step-by-step protocol

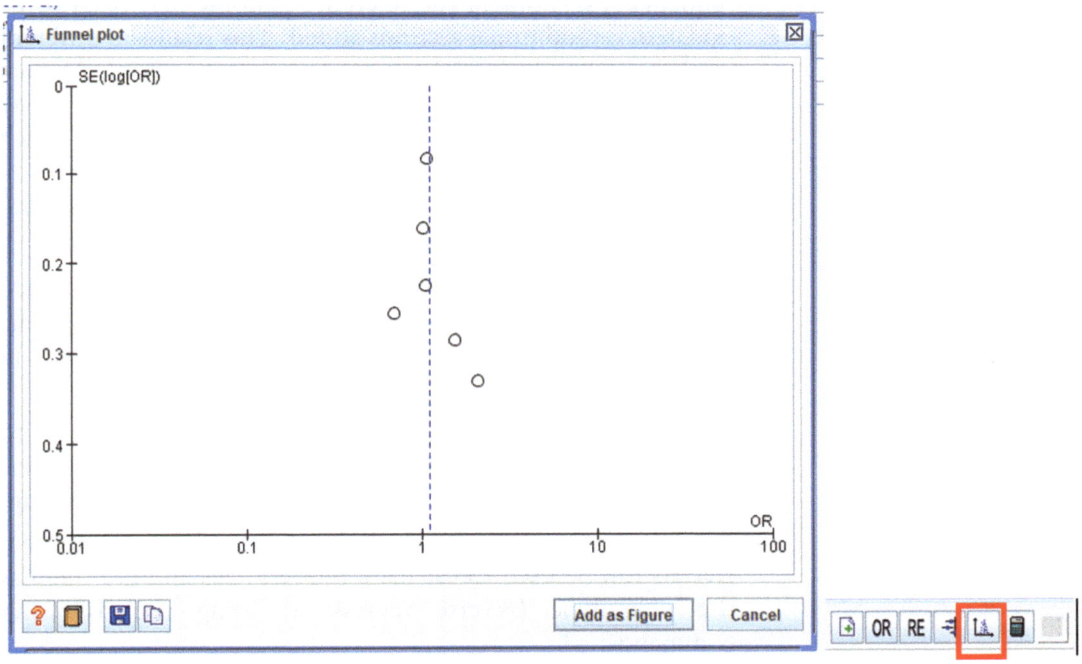

Fig. 38 Screenshots illustrating the RevMan step-by-step protocol

(a) Per-individual QC: exclude samples with missing data rate >20%.

(b) Per-marker QC: exclude SNPs with a missing rate of >5%, a MAF <1%, or an HWE *p*-value $<1 \times 10^{-4}$.

2. Genome-wide genotypes must be on the correct build for all the individual studies (e.g., 37/hg19) and correct strand (forward). If different batches of genotypes do not appear to "match," then check if there were version updates to the genotyping array employed and/or the same imputation approach was used across cohorts.

3. HUGO Gene Nomenclature Committee (HGNC) gene names and symbols should be used in the reporting of results. Unique names and symbols are given to human loci to prevent mis-communication and promote unambiguous reporting of results. Approved gene names should be obtained from the HUGO Gene Nomenclature Committee, https://beta.genenames.org/.
4. As well as unique loci annotations, unique SNP names should be used to refer to specific SNPs, with official base positions and SNP names listed at https://www.ncbi.nlm.nih.gov/projects/SNP/. It is important to note which genome build was used. A genome build is the construction of a reference genome using an array of different sequencing techniques. As these techniques improve and more of the genome is sequenced, sections of the reference genome may need to be updated, or additional sections added. This results in different versions or "builds" of the genome being produced. As such the base position of SNPs may change or merge between one genome build to the next, so it is important to note which genome build has been used.
5. For imputed variants, the association analysis can be carried on dosage instead of genotyped values.
6. Association analyses on sex chromosomes should be performed in males and females separately. Analysis of the mitochondrial genome requires specific analyses that are not covered in this text.
7. Association analyses should be stratified by ancestry. In order to do that, split the dataset in several files according to the different genetic background and repeat the analysis for each group.
8. For a quantitative trait which is not normally distributed, Rvtests can be used to calculate the residuals and use them as the phenotype (reverse regression) using the following commands:
   (a) *--useResidualAsPhenotype*\ to calculate the residuals before testing variants.
   (b) *--inverseNormal*\ to inverse normalize the residual distribution.
9. When no meta-analysis is planned, the *--meta* command in Rvtests can be substituted by the flag *--single,wald*, which generates single-variant Wald and score test for association tests for every variant.
10. RAREMETAL can carry out conditional analyses using the summary statistics in summary files and covariance files. To carry out a conditional analysis, it is necessary to create a text file that specifies the variant to condition on. The flag --

condition indicating the name of such file should be added to the command line.

11. RAREMETAL can also generate gene-level meta-analysis results in annotated files using rare variant-specific tests, as simple burden test, variable threshold test, Madson-Browning weighted burden test, and/or SKAT, and tabulates significant genes with detailed single-variant results included.
12. It is important to include GWAS data in a literature review and subsequent meta-analysis for targeted SNPs. Differences between reported and calculated *p*-values for some studies are frequently due to differences in handling of covariates or quality control filters. There are online tools to evaluate the quality of genetic association studies included in meta-analyses such as Q-GENIE [21].
13. If conducting a systematic review and meta-analysis separately to a primary genetic association study, then it is often possible to register a protocol prior to actually commencing the study. For example, https://www.biorxiv.org/; https://osf.io; https://www.crd.york.ac.uk/prospero/.
14. Be careful of data protection regulations as transitioning from directly typed SNPs in a GWAS to high-density imputed GWAS and next-generation sequencing datasets with associated clinical and demographic information raises privacy concerns with potentially identifiable data, particularly when rare and/or clinically actionable variants are considered.

References

1. McKnight AJ, Duffy S, Maxwell AP (2015) Genetics of diabetic nephropathy: a long road of discovery. Curr Diab Rep 15(7):41. https://doi.org/10.1007/s11892-015-0610-9
2. Chan Y, Lim ET, Sandholm N, Wang SR, McKnight AJ, Ripke S, Consortium D, Consortium G, Consortium G, Consortium I, Consortium PGC, Daly MJ, Neale BM, Salem RM, Hirschhorn JN (2014) An excess of risk-increasing low-frequency variants can be a signal of polygenic inheritance in complex diseases. Am J Hum Genet 94(3):437–452. https://doi.org/10.1016/j.ajhg.2014.02.006
3. Germain M, Pezzolesi MG, Sandholm N, McKnight AJ, Susztak K, Lajer M, Forsblom C, Marre M, Parving HH, Rossing P, Toppila I, Skupien J, Roussel R, Ko YA, Ledo N, Folkersen L, Civelek M, Maxwell AP, Tregouet DA, Groop PH, Tarnow L, Hadjadj S (2015) SORBS1 gene, a new candidate for diabetic nephropathy: results from a multi-stage genome-wide association study in patients with type 1 diabetes. Diabetologia 58 (3):543–548. https://doi.org/10.1007/s00125-014-3459-6
4. Sandholm N, Forsblom C, Makinen VP, McKnight AJ, Osterholm AM, He B, Harjutsalo V, Lithovius R, Gordin D, Parkkonen M, Saraheimo M, Thorn LM, Tolonen N, Waden J, Tuomilehto J, Lajer M, Ahlqvist E, Mollsten A, Marcovecchio ML, Cooper J, Dunger D, Paterson AD, Zerbini G, Groop L, Consortium S, Tarnow L, Maxwell AP, Tryggvason K, Groop PH, FinnDiane Study G (2014) Genome-wide association study of urinary albumin excretion rate in patients with type 1 diabetes. Diabetologia 57(6):1143–1153. https://doi.org/10.1007/s00125-014-3202-3
5. Sandholm N, McKnight AJ, Salem RM, Brennan EP, Forsblom C, Harjutsalo V, Makinen VP, McKay GJ, Sadlier DM, Williams WW, Martin F, Panduru NM, Tarnow L, Tuomilehto J, Tryggvason K, Zerbini G, Comeau ME, Langefeld CD, Consortium F, Godson C, Hirschhorn JN, Maxwell AP, Florez

JC, Groop PH, FinnDiane Study Group and the GENIE Consortium (2013) Chromosome 2q31.1 associates with ESRD in women with type 1 diabetes. J Am Soc Nephrol 24 (10):1537–1543. https://doi.org/10.1681/ASN.2012111122

6. Sandholm N, Salem RM, McKnight AJ, Brennan EP, Forsblom C, Isakova T, McKay GJ, Williams WW, Sadlier DM, Makinen VP, Swan EJ, Palmer C, Boright AP, Ahlqvist E, Deshmukh HA, Keller BJ, Huang H, Ahola AJ, Fagerholm E, Gordin D, Harjutsalo V, He B, Heikkila O, Hietala K, Kyto J, Lahermo P, Lehto M, Lithovius R, Osterholm AM, Parkkonen M, Pitkaniemi J, Rosengard-Barlund M, Saraheimo M, Sarti C, Soderlund J, Soro-Paavonen A, Syreeni A, Thorn LM, Tikkanen H, Tolonen N, Tryggvason K, Tuomilehto J, Waden J, Gill GV, Prior S, Guiducci C, Mirel DB, Taylor A, Hosseini SM, Group DER, Parving HH, Rossing P, Tarnow L, Ladenvall C, Alhenc-Gelas F, Lefebvre P, Rigalleau V, Roussel R, Tregouet DA, Maestroni A, Maestroni S, Falhammar H, Gu T, Mollsten A, Cimponeriu D, Ioana M, Mota M, Mota E, Serafinceanu C, Stavarachi M, Hanson RL, Nelson RG, Kretzler M, Colhoun HM, Panduru NM, Gu HF, Brismar K, Zerbini G, Hadjadj S, Marre M, Groop L, Lajer M, Bull SB, Waggott D, Paterson AD, Savage DA, Bain SC, Martin F, Hirschhorn JN, Godson C, Florez JC, Groop PH, Maxwell AP (2012) New susceptibility loci associated with kidney disease in type 1 diabetes. PLoS Genet 8(9): e1002921. https://doi.org/10.1371/journal.pgen.1002921

7. Sandholm N, Van Zuydam N, Ahlqvist E, Juliusdottir T, Deshmukh HA, Rayner NW, Di Camillo B, Forsblom C, Fadista J, Ziemek D, Salem RM, Hiraki LT, Pezzolesi M, Tregouet D, Dahlstrom E, Valo E, Oskolkov N, Ladenvall C, Marcovecchio ML, Cooper J, Sambo F, Malovini A, Manfrini M, McKnight AJ, Lajer M, Harjutsalo V, Gordin D, Parkkonen M, FinnDiane Study Group JT, Lyssenko V, McKeigue PM, Rich SS, Brosnan MJ, Fauman E, Bellazzi R, Rossing P, Hadjadj S, Krolewski A, Paterson AD, Dcct/Edic Study Group JCF, Hirschhorn JN, Maxwell AP, Genie Consortium DD, Cobelli C, Colhoun HM, Groop L, McCarthy MI, Groop PH, Consortium S (2017) The genetic landscape of renal complications in type 1 diabetes. J Am Soc Nephrol 28(2):557–574. https://doi.org/10.1681/ASN.2016020231

8. Todd JN, Dahlstrom EH, Salem RM, Sandholm N, Forsblom C, FinnDiane Study G, McKnight AJ, Maxwell AP, Brennan E, Sadlier D, Godson C, Groop PH, Hirschhorn JN, Florez JC (2015) Genetic evidence for a causal role of obesity in diabetic kidney disease. Diabetes 64(12):4238–4246. https://doi.org/10.2337/db15-0254

9. van Zuydam NR, Ahlqvist E, Sandholm N, Deshmukh H, Rayner NW, Abdalla M, Ladenvall C, Ziemek D, Fauman E, Robertson NR, McKeigue PM, Valo E, Forsblom C, Harjutsalo V, Finnish Diabetic Nephropathy S, Perna A, Rurali E, Marcovecchio ML, Igo RP Jr, Salem RM, Perico N, Lajer M, Karajamaki A, Imamura M, Kubo M, Takahashi A, Sim X, Liu J, van Dam RM, Jiang G, Tam CHT, Luk AOY, Lee HM, Lim CKP, Szeto CC, So WY, Chan JCN, Hong Kong Diabetes Registry Theme-based Research Scheme Project G, Ang SF, Dorajoo R, Wang L, Clara TSH, McKnight AJ, Duffy S, Warren, Genetics of Kidneys in Diabetes Study G, Pezzolesi MG, Consortium G, Marre M, Gyorgy B, Hadjadj S, Hiraki LT, Diabetes C, Complications Trial/Epidemiology of Diabetes I, Complications Research G, Ahluwalia TS, Almgren P, Schulz CA, Orho-Melander M, Linneberg A, Christensen C, Witte DR, Grarup N, Brandslund I, Melander O, Paterson AD, Tregouet D, Maxwell AP, Lim SC, Ma RCW, Tai ES, Maeda S, Lyssenko V, Tuomi T, Krolewski AS, Rich SS, Hirschhorn JN, Florez JC, Dunger D, Pedersen O, Hansen T, Rossing P, Remuzzi G, Micro SUmf, Macrovascular hard endpoints for Innovative diabetes Tools C, Brosnan MJ, Palmer CNA, Groop PH, Colhoun HM, Groop LC, McCarthy MI (2018) A genome-wide association study of diabetic kidney disease in subjects with type 2 diabetes. Diabetes 67(7):1414–1427. https://doi.org/10.2337/db17-0914

10. Williams WW, Salem RM, McKnight AJ, Sandholm N, Forsblom C, Taylor A, Guiducci C, McAteer JB, McKay GJ, Isakova T, Brennan EP, Sadlier DM, Palmer C, Soderlund J, Fagerholm E, Harjutsalo V, Lithovius R, Gordin D, Hietala K, Kyto J, Parkkonen M, Rosengard-Barlund M, Thorn L, Syreeni A, Tolonen N, Saraheimo M, Waden J, Pitkaniemi J, Sarti C, Tuomilehto J, Tryggvason K, Osterholm AM, He B, Bain S, Martin F, Godson C, Hirschhorn JN, Maxwell AP, Groop PH, Florez JC, Consortium G (2012) Association testing of previously reported variants in a large case-control meta-analysis of diabetic nephropathy. Diabetes 61(8):2187–2194. https://doi.org/10.2337/db11-0751

11. Iyengar SK, Sedor JR, Freedman BI, Kao WH, Kretzler M, Keller BJ, Abboud HE, Adler SG, Best LG, Bowden DW, Burlock A, Chen YD, Cole SA, Comeau ME, Curtis JM, Divers J, Drechsler C, Duggirala R, Elston RC, Guo X, Huang H, Hoffmann MM, Howard BV, Ipp E, Kimmel PL, Klag MJ, Knowler WC, Kohn OF, Leak TS, Leehey DJ, Li M, Malhotra A, Marz W, Nair V, Nelson RG, Nicholas SB, O'Brien SJ, Pahl MV, Parekh RS, Pezzolesi MG, Rasooly RS, Rotimi CN, Rotter JI, Schelling JR, Seldin MF, Shah VO, Smiles AM, Smith MW, Taylor KD, Thameem F, Thornley-Brown DP, Truitt BJ, Wanner C, Weil EJ, Winkler CA, Zager PG, Igo RP Jr, Hanson RL, Langefeld CD, Family Investigation of N, Diabetes (2015) Genome-wide association and trans-ethnic meta-analysis for advanced diabetic kidney disease: family investigation of nephropathy and diabetes (FIND). PLoS Genet 11(8):e1005352. https://doi.org/10.1371/journal.pgen.1005352
12. Chang CC, Chow CC, Tellier LC, Vattikuti S, Purcell SM, Lee JJ (2015) Second-generation PLINK: rising to the challenge of larger and richer datasets. Gigascience 4:7. https://doi.org/10.1186/s13742-015-0047-8
13. Purcell S, Neale B, Todd-Brown K, Thomas L, Ferreira MA, Bender D, Maller J, Sklar P, de Bakker PI, Daly MJ, Sham PC (2007) PLINK: a tool set for whole-genome association and population-based linkage analyses. Am J Hum Genet 81(3):559–575. https://doi.org/10.1086/519795
14. Zhan X, Hu Y, Li B, Abecasis GR, Liu DJ (2016) RVTESTS: an efficient and comprehensive tool for rare variant association analysis using sequence data. Bioinformatics 32 (9):1423–1426. https://doi.org/10.1093/bioinformatics/btw079
15. Feng S, Liu D, Zhan X, Wing MK, Abecasis GR (2014) RAREMETAL: fast and powerful meta-analysis for rare variants. Bioinformatics 30(19):2828–2829. https://doi.org/10.1093/bioinformatics/btu367
16. Copenhagen: The Nordic Cochrane Centre TCC (2014) Review Manager (RevMan). 5 edn
17. Higgins JP, Thompson SG, Deeks JJ, Altman DG (2003) Measuring inconsistency in meta-analyses. BMJ 327(7414):557–560. https://doi.org/10.1136/bmj.327.7414.557
18. Nedovic D, Panic N, Pastorino R, Ricciardi W, Boccia S (2016) Evaluation of the endorsement of the strengthening the reporting of genetic association studies (STREGA) statement on the reporting quality of published genetic association studies. J Epidemiol 26 (8):399–404. https://doi.org/10.2188/jea.JE20150173
19. von Elm E, Moher D, Little J, Collaboration S (2009) Reporting genetic association studies: the STREGA statement. Lancet 374 (9684):98–100. https://doi.org/10.1016/S0140-6736(09)61265-4
20. Stroup DF, Berlin JA, Morton SC, Olkin I, Williamson GD, Rennie D, Moher D, Becker BJ, Sipe TA, Thacker SB (2000) Meta-analysis of observational studies in epidemiology: a proposal for reporting. Meta-analysis of observational studies in epidemiology (MOOSE) group. JAMA 283(15):2008–2012
21. Sohani ZN, Meyre D, de Souza RJ, Joseph PG, Gandhi M, Dennis BB, Norman G, Anand SS (2015) Assessing the quality of published genetic association studies in meta-analyses: the quality of genetic studies (Q-Genie) tool. BMC Genet 16:50. https://doi.org/10.1186/s12863-015-0211-2

Chapter 17

Assessment of Urinary MicroRNAs by Quantitative Polymerase Chain Reaction in Diabetic Nephropathy Patients

Lucy Jade Newbury, Alexa Wonnacott, Kate Simpson, Timothy Bowen, and Donald Fraser

Abstract

Urinary microRNAs show promise as noninvasive biomarkers in renal disease. Here, we describe a detailed protocol for the column-based extraction and quantification of miRNAs by reverse-transcription quantitative polymerase chain reaction (RT-qPCR) from urine samples.

Key words MicroRNAs, Urine, Biomarker, Diabetic nephropathy, Chronic kidney disease, RT-qPCR

1 Introduction

Diabetic nephropathy (DN) is the leading cause of kidney failure requiring renal replacement therapy worldwide, but effective methods to identify and halt progression of disease-specific pathophysiological changes remain elusive [1–3]. Currently, monitoring of DN progression is carried out by detection of urinary microalbuminuria, but since not all microalbuminuric patients progress to overt nephropathy prognosis is complicated [4].

While numerous novel DN biomarkers have been analyzed, none are currently in routine clinical use, and they may lack specificity and sensitivity to predict individual DN patient outcomes. Novel markers that can discriminate etiology, DN progression, or response to treatment therefore remain highly desirable.

The majority of the protein-coding genes encoded by the human genome are regulated by microRNAs (miRNAs), ubiquitously expressed short noncoding RNAs. Detection of miR-192, miR-194, miR-215, miR-216, miR-146a, miR-204, and miR-886 is elevated in the kidney [5]. Successful reverse-transcription quantitative polymerase chain reaction (RT-qPCR) detection of circulating miRNAs has been described [6] and we have shown that urinary

Luigi Gnudi and David A. Long (eds.), *Diabetic Nephropathy: Methods and Protocols*, Methods in Molecular Biology, vol. 2067, https://doi.org/10.1007/978-1-4939-9841-8_17,

miRNAs represent a highly promising novel source of noninvasive biomarkers that are stabilized via association with argonaute 2 protein and/or extracellular vesicle exosomes and are rapidly and precisely detected by RT-qPCR [7].

One key criterion for potential biomarker evaluation is the ease with which it can be integrated into existing care pathways. In this context, urinary miRNA biomarkers have several potential significant advantages over circulating miRNAs for adoption, including speed and cost of noninvasive sample access [8]. However, few urinary miRNA DN biomarker candidates have so far been reported. We provide here practical protocols for detection of urinary miRNAs by RT-qPCR, together with notes on the applicability of our technique for analyzing other liquid biopsies. We also consider the potential impact of emerging technologies, including RNA sequencing, on biomarker identification.

Roles for miRNAs in DN pathology have been identified [9, 10], including previous work from this laboratory showing decreased miR-192 detection in biopsies from late-stage diabetic kidney disease (DKD) patients with diminished renal function [11]. This underlines the potential of miRNAs as DN biomarkers, which will best be selected on the basis of function in addition to differences in abundance [12]. In conclusion, urinary miRNAs have considerable potential as biomarkers for DN and other renal diseases. Indeed, selected miRNA detection might be used in conjunction with existing and other novel markers as part of a DN biomarker panel.

2 Materials

2.1 Urine Sample Collection and Storage

1. Universal Collection (UC) tubes.
2. Centrifuge compatible with 20 mL UC and 2000 × *g*.
3. 1.5 mL Microcentrifuge tubes.

2.2 Total RNA Isolation from Urine (see Note 1)

1. Carrier RNA (*see* **Note 2**).
2. Spike-in extraction control—*Caenorhabditis elegans*, cel-miR-39, dilute stock to 0.5pM/μL (*see* **Note 3**).
3. Extraction columns—optimized for Qiagen miRNeasy mini kit (*see* **Note 4**).
4. 1.5 mL Microcentrifuge.

2.3 miRNA Quantification Using RT-qPCR

1. miRNA PCR assays, either commercially available or designed using bioinformatics tools (*see* **Note 5**): We recommend TaqMan™ miRNA Assay, ThermoFisher Scientific Catalog No. 4427975 (assay ID for miR-191 = 002299, cel-miR-39 = 000200).

2. Thermal cycler for reverse-transcription (RT) reaction.
3. qPCR machine: We routinely use VIA7 with a 96-well fast block.
4. Plastics: PCR tubes/strips, PCR plates (compatible with qPCR machine), pipette tips, 1.5 mL microcentrifuge tube.
5. PCR reagents appropriate for PCR assays used: We routinely use TaqMan™ Universal Master Mix II (no UNG) Catalog No. 4440040.

3 Methods

3.1 Urine Sample Collection and Storage

1. Collect urine sample and immediately place on ice (*see* **Note 6**).
2. Centrifuge samples at 4 °C at 2000 × *g* (RCF) for 10 min (*see* **Note 7**).
3. Aliquot the supernatant for RNA extraction and biochemistry analysis to avoid repeated freeze-thaw cycles. Store the remaining spun urine in a universal container (20 mL) (*see* **Note 8**).
4. Store at −80 °C until needed or proceed immediately to Subheading 3.2 for RNA extraction.

3.2 Total RNA Isolation from Urine

This protocol is adapted from Qiagen miRNeasy kit Catalog No. 217004 (*see* **Note 4**). Although this protocol is developed for miRNA extraction from urine, it may be easily adapted for other biofluids (*see* **Note 9**). This protocol has been validated to confirm that the presence of proteinuria does not impact the efficiency of the reaction (*see* **Note 10**).

1. Defrost urine sample on ice, if required.
2. On ice, add 1 μg of MS2 bacteriophage carrier RNA to 350 μL of urine sample (*see* **Note 2**).
3. On ice, add 0.5 pM spike-in of *Caenorhabditis elegans* (cel--miR-39) to each urine sample/carrier mix (*see* **Note 3**).
4. On ice, add 750 μL of QIAzol. Invert tube to mix. Incubate at room temperature for 5 min.
5. Under a fume hood, add 200 μL of chloroform to each sample and mix vigorously. Incubate at room temperature for 2–3 min.
6. Centrifuge the samples at 4 °C at 12,000 × *g* for 15 min.
7. Transfer the upper aqueous phase (600 μL) to a new collection tube. Avoid transferring any interphase. Add 1.5× volumes (900 μL) of 100% ethanol, and mix thoroughly by pipetting (*see* **Note 11**).
8. From this point, revert to the manufacturer's protocol. If using a different kit, adapt appropriately.

9. Add 700 μL of ethanol/aqueous phase mix onto a single affinity column. Centrifuge for 15 s at 12,000 × *g*. Discard the flow-through. Repeat until all samples are bound to affinity column.
10. Add 700 μL buffer RWT to the RNeasy Mini column. Close the lid, and centrifuge for 15 s at 12,000 × *g*. Discard the flow-through.
11. Add 500 μL buffer RPE to the RNeasy Mini column. Close the lid, and centrifuge for 15 s at 12,000 × *g*. Discard the flow-through. Repeat this step.
12. Spin for 2 min at full speed to dry the column.
13. Elute samples in 50 μL of RNase-free water and store at −80 °C until analysis (*see* **Note 11**).

3.3 miRNA Quantification: RT-qPCR

1. Our preferred method of individual miRNA quantification is a two-step RT-qPCR, using a specific miRNA RT for each miRNA, followed by relative qPCR quantification. We routinely use TaqMan™ miRNA assays (*see* **Notes 5** and **12**) but other methods of miRNA quantification may be used (*see* **Note 13**).
2. Add between 1 and 5 μL of eluted RNA sample from Subheading 3.2, deoxynucleotide (DNTPs), reverse transcriptase, reaction buffer, specific miRNA primer, RNase inhibitor, and molecular grade water to a 200 μL PCR tube as per the manufacturer's instructions. We routinely use high-capacity cDNA reverse transcription (*see* **Note 14**).
3. Place RT reaction on a thermal cycler and run on appropriate RT settings, for example: 13 min at 16 °C (for RT primer annealing), 30 min at 42 °C (for random DNTP extension), 5 min at 85 °C (to dissociate the annealing primer), and at 4 °C for infinity. After RT reaction samples can be stored at −20 °C.
4. To normalize the target miRNA data, a reference miRNA is also measured. We most frequently use miR-191 (*see* **Note 12**).
5. Cel-miR-39 was added during the extraction process and may also be measured at this point using a specific RT reaction, to control for RNA extraction efficiency (*see* **Note 3**).
6. Dilute the RT reactions for each miRNA with 30 μL of molecular grade water to a total volume of 45 μL prior to qPCR analysis (*see* **Notes 9** and **15**).
7. In a 1.5 mL microcentrifuge tube, add DNTPs, DNA polymerase enzyme, reaction buffer, and specific miRNA primer probe. This is normally commercially provided in an easy-to-use master mix; we routinely use TaqMan™ Universal Master Mix II (no UNG), according to the manufacturer's instructions.

8. Pipette 4 μL of diluted RT reaction (cDNA) along with 16 μL of master mix into a 96-well plate (appropriate for machine and block used, *see* **Note 16**). We routinely perform qPCR reactions in triplicate (*see* **Note 17**).
9. Place plate on qPCR machine and run qPCR reaction. The PCR reaction we routinely use is as follows: 10 min at 95 °C, for 40 cycles: 15 s at 95 °C (denature) and 60 s at 60 °C (anneal/extend).
10. When running multiple plates or combining data/cohorts from different time points, use inter-run calibrators (ICR) to normalize between plates. Additional RT reactions of chosen ICR samples should be performed and run on each plate (*see* **Note 18**).
11. Analyze data using the $2^{\wedge -ddct}$ method, displayed as fold change relative to the control group (*see* **Note 19**).

4 Notes

Urine Sample Collection and Storage

1. Our protocol describes miRNA extraction from total urine samples. It is also possible to apply this protocol to urinary fractions obtained from, e.g., sucrose density gradient centrifugation, and thereby compare extracellular vesicle- and non-extracellular vesicle-miRNA populations. We have shown that urinary miRNAs are associated with exosomes isolated by this method [7].
2. As mentioned in **Note 4**, the yield of RNA from urine samples is low and we have therefore recommended the addition of an RNA carrier to maximize efficient RNA recovery. Our protocol uses MS2 RNA carrier from bacteriophage, but other RNA carriers may be used. A limitation of the addition of RNA carrier is its interference with quantification, quality measurements, and downstream techniques such as sequencing. During sequencing, the carrier itself will be sequenced, thus wasting a large proportion of sequencing reads. This will impact the depth of sequencing of miRNAs present in the sample.
3. We recommend addition of a spike-in control to control for RNA efficiency. This is particularly important when extractions are batched over time. Our recommended spike-in control is *C. elegans* miRNA cel-miR-39, a transcript not present in human-derived samples. However, as in **Note 2** above, the addition of a spike-in control limits accurate quantification of RNA samples.

4. RNA extraction is generally performed in one of the two ways: using a column-based extraction method, or by isopropanol RNA precipitation of the RNA. As the RNA yield from urine samples is very low, we favor column-based extraction in this setting. In this protocol we describe a column-based extraction technique specifically optimized for use with the miRNeasy mini kit, but this protocol may be adapted for use with other commercially available column-based kits.

Total RNA Isolation from Urine

5. Numerous kits are commercially available for miRNA quantification by RT-qPCR that use either a miRNA-specific primer as part of a miRNA-specific RT reaction, or a universal primer, prior to qPCR. Our preferred kit is TaqMan™ miRNA assay Catalog No. 4427975. These kits use a miRNA-specific RT primer. For researchers wishing to use their own miRNA RT-qPCR protocols, Internet-accessible primer design software is available. In our experience this process is not straightforward.
6. We recommend that urine samples are placed on ice or at 4 °C post-collection, aliquoted, and frozen as soon as possible. We have detected miRNAs following 24 h of room temperature storage, at approximately 60% of signal seen at time zero [7].
7. We recommend sample centrifugation at 2000 × *g* for 10 min to maximize the yield of the subsequent RNA extraction from the supernatant. The pellet collected by this process may also be analyzed for miRNA content. If desired, this step may be performed using the same RNA extraction protocol described in Subheading 3.2. Since we focus on streamlining miRNA detection for use in the point-of-care clinical environment, we do not routinely analyze pellets.
8. Repeated freeze-thaw cycles are not encouraged for RNA samples, but may be unavoidable. We have detected miRNAs following four freeze-thaw cycles, but at reduced relative expression.
9. The protocol described in this chapter focuses on the miRNA extraction from urine samples. However, this protocol may also be applied to other biofluids including blood and dialysis fluid, with minimal adjustment. Indeed, we have described the extraction of miRNAs from peritoneal dialysis effluent using a related protocol [13].
10. In our cohorts to date, proteinuria up to 3G/24h or equivalent has not affected the extraction process; however the effect of higher levels of proteinuria and/or other urinary abnormalities are yet to be tested.

miRNA Quantification Using RT-qPCR

11. Throughout this protocol it is critical to maintain equivalent input volume, aqueous volume, and elution volume for processing of each urine sample. This is particularly important when RNA carrier and/or spike-in control are employed, since the eluted RNA cannot be quantified.
12. The choice of reference selection to normalize miRNA data is an ongoing debate. For a miRNA to act as a good reference, its expression should not change between, for example, control and disease groups. The situation is complicated further in urine sample analysis since we must also account for variability in hydration levels, and therefore urine concentration, irrespective of the presence or absence of disease. When selecting a reference miRNA, it is therefore important to demonstrate *equivalent* variability in both control and disease groups. In our experience, miR-191 has proved suitable for the analysis of diabetic nephropathy and acute kidney injury cohorts compared to control groups. A functional role of miR-191 in renal disease has not been reported.
13. Other techniques for miRNA detection include TaqMan™ Low Density Arrays (TLDAs), miRNA hybridization arrays, and next-generation sequencing (NGS)—RNA-seq. These techniques allow the simultaneous quantification of multiple miRNAs. A TLDA card uses qPCR-based technology to reproducibly detect over 350 miRNAs. TLDA card analysis involves a pre-amplification step, and we have generated robust data from low RNA yields such as urine using this technique. miRNA hybridization arrays permit the detection of 1500–2000 miRNAs, depending on the array used. NGS is capable of detecting all miRNAs in the cell using sequence-by-synthesis technology, most commonly undertaken using the Illumina platform. This powerful technology has been optimized for use with high-yield, high-quality RNA samples, but newer kits are emerging that extend to the use of lower yield samples.
14. The addition of RNA carrier and spike-in control means that RNA quantification and analysis of RNA integrity are not possible. These reagents can be removed from the protocol, but this decreases RNA yield.
15. Dilution of each sample following reverse transcription (RT) is recommended to prevent the enzymes/reagents used in the RT reaction from inhibiting the efficiency of the downstream qPCR. It is of particular importance that the samples are diluted with a standardized volume of water due to the inability to quantify the amount of input RNA (*see* **Note 11**).

16. Many different qPCR machines and blocks are available commercially and would be applicable to this protocol; we routinely use a VIA7 with a fast 96-well block.
17. Accurate pipetting is crucial for validity and reproducibility of the results, both at RT and qPCR stages of the protocol. It is recommended that qPCR reactions should be replicated in triplicate to demonstrate accurate pipetting.
18. Inter-run calibrators (IRCs) are samples replicated on all PCR plates to control for inter-plate variability. IRCs can either be a set of predefined control samples or a set of chosen samples from initial plate runs that are then repeated on all subsequent plates. IRCs are critically important in biomarker studies/large patient cohorts when miRNA analyses for single miRNAs must be carried out using multiple plates, and when combining analyses from multiple cohorts. When making a set of IRCs, it is important to ensure that there is sufficient quantity to be used throughout the entire project. Therefore, we recommend combining multiple RT reactions to insure adequate volumes of IRC stock. In addition, to avoid repeated freeze-thaw, aliquot IRCs. IRC samples should have equivalent miRNA abundance as test samples, ideally from the same starting material. We routinely run nine IRCs per plate, derived from three urine samples, analyzing three different miRNAs that represent low, average, and high abundance in control samples.
19. For miRNA biomarker discovery we recommend the use of relative quantification, allowing a cost-effective way to compare many different miRNAs in the context of disease versus control, without the relatively cumbersome requirement of an individual standard curve for each miRNA analyzed on each PCR plate. However, absolute quantification would be warranted at the point of implementation as a diagnostic tool in the clinical setting.

References

1. Jha V, Garcia-Garcia G, Iseki K, Li Z, Naicker S, Plattner B, Saran R, Wang AY, Yang CW (2013) Chronic kidney disease: global dimension and perspectives. Lancet 382(9888):260–272. Elsevier Ltd, England. https://doi.org/10.1016/s0140-6736(13)60687-x
2. Cowie CC, Port FK, Wolfe RA, Savage PJ, Moll PP, Hawthorne VM (1989) Disparities in incidence of diabetic end-stage renal disease according to race and type of diabetes. N Engl J Med 321(16):1074–1079. https://doi.org/10.1056/nejm198910193211603
3. Regele F, Jelencsics K, Shiffman D, Pare G, McQueen MJ, Mann JF, Oberbauer R (2015) Genome-wide studies to identify risk factors for kidney disease with a focus on patients with diabetes. Nephrol Dial Transplant 30(Suppl 4):iv26–iv34. The Author 2015. Published by Oxford University Press on behalf of ERA-EDTA, England. https://doi.org/10.1093/ndt/gfv087
4. Parving HH, Persson F, Rossing P (2015) Microalbuminuria: a parameter that has changed diabetes care. Diabetes Res Clin Pract 107(1):1–8. Elsevier Ireland Ltd,

Ireland. https://doi.org/10.1016/j.diabres.2014.10.014

5. Landgraf P, Rusu M, Sheridan R, Sewer A, Iovino N, Aravin A, Pfeffer S, Rice A, Kamphorst AO, Landthaler M, Lin C, Socci ND, Hermida L, Fulci V, Chiaretti S, Foa R, Schliwka J, Fuchs U, Novosel A, Muller RU, Schermer B, Bissels U, Inman J, Phan Q, Chien M, Weir DB, Choksi R, De Vita G, Frezzetti D, Trompeter HI, Hornung V, Teng G, Hartmann G, Palkovits M, Di Lauro R, Wernet P, Macino G, Rogler CE, Nagle JW, Ju J, Papavasiliou FN, Benzing T, Lichter P, Tam W, Brownstein MJ, Bosio A, Borkhardt A, Russo JJ, Sander C, Zavolan M, Tuschl T (2007) A mammalian microRNA expression atlas based on small RNA library sequencing. Cell 129(7):1401–1414
6. Arroyo JD, Chevillet JR, Kroh EM, Ruf IK, Pritchard CC, Gibson DF, Mitchell PS, Bennett CF, Pogosova-Agadjanyan EL, Stirewalt DL, Tait JF, Tewari M (2011) Argonaute 2 complexes carry a population of circulating microRNAs independent of vesicles in human plasma. Proc Natl Acad Sci U S A 108 (12):5003–5008
7. Beltrami C, Clayton A, Newbury LJ, Corish P, Jenkins RH, Phillips AO, Fraser DJ, Bowen T (2015) Stabilization of urinary microRNAs by association with exosomes and argonaute 2 protein. Noncoding RNA 1(2):151–166. https://doi.org/10.3390/ncrna1020151
8. Smith DA, Newbury LJ, Drago G, Bowen T, Redman JE (2017) Electrochemical detection of urinary microRNAs via sulfonamide-bound antisense hybridisation. Sensors Actuators B Chem 253. (Suppl C:335–341. https://doi.org/10.1016/j.snb.2017.06.069
9. Trionfini P, Benigni A, Remuzzi G (2015) MicroRNAs in kidney physiology and disease. Nat Rev Nephrol 11(1):23–33. England. https://doi.org/10.1038/nrneph.2014.202
10. Simpson K, Wonnacott A, Fraser DJ, Bowen T (2016) MicroRNAs in diabetic nephropathy: from biomarkers to therapy. Curr Diab Rep 16(3):35. https://doi.org/10.1007/s11892-016-0724-8
11. Krupa A, Jenkins R, Luo DD, Lewis A, Phillips A, Fraser D (2010) Loss of MicroRNA-192 promotes fibrogenesis in diabetic nephropathy. J Am Soc Nephrol 21 (3):438–447. https://doi.org/10.1681/ASN.2009050530
12. Heinzel A, Muhlberger I, Stelzer G, Lancet D, Oberbauer R, Martin M, Perco P (2015) Molecular disease presentation in diabetic nephropathy. Nephrol Dial Transplant 30 (Suppl 4):iv17–iv25. The Author 2015. Published by Oxford University Press on behalf of ERA-EDTA, England. https://doi.org/10.1093/ndt/gfv267
13. Lopez-Anton M, Lambie M, Lopez-Cabrera-M, Schmitt CP, Ruiz-Carpio V, Bartosova M, Schaefer B, Davies S, Stone T, Jenkins R, Taylor PR, Topley N, Bowen T, Fraser D (2017) miR-21 promotes fibrogenesis in peritoneal dialysis. Am J Pathol 187(7):1537–1550. https://doi.org/10.1016/j.ajpath.2017.03.007

Chapter 18

Metabolomic and Proteomic Techniques for Establishing Biomarkers and Improving Our Understanding of Pathophysiology in Diabetic Nephropathy

Justyna Siwy, Linda Ahonen, Pedro Magalhães, Maria Frantzi, and Peter Rossing

Abstract

Molecular studies of the proteome and metabolome in readily available body fluids such as urine and blood performed in a comprehensive qualitative and quantitative way are a valuable source of information for kidney disease research. They provide potential biomarkers of disease progression, markers of efficacy of interventions, as well as information on the underlying pathophysiology. Identified proteins and metabolites may point to dysregulated biological pathways and this knowledge may be useful in the identification of new treatment targets.

Many studies, focusing on chronic kidney disease as well as diabetic nephropathy, demonstrate that peptidome and metabolome analysis can substantially contribute to early detection and prediction of disease progression, but also stratification of kidney disease in clinical practice. An innovative, well-explored application of urinary peptidome analysis is the back-translation of results obtained in humans to animals, for animal model validation and improvement of the preclinical readouts. In this chapter, we provide an overview of urinary proteomic analysis with the CE-MS analytical platform, a strategy that has been successfully employed in several studies for the identification and validation of biomarkers in kidney diseases. We describe how to obtain the orthology between the animal model and humans. We also deliver an overview of the analysis of the metabolome with the GC×GC-TOF-MS and UHPLC-Q-TOF-MS analytical platforms for blood and serum as new methods being applied in kidney disease.

It is expected that a systems medicine approach to kidney disease including multiple omics methods will provide us with the best way to understand and treat diabetic kidney disease in the future.

Key words Capillary electrophoresis, Mass spectrometry, Urine, Rodent, Clinical proteomics, Peptidomics

1 Introduction

Diabetes is a disease with an increasing prevalence and therefore it is of high importance to investigate the possible metabolic pathways

Justyna Siwy and Linda Ahonen have contributed equally.

Luigi Gnudi and David A. Long (eds.), *Diabetic Nephropathy: Methods and Protocols*, Methods in Molecular Biology, vol. 2067, https://doi.org/10.1007/978-1-4939-9841-8_18,

affected by this disease. It is, however, equally important to investigate the complications caused by diabetes. Diabetic nephropathy (DN) or diabetic kidney disease (DKD) is one of the complications caused by diabetes [1–4], and single biomarkers, or multiple markers measured with proteomic and metabolomic methods in blood or urine, have been used in order to achieve a broader understanding of this diabetes-related complication and the progress thereof [1–6].

Urine is considered a very good source of biomarkers for kidney diseases, being often explored via different -omics methods [7]. The protein and peptide molecules that are present in urine show high stability, and as they are in direct proximity with the kidney, they can provide information about the pathophysiology of kidney disease [8]. Moreover, urinary peptidomics analysis, as being performed in a holistic manner, can display both acute and long-term events, providing a "snapshot" of the peptidome at a given time point. In addition, taking into consideration that the majority of current and new drugs target protein functions and networks, in this context, an efficient translation of the knowledge obtained using animal models to the clinic via the application of peptidomics analysis would be beneficial. As such, a humanized readout for a disease can ease the transition from preclinical to clinical drug discovery phase (Fig. 1). Research toward this direction has already been advanced for rodents. As such, Klein et al. were able to improve the translatability of the results obtained in an animal model for DN (diabetes *db/db* mice and BTBR*ob/ob* mice), showing the possibility of identifying a panel of identical molecular features in both humans and animal models [9]. In this study, for the detection of the identical disease-associated urinary peptides in mice and human, capillary electrophoresis coupled online to an electrospray ionization time-of-flight mass spectrometer (CE-MS) technology was performed [9, 10]. In another study, involving rats, the same technology was successfully applied for the comparison of disease-associated peptides in human and Zucker diabetic rats to investigate whether this animal model was able to display similar features of human disease [11].

The CE-MS is a powerful proteomic technology that enables the analysis of naturally occurring peptides and has been successfully applied in multiple clinical proteomics studies, as recently reviewed [12, 13]. The principle of the analysis lies in the coupling of a separation platform (capillary electrophoresis) to a time-of-flight mass spectrometer. During the first step of the analysis, the separation through fused silica capillaries is based on the differences in the electrophoretic mobility of the peptides, which is dependent on the charge and size of the molecule. Directly after the separation, the peptides are ionized and entered to migrate in the time-of-flight mass spectrometer, where the ion peaks are eventually detected. This technology showed very high reproducibility and

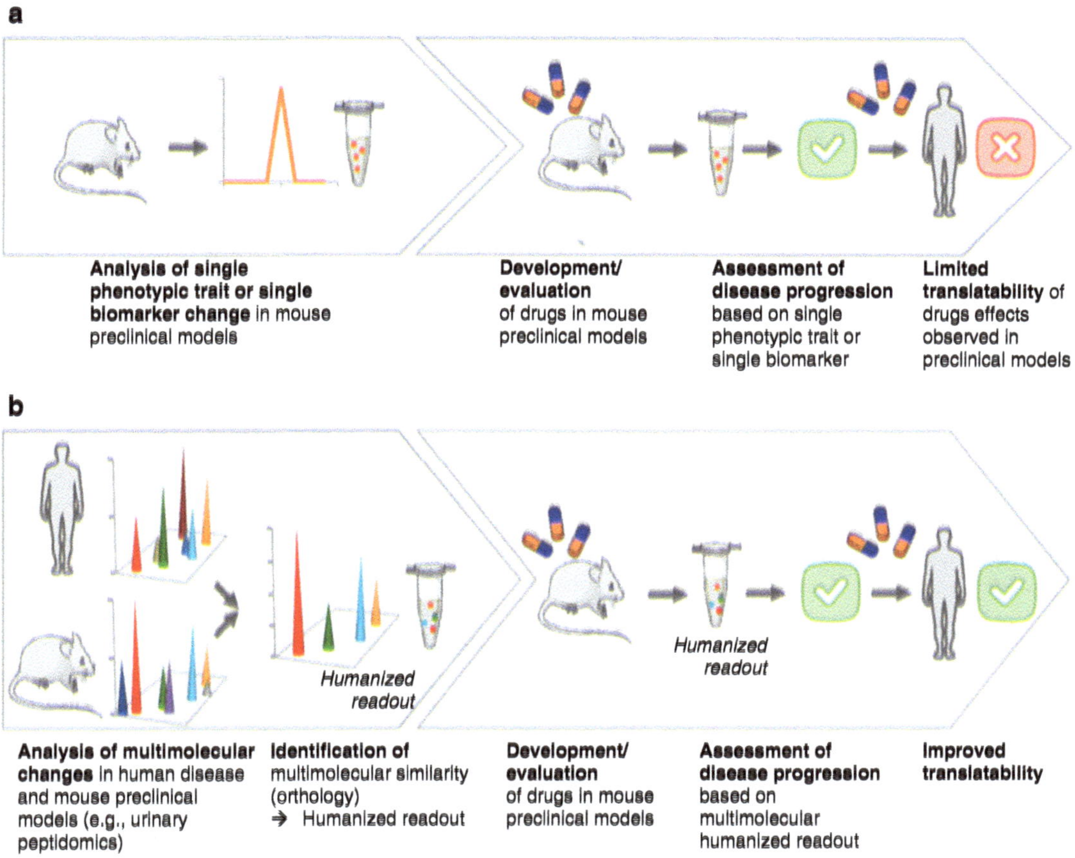

Fig. 1 Improvement of the translatability between human and animal models of disease for treatment development. (**a**) Limited translatability of a single phenotypic trait or biomarker in animals and humans. A single feature is not able to determinate the complexity of most disorders. Therefore, novel drugs, although successful in the preclinical phase, often fail in humans, when only based on such single-feature readout. (**b**) In contrast, the analysis of multimolecular changes using omics approaches (e.g., urinary peptidomics) gives the possibility for more complete description of complex phenotypes. Furthermore, the combination of these multiple features similar (ortholog) in human disease and animal models, leading to a "humanized" readout, most likely will more efficiently translate the effects of new drugs in preclinical models to the clinic (reprinted from Kidney International, 2016, Vol. 90, Issue 5, Julie Klein, Adela Ramirez-Torres, Anette Ericsson, Yufeng Huang, Benjamin Breuil, Justyna Siwy, Harald Mischak, Xiao-Rong Peng, Jean-Loup Bascands and Joost P. Schanstra, "Urinary peptidomics provides a noninvasive humanized readout of diabetic nephropathy in mice." 1045-55, with permission from Elsevier)

accuracy [14], particularly in urine. The high reproducibility of CE-MS is achieved in our hands by the careful selection of the analyzed body fluid and by profiling all samples under highly standardized preparation/analysis conditions and stringent quality control steps. Recently, all necessary steps to carry out the urinary proteome analysis using CE-MS technology in kidney disease of humans were described [15].

The term metabolomics was defined by Oliver Fiehn in 2002 as *the comprehensive analysis in which all the metabolites of a biological system are identified and quantified* [16]. Within metabolomics (and proteomics) the field is mainly divided into targeted and non-targeted analysis. The non-targeted approach is usually based on rapid high-throughput analysis of all possible metabolites present in a given set of samples without prior knowledge of the metabolites [17, 18]. Often, little or no effort is put into quantifying any of the metabolites when utilizing a non-targeted approach as there is a big uncertainty due to multiple variables and unidentified metabolites present in the samples [18–21]. The key advantage with this approach is, however, that it enables novel metabolites to be identified [18, 22, 23]. The targeted approach, on the other hand, is usually built upon exact quantification of one or a set of known metabolites, which are related for example to a specific pathway, biological activity, or disease [16–18, 22, 24]. Therefore, metabolomics can provide a wide variety of information on biological systems. Consequently, also the interest in using metabolomics for research purposes and as a tool in clinical diagnostics has increased remarkably during the past decades [22, 23, 25].

Numerous methodologies used for metabolomics analyses have been developed globally by different research groups [1–4, 22–24, 26–29]. The most common techniques are based on nuclear magnetic resonance spectroscopy (NMR) or mass spectrometry either coupled to different separation techniques or using direct infusion [1–4, 18, 22–27, 30, 31]. Mass spectrometry-based metabolomics offers analyses with high selectivity and sensitivity especially in combination with a separation technique, e.g., liquid chromatography (LC), gas chromatography (GC), or capillary electrophoresis [3, 18, 20, 25]. However, the large diversity in physicochemical properties of the different metabolites found in different biological systems usually means that no single analytical approach can cover the entire metabolome and consequently many metabolomics laboratories utilize different sample preparation protocols and multiple platforms (e.g., different platforms for polar metabolomics and lipidomics) in order to acquire a comprehensive amount of data from each sample set [18, 20, 31–35].

The most common metabolomics analyses are performed on minimally invasive sample types (e.g., serum/plasma or urine) as these are easily accessible [1–4, 18, 22, 26–29, 31]. The results from such analyses have provided important information about many different diseases and the progression of diseases such as diabetes and complications resulted from diabetes.

In the following section, the step-by-step CE-MS method for a reproducible peptidomics analysis of rodent (mice or rat) urine samples is described. Special emphasis is placed on the detailed protocols of sample handling, preparation, system configuration, and data processing. In addition, further workflows on the identification of the peptide biomarkers are also included. Ultimately, the scope of the analysis is the comparison of the peptides identified in the animal models to human peptides with the aim to exploit similarities among them. Additionally, two different platforms for performing metabolomics studies are presented: polar metabolites are analyzed using comprehensive two-dimensional gas chromatography combined with time-of-flight mass spectrometry (GCxGC-TOFMS) [28, 36, 37] and molecular lipids are analyzed using ultrahigh-performance liquid chromatography coupled to quadrupole time-of-flight mass spectrometry (UHPLC-Q-TOF-MS) [28, 29]. These metabolomics methods are currently used in our laboratory and could also be implemented for metabolomics research in relation to DN.

2 Materials

2.1 CE-MS Proteomics

The materials that are required for the sample preparation as well as the composition of the buffer are explained in detail below:

2.1.1 Sample Preparation

- Rat, mice, or human urine samples are stored at −20 °C and are thawed immediately prior to sample preparation.
- Buffer for sample dilution consisting of 2 M urea, 100 mM NaCl, 0.0125% NH_3, and 0.01% SDS, pH 10–12 (*see* **Note 1**).
- Centrisart ultrafilter tubes 20 kDa, 0.62 cm^2 tubes.
- Desalting columns (sample volume 0.5 mL).
- Elution buffer/ammonia buffer consisting of 0.04% NH_3, pH 10.5–11.
- Lyophilization Christ Speed-Vac RVC 2–18/Alpha 1–2.

2.1.2 CE-MS Analysis

- Capillary electrophoresis (CE) system.
- Capillary: 90 cm, 50 μm internal diameter fused silica capillary.
- Capillary equilibration buffer, consisting of 1 mol/l NaOH.
- Ammonium hydroxide buffer, consisting of 1.88% ammonium solution.
- CE-running buffer consisting of 20% acetonitrile (ACN) in 1 M formic acid (98–100%) (*see* **Note 2**).
- Sheath liquid, consisting of 30% (v/v) isopropanol and 0.04% (v/v) formic acid in HPLC-grade water (flow rate: 2 μL/min).
- Electro-ionization sprayer kit (*see* **Note 3**).
- Micro-TOF mass spectrometer (ESI-TOF).

- Cole-Parmer single-syringe infusion pump.
- Hamilton syringe 2.5 mL.
- Standard protein/peptide solution (0.5 pmol/mL) for the calibration of CE-MS: lysozyme (14,303 Da), ribonuclease (13,681 Da), aprotinin (6513 Da), and four synthetic peptides: ELMTGELPYSHINNRDQIIFMVGR (2832 Da), TGSLPYSHIGSRDQIIFMVGR (2333 Da), GIVLYELMTGELPYSHIN (2048 Da), and REVQSKIGYGRQIIS (1733 Da).

2.1.3 Data Processing and Statistical Analysis

- Software for peak detection: MosaiquesVisu.
- Commercial statistical package: SAS (www.sas.com) and MedCalc (www.medcalc.be) available at www.bioconductor.org.

2.2 GC×GC-TOFMS

2.2.1 Sample Preparation

- Eppendorf tubes and glass vials.
- Centrifuge.
- LC-MS-grade methanol (MeOH).
- Internal standards: DL-valine-d_8, heptadecanoic acid-d_{33}, succinic acid-d_4, and DL-glutamic acid-d_5.

2.2.2 Derivatization and Analyses

- Leco Pegasus 4D GC×GC-TOFMS instrument with two different capillary columns:
  - 10 m RTX-5 (inner diameter (i.d.) 0.18 mm, stationary-phase thickness 0.20 μm) - a methyl-deactivated retention gap (length 1.5 m, i.d. 0.53 mm) is used in front of this first column:
  - 1.5 m BPX-50 (i.d. 100 μm, stationary-phase thickness 0.1 μm).
- For derivatization of the analytes: 2% methoxyamine-hydrochloride in pyridine and *N*-methyl-*N*-(trimethylsilyl) trifluoroacetamide (MSTFA).
- Retention index standard mixture including *n*-alkanes (8 mg L^{-1}) with 4,4′-dibromooctafluorobiphenyl (10 mg L^{-1}) in hexane.
- High-purity helium as the carrier gas for the chromatographic separation.

2.2.3 Data Preprocessing and Statistical Analysis

- Within-sample data processing: ChromaTOF.
- Data preprocessing: Guineu software.
- Metabolite identification: NIST Mass Spectral Library and the Golm database.

Table 1
Exogenous lipids present in the standard mixture

Lipid	Abbreviation
1,2-Diheptadecanoyl-*sn*-glycero-3-phosphoethanolamine	PE (17:0/17:0)
N-heptadecanoyl-D-*erythro*-sphingosylphosphorylcholine	SM (d18:1/17:0)
N-heptadecanoyl-D-*erythro*-sphingosine	Cer (d18:1/17:0)
1,2-Diheptadecanoyl-*sn*-glycero-3-phosphocholine	PC (17:0/17:0)
1-Heptadecanoyl-2-hydroxy-*sn*-glycero-3-phosphocholine	LPC (17:0)
1,2-Dimyristoyl-*sn*-glycero-3-phospho(choline-d_{13})	PC (14:0/d13)
Tripalmitin-1,1,1-13C3	TG (16:0/16:0/16:0)-13C3
Trioctanoin-1,1,1-13C3	TG (8:0/8:0/8:0)-13C3
1-Palmitoyl-d31-2-oleoyl-*sn*-glycero-3-phosphocholine	PC (16:0/d31/18:1)

2.3 UHPLC-Q-TOF-MS

2.3.1 Sample Preparation

- Eppendorf tubes and glass vials with glass inserts.
- Centrifuge.
- 0.9% Sodium chloride, standard mixture containing nine exogenous lipids (Table 1), analytical grade chloroform, and LC-MS-grade methanol in a 2:1 (v/v) mixture.

2.3.2 Sample Analysis

- A 1290 Infinity UHPLC system connected to a 6550 iFunnel Q-TOF is used for sample analysis.
- 10% Dichloromethane (analytical grade) in methanol and acetonitrile:methanol:isopropanol:water (1:1:1:1, v/v/v/v, LC-MS grade) + 0.1% formic acid (reagent grade) are used as wash solutions between consecutive sample injections.
- Chromatographic separations are performed on an ACQUITY UPLC® BEH C18 column (2.1 × 100 mm, particle size: 1.7 μm).
- Eluent A: Water + 1% ammonium acetate (1 M) + 0.1% formic acid and eluent B: acetonitrile:isopropanol (1:1, v/v) + 1% ammonium acetate (1 M) + 0.1% formic acid.
- Nitrogen from:
  - A nitrogen generator.
  - A gas cylinder (purity 6.0).

2.3.3 Data Preprocessing and Statistical Analysis

- Data acquisition: MassHunter B.06.01.
- Data preprocessing: MZmine2 and R.

3 Methods

3.1 Proteomic Analysis

3.1.1 Sample Preparation

Urine samples are processed in order to be enriched for small proteins and peptides (<20 kDa) and to remove any salts and electrolytes that may interfere with the CE-MS analysis. The detailed protocol for sample preparation is presented below. Given the small volume of the samples that can be retrieved from the animal models, a sample preparation is adjusted on a smaller scale, and the so-called mini-preparation is attempted.

- Defrost the urine samples at room temperature (*see* **Note 4**).
- Remove the internal filters from the Centrisart tubes and store them in a dry and clean place.
- Pipette 150 μL of urea buffer and 150 μL of urine in the Centrisart tubes, and mix both solutions carefully using the pipette.
- Place back the filter unit into the Centrisart tubes and start a centrifugation at 3400 × *g* for 45 min at 4 °C.
- During the sample centrifugation the NAP columns must be opened as specified by the manufacturer. Each column should be placed in 50 mL collection tubes with pierced lids.
- For the equilibration of NAP5 columns, add 15 mL of elution buffer. Thereafter and until urine samples are ready the columns should be kept filled with a few ml of buffer and sealed with their lids to avoid drying out.
- Once the centrifugation of urine samples is finished, open the NAP5 columns, and wait until the elution buffer has run out. Then add 200 μL of the Centrisart filtrate in NAP5 column and wait until the whole amount of loaded sample has been transferred inside the column.
- Add 300 μL of elution buffer into the column.
- Once the elution buffer is also inside the column, place the NAP5 columns in 15 mL collection tubes and elute by adding 700 μL of elution buffer.
- Freeze the eluted samples at −80 °C prior to lyophilization overnight.
- After the overnight lyophilization and before the CE-MS analysis, the samples are resuspended in 10 μL of deionized water.
- Centrifuge the samples prior to the run for 20 min at 4 °C (this helps to avoid blocking the capillary).

3.1.2 CE-MS Analysis

CE-MS analysis is performed using a Beckmann P/ACE MDQ capillary electrophoresis system online coupled to a MicroTOF MS. The samples are injected hydrodynamically and separation of the peptides is achieved by reverse polarity. The cartridge temperature is maintained at 25 °C. The detailed protocol is provided below:

- First, install the capillary carefully only into the CE. Before connecting the capillary to the MS, condition the capillary with 1 M NaOH (pressure 50 psi) for 10 min. Then wash the capillary with NH_4OH solution (50 psi) for 10 min and directly after that with CE-running buffer (50 psi) for 20 min.
- After this conditioning has been completed, connect the capillary to the MS.
- Every week and each time the capillary is changed, the MS should be recalibrated using the standard protein/peptide solution (0.5 pmol μL^{-1}) for CE-MS.
- The Beckmann CE must be set to run in "reverse mode" when connected to the MS system using the external detector adapter (EDA) (*see* **Note 5**).
- Rinse the capillary with CE-running buffer (pressure applied 50 psi) for 2 min before each sample injection. Inject 290 nL of sample (pressure of 2.0 psi for 99 s). Separation is carried out by reverse polarity at +25 kV at the injection side for 30 min with a capillary set temperature of 35 °C. Then, apply pressure of 0.1 psi for 1 min, 0.2 psi for 1 min, 0.3 psi for 1 min, 0.4 psi for 1 min, and 0.5 psi for the following 30 min.
- Apply coaxially sheath liquid at a running speed of 0.02 mL h^{-1}.
- After each run, rinse the capillary with deionized water with 50 psi for 1 min followed by a washing step with NH_4OH solution with 50 psi for 3 min, and then by a flushing step with deionized water with 50 psi for 3 min.
- ESI sprayer is grounded to achieve electric potential zero and the electrospray interface potential is set between −4000 and −5000 V.
- MS spectra are accumulated every 3 s, over a mass-to-charge range from 400 to 3000 *m/z* for about 60 min, depending on the analysis requirements.

3.1.3 Data Processing: Peak Detection, Deconvolution, Calibration, and Peptide Annotation

- Mass spectral ion peaks are deconvoluted into single masses using MosaiquesVisu software [38] (www.proteomiques.com) and combined, if they represent identical molecules at different charge states. In a first step, MosaiquesVisu identifies all peaks within each single spectrum. Only signals observed in a minimum of two consecutive spectra with a signal-to-noise ratio of at least 4 are considered. Signals with a calculated charge of +1 are automatically discarded. Mass spectral ion peaks representing identical molecules at different charge states are deconvoluted into single masses either using the distance between resolved isotope peaks of the ion or according to conjugated signals for unresolved isotope peaks.

- TOF-MS data of mice and rat urine samples are calibrated utilizing 150 internal reference masses for mice or 108 for rat by applying linear regression.
- Furthermore, CE migration time and ion signal intensity are normalized, as migration time and ion counts show significant variability between samples mainly due to different salt and peptide concentrations. For mice, reference signals of 452 urinary entities are used for CE migration time calibration by local regression. In the case of rat urines, 545 reference signals are used. For normalization of MS signal intensities in the case of mice urine samples 41 internal peptides are used whereas 37 internal peptides are employed in the case of rat urine samples. These specific peptides display a small relative standard deviation. For calibration, linear regression is performed [39, 40]. The resulting peak list contains the molecular mass (Da) and normalized CE migration time (min) for each feature. Normalized signal intensity can be used as a measure of relative abundance.
- Data sets are accepted only if the following quality control criteria are met: a minimal MS resolution of 8000 (required resolution to resolve ion signals with $z = 6$) in a minimal migration time interval (the time window, in which separated signals can be detected) of 10 min. After calibration, the mean deviation of migration time (compared to reference standards) must be below 0.35 min.
- All detected peptides are deposited, matched, and annotated in a Microsoft SQL database, enabling digital data compilation. Proteins and peptides within different samples of one species are considered identical, if the absolute mass deviation is linearly increased from 50 ppm (0.8 kDa) to 100 ppm (20 kDa). The CE migration time deviation was linearly increased over the entire electropherogram from 2 to 5%. This process allows for the comparison of a specific "disease group" to any desired "control group," enabling the identification of statistically significant changes and the definition of potential biomarkers.

3.1.4 Statistical Analysis

- For biomarker definition, the *p*-values are calculated using the natural logarithm-transformed intensities for variance stabilization and the Gaussian approximation to the t-distribution. To account for the false discovery rate and as a safety measure against multiple tests of statistical significance on the same data, multiple testing adjustments of *p*-values have to be applied (e.g., Benjamini-Hochberg) to the subset of markers that passed a certain frequency threshold (usually 70% at least in one of the two groups). The adjustment for multiple testing is one of the requirements to identify significant proteomics biomarkers and seems to be best suited for the challenge: how to improve the detection of biomarkers clearly associated to disease.

Considerations in the challenges of defining valid biomarkers and classifiers have been well described recently [41]. They apply to the following:

- Is the change (frequency or abundance) of a certain molecule observed in a omics study of disease, or the result of the disease, or does it merely reflect an artifact due to technical variability in the pre-analytical steps or in the analysis, biological variability, or bias introduced in the study (e.g., due to lifestyle, age, and gender)?
- How should we estimate the number of samples required for the definition of likely valid biomarkers?
- Which algorithms can be employed to combine biomarkers into a multi-marker classifier, and how can the validity of a multi-marker classifier be assessed? Is validation in an independent test set necessary?
- Importantly, the assessment of the performance of any biomarker pattern for kidney or any other disease needs to be validated on an independent test set as the results obtained from the training set even when performing "leave-one-out cross validation" may be misleading [41].

3.1.5 Mass Spectrometry for Peptide Identification

There are several techniques available for the estimation of the amino acid sequences of the defined specific peptides. Zürbig et al. described in detail a combination of various separation techniques with different MS approaches for peptide identification [42]. Nevertheless, in the last few years, the CE-MS-defined peptide biomarkers for different diseases were almost identified exclusively using CE or liquid chromatography (LC) coupled to tandem-MS instruments [43–46]. The advantages and drawbacks of these methods have been extensively discussed [47–49]. The main advantage of CE-MS/MS in this context is the possibility to perform a direct matching of the obtained sequences to the peptides defined by CE-MS analysis. Here both mass and CE migration time can be directly correlated. In the case of LC-MS/MS the approximate retention time can be only predicted based on the number of basic and neutral polar amino acids in the peptide sequence [42]. On the other hand, due to the larger loading capacity of LC columns, via LC-MS/MS, a higher sensitivity can be reached. To obtain better and higher sequence coverage, the best option is the usage of both technologies [48].

3.1.6 Orthology

The specific peptide biomarkers identified by their amino acid sequence in rodent models can be by now compared with the human disease-specific peptides. In this step, the orthology of the peptides between the species has to be estimated. This will help to clarify whether the biomarkers defined in animal model may consistently reflect the human disease. In the context of DN, the translation of animal-specific biomarkers in urine into the human biomarkers was already described in two articles [9, 11]. Furthermore, a study concentrated in aging processes also investigated the orthology between mouse and human urinary peptides specific for aging [12]. In all these publications the orthology was examined by using the following three criteria:

- Identical fragments defined by the amino acid sequence
- Peptide sequences with one identical cleavage site (N- or C-term)
- Peptide sequence from the same protein area with an overlap in two or six amino acids

The identification of ortholog peptides can have a dual application, either in the perspective of drug development described in Klein et al. [9] for example to monitor drug efficacy and toxicity or for animal model characterization to demonstrate if the selected animal model translates the human disease-specific features [11, 50].

3.2 Metabolomics

3.2.1 GCxGC-TOFMS Sample Preparation

The plasma/serum samples are prepared for the analysis of polar metabolites on the GCxGC-TOFMS platform using protein precipitation with methanol (MeOH) as explained below.

- The sample set is randomized before sample preparation.
- The samples, which have been stored at −80 °C, are thawed on crushed ice immediately prior to the sample preparation.
- 30 μL of plasma/serum from each sample is pipetted into Eppendorf tubes.
- 410 μL of MeOH including four internal standards is added to each sample. The internal standards are the following: DL-valine-d_8, heptadecanoic acid-d_{33}, succinic acid-d_4, and DL-glutamic acid-d_5 and their concentrations in the mixture are 0.9 μg mL^{-1}, 4.3 μg mL^{-1}, 1.4 μg mL^{-1}, and 2.7 μg mL^{-1}, respectively.
- The samples are vortex-mixed and incubated on ice for 30 min after which they are centrifuged at 4 °C (9400 × *g*, 3 min).
- 180 μL of the supernatant is transferred to a glass vial and stored at −80 °C until analysis.

GC×GC-TOFMS Analysis

For the analysis of the polar metabolites, a Leco Pegasus 4D GC×GC-TOFMS instrument, equipped with a consumable-free modulator, was utilized. The gas chromatographic separation was performed on a gas chromatograph equipped with a MultiPurpose Sampler (MPS) for automatized sample derivatization and infusion. The analyses of the samples are performed according to the following procedure:

- The sample set is re-randomized, thawed, and evaporated to dryness (under N_2).
- The metabolites are converted into their trimethylsilyl (TMS) and methoxime (MEOX) derivatives in a two-step derivatization procedure immediately prior to analysis: (1) 25 μL of 2% methoxyamine-hydrochloride in pyridine is added to the sample residue and the mixture is incubated at 45 °C for 60 min and (2) 25 μL of *N*-methyl-*N*-(trimethylsilyl) trifluoroacetamide (MSTFA) is added to the mixture, which is again incubated at 45 °C for 60 min.
- 50 μL of a retention index standard mixture (*n*-alkanes, 8 mg L^{-1}) with an injection standard (4,4′-dibromooctafluorobiphenyl, 10 mg L^{-1}), both in hexane, is added before sample analysis.
- Splitless injection (1 μL) at 250 °C is utilized for sample introduction.
- The metabolites are separated in two dimensions using two different capillary columns. The first-dimension column is a 10 m long RTX-5 capillary column (i.d. 0.18 mm, stationary-phase thickness 0.20 μm) and the second-dimension column is a 1.5 m long BPX-50 capillary column (i.d. 100 μm, stationary-phase thickness 0.1 μm). Additionally, a methyl-deactivated retention gap (length 1.5 m, i.d. 0.53 mm) is used in front of the first column and high-purity helium is utilized as the carrier gas at a constant pressure of 40 psig. The temperature program is presented in Table 2 and the second-dimension column temperature is maintained at 15 °C higher than the first-dimension

Table 2
Temperature program used for analyzing polar metabolites on the GC×GC-TOFMS platform

Rate (°C min^{-1})	Temperature (°C)	Duration (min)
Initial	50	2
7	240	0
25	300	3

column. A 4 s separation time is used for separation of the analytes in the second dimension.

- Electron impact ionization is applied, and mass spectra are acquired at *m/z* 45–700 with 100 spectra s^{-1}.

Quality Control

In order to ensure high-quality data analyzing polar metabolites on the GC×GC-TOFMS system, blank and control samples are introduced regularly along with the real samples. Additionally, the standards added to the samples are used for quality control. The blank samples consist of a mixture of methanol and internal standards, while the control samples are based on a pool created out of all samples present in the particular study. This excludes the possibility of detecting features originating from solvents or the equipment instead of from the samples.

Data Preprocessing and Statistical Analysis

Once the raw data has been acquired, the next step is to preprocess the data. For data acquired on the GC×GC-TOFMS platform, the vendor software ChromaTOF is used for within-sample data processing. Here automatic peak detection and mass spectrum deconvolution are performed. The peak width threshold is set to 0.2 s for this process and peaks with signal-to-noise (*S/N*) values lower than 10 are rejected. Further data preprocessing is then performed in the Guineu software [37]. Here mass spectra are aligned and normalization (in order to minimize the effects caused by analytical variance) of the data is performed by correcting for the added internal standards. Guineu can also be used for quantifying specific targeted metabolites using external calibration curves. Additionally, the NIST Mass Spectral Library and the Golm database are used for metabolite identification.

3.2.2 UHPLC-Q-TOF-MS

Sample Preparation

The plasma/serum samples are prepared for the lipidomics analyses on the UHPLC-Q-TOF-MS platform using a modified Folch extraction procedure as explained below.

- The sample set is randomized before sample preparation.
- The samples, which have been stored at −80 °C, are thawed on crushed ice immediately prior to the sample preparation.
- 10 μL of plasma/serum from each sample is pipetted into Eppendorf tubes.
- 10 μL of 0.9% sodium chloride, 28 μL of a standard mixture containing nine exogenous lipids (Table 1) in a concentration of 10 μg mL^{-1}, and 92 μL of a chloroform ($CHCl_3$):MeOH (2:1, v/v) mixture are added to each sample.
- The samples are vortex-mixed and incubated on ice for 30 min after which they are centrifuged at 4 °C (9400 × *g*, 3 min).

- 60 μL of the lower phase is transferred into glass vials with glass inserts and 60 μL of the previously mentioned $CHCl_3$:MeOH (2:1, v/v) mixture is added to each sample.
- The samples are stored at −80 °C until analysis.

UHPLC-Q-TOF-MS Analysis

A UHPLC-Q-TOF-MS system is utilized for performing the lipidomics analyses. A 1290 Infinity UHPLC system is used for chromatographic separation of the lipids and a 6550 iFunnel Q-TOF, interfaced with a dual-jet stream electrospray (dual-ESI) ion source, for the mass spectrometric detection.

- The sample set is re-randomized before analysis.
- The multisampler (maintained at 10 °C) uses 10% dichloromethane in MeOH and acetonitrile:methanol:isopropanol: water (1:1:1:1, v/v/v/v) + 0.1% formic acid as needle wash solutions after each injection for 8 s each. The injection volume is 1 μL.
- The column thermostat is maintained at 50 °C throughout the analyses.
- Separations are performed on an ACQUITY UPLC® BEH C18 column (2.1 × 100 mm, particle size 1.7 μm).
- The flow rate, using a quaternary solvent manager, is kept at 0.4 mL min^{-1} and water + 1% ammonium acetate (1 M) + 0.1% formic acid (A) and acetonitrile:isopropanol (1:1, v/v) + 1% ammonium acetate (1 M) + 0.1% formic acid (B) are used as the mobile phases for gradient elution according to Table 3.
- Nitrogen, generated by a nitrogen generator, is used as the nebulizing gas at a pressure of 21 psi, as the drying gas at a flow rate of 14 L min^{-1} (at 193 °C), and as the sheath gas at a flow rate of 11 L min^{-1} (at 379 °C).

Table 3
Gradient elution program used for lipidomics analyses on the UHPLC-Q-TOF equipment

Time (min)	%B
0	35% B
2	80% B
7	100% B
14	100% B
14.1	35% B
18	35% B (re-equilibration)

- High-purity nitrogen (6.0) is used as the collision gas.
- The capillary voltage and nozzle voltage are kept at 3643 V and 1500 V, respectively.
- A reference mass solution, which includes ions at *m/z* 121.0509 and 922.0098 and which is prepared according to instructions, is introduced into the mass spectrometer through the second nebulizer in the dual-ESI ion source. This is performed by a separate 1290 isocratic pump at a constant flow rate of 4 mL min^{-1} (split 1:100 before the nebulizer).
- Mass spectra are acquired using MassHunter B.06.01 at a mass range of *m/z* 100–1700 using extended dynamic range with an approximate resolution of 30,000 FWHM (measured during calibration of the instrument at *m/z* 1521.9715, which is included in the calibration mixture).

Quality Control

Quality control of the lipidomics data, acquired on the UHPLC-Q-TOF-MS system, is slightly more demanding than GC×GC-TOFMS due to interferences originating from the matrix (i.e., matrix effects). To adjust for this confounder, additional quality control samples are introduced along with the actual samples: solvent samples, blank samples, NIST (National Institute of Standards and Technology) Standard Reference Material 1950, pure standard mixture, extracted standard mixture, and pooled samples. The solvent samples are used to ensure that no carryover from the previous analysis is affecting the next sample analysis. The blank samples are solvent samples, which have been prepared in the same way as the actual samples to be able to determine the background originating from the chemicals used in the sample preparation step. The NIST samples are used for interlaboratory purposes to ensure that the data is comparable with data acquired in other laboratories worldwide. The two different standard mixtures are measured to ensure stabile response of the lipid standards as well as calculate the extraction efficiency without any interfering matrix effect. The pooled samples are used similarly as it is for the analyses of polar metabolites. At the end of each sample set the relative standard deviations (%RSDs) for the retention times and the peak areas for the added lipid standards are calculated for each group of quality control samples. This is done in order to ensure that our methods run according to generally accepted analytical requirements with respect to reliability and repeatability.

Data Preprocessing and Statistical Analysis

The lipidomics data acquired on the UHPLC-Q-TOF-MS system is mainly preprocessed using MZmine2. All raw data files are converted into mzML format and imported into MZmine2. The data is then processed using the following features of MZmine in order to clean up the mass spectrum and identify the lipids present in each sample: mass detection, chromatogram builder, chromatogram deconvolution, isotopic peak grouper, peak filter, peak list row filter, join aligner, peak list row filter, gap filling, peak list filter, and identification with custom database search. Each of these steps requires careful inspection of the chromatograms in order to ensure that nothing relevant is left out and that the quality of the data remains acceptable. The last data preprocessing step is performed in R. Here we normalize the peak areas by chosen lipid class-specific internal standards and perform semi-quantification on lipids found in our internal peak library. After the data preprocessing is done, data analysis is performed in various ways. This is an important step in metabolomics (for both lipidomics and polar metabolite data) and it requires in-depth knowledge of the biological systems and/or the disease being investigated. The results have to be critically viewed and the process thereof differs tremendously depending on different variables (e.g., the acquired data, the presented research question). Therefore, there is no uniform pipeline for performing this step and the approach is chosen case dependently.

4 Notes related to CE-MS analysis

1. Buffers for sample preparation should be freshly prepared on the day of analysis.
2. Buffers for CE-MS analysis should be freshly prepared every week.
3. The ESI sprayer tip should be cleaned once a week with methanol in an ultrasonic bath. Once a month, it is advised to disassemble the ESI sprayer and clean the parts separately with methanol in an ultrasonic bath. It is important that the inner steel capillary is placed centrally and aligned with the tip of the ESI sprayer.
4. From time to time samples have to be mixed gently by inversion.
5. A description of how to create a method is described in the 32 Karat™ Software User's Guide.

   There are some basic settings that all methods have in common:

   (a) Maximum current: 20 μA
   (b) Cartridge temperature: 35 °C
   (c) Sample storage temperature: 5 °C
   (d) Trigger settings: wait until cartridge coolant temperature is reached
   (e) Analog output scaling: factor 1
   (f) Inlet trays: buffer - 36 vials; sample - no tray
   (g) Outlet trays: buffer - 36 vials; sample - 48 vials

5 Conclusions

We have provided examples on how mass spectrometry can be used for analysis of the proteome and metabolome of body fluids such as urine and blood. Both metabolomics and proteomics have been used to identify markers or panels of markers identifying subjects at increased risk for progression of diabetic kidney disease [5, 51]. Currently most data have been developed using the proteomic analyses. A systems medicine approach for understanding dysregulated biological pathways and how drug interventions affect them is needed to improve the discovery of new intervention strategies [52]. The methods also help providing insight into the underlying pathophysiology and as discussed will also help in the translation of findings between species. As we are struggling with identifying a good experimental model for human diabetic nephropathy, finding ways to translate findings from available models to humans and back is very important.

References

1. van der Kloet FM et al (2012) Discovery of early-stage biomarkers for diabetic kidney disease using ms-based metabolomics (FinnDiane study). Metabolomics 8(1):109–119
2. Liu X et al (2015) A systematic review of metabolite profiling in diabetic nephropathy. J Endocrinol Diab 2(3):1–11
3. Darshi M, Van Espen B, Sharma K (2016) Metabolomics in diabetic kidney disease: unraveling the biochemistry of a silent killer. Am J Nephrol 44(2):92–103
4. Pena MJ et al (2014) Urine and plasma metabolites predict the development of diabetic nephropathy in individuals with type 2 diabetes mellitus. Diabet Med 31(9):1138–1147
5. Sharma K et al (2013) Metabolomics reveals signature of mitochondrial dysfunction in diabetic kidney disease. J Am Soc Nephrol 24 (11):1901–1912
6. Niewczas MA et al (2017) Circulating modified metabolites and a risk of ESRD in patients with type 1 diabetes and chronic kidney disease. Diabetes Care 40(3):383
7. Mischak H et al (2015) Proteomic biomarkers in kidney disease: issues in development and implementation. Nat Rev Nephrol 11 (4):221–232
8. Lacroix C et al (2014) Label-free quantitative urinary proteomics identifies the arginase pathway as a new player in congenital obstructive nephropathy. Mol Cell Proteomics 13 (12):3421–3434
9. Klein J et al (2016) Urinary peptidomics provides a noninvasive humanized readout of diabetic nephropathy in mice. Kidney Int 90 (5):1045–1055
10. Good DM et al (2010) Naturally occurring human urinary peptides for use in diagnosis of chronic kidney disease. Mol Cell Proteomics 9 (11):2424–2437
11. Siwy J et al (2012) Evaluation of the Zucker Diabetic Fatty (ZDF) rat as a model for human disease based on urinary peptidomic profiles. PLoS One 7(12):e51334
12. Nkuipou-Kenfack E et al (2017) The use of urinary proteomics in the assessment of suitability of mouse models for ageing. PLoS One 12(2):e0166875
13. Pontillo C et al (2015) CE-MS-based proteomics in biomarker discovery and clinical application. Proteomics Clin Appl 9 (3-4):322–334
14. Mischak H, Vlahou A, Ioannidis JP (2013) Technical aspects and inter-laboratory variability in native peptide profiling: the CE-MS experience. Clin Biochem 46(6):432–443
15. Albalat A et al (2013) Urinary proteomics based on capillary electrophoresis coupled to mass spectrometry in kidney disease. Methods Mol Biol 919:203–213
16. Fiehn O (2002) Metabolomics—the link between genotypes and phenotypes. Plant Mol Biol 48(1):155–171

17. Fiehn O (2001) Combining genomics, metabolome analysis, and biochemical modelling to understand metabolic networks. Comp Funct Genomics 2(3):155–168
18. Naz S et al (2014) Method validation strategies involved in non-targeted metabolomics. J Chromatogr A 1353:99–105
19. Sana TR et al (2008) Molecular formula and METLIN personal metabolite database matching applied to the identification of compounds generated by LC/TOF-MS. J Biomol Tech 19 (4):258–266
20. Draper J et al (2009) Metabolite signal identification in accurate mass metabolomics data with MZedDB, an interactive m/z annotation tool utilising predicted ionisation behaviour rules. BMC Bioinformatics 10(1):227
21. Kind T, Fiehn O (2006) Metabolomic database annotations via query of elemental compositions: mass accuracy is insufficient even at less than 1 ppm. BMC Bioinformatics 7(1):234
22. Chen C et al (2008) Identification of novel toxicity-associated metabolites by metabolomics and mass isotopomer analysis of acetaminophen metabolism in wild-type and Cyp2e1-null mice. J Biol Chem 283(8):4543–4559
23. Viant MR, Rosenblum ES, Tjeerdema RS (2003) NMR-based metabolomics: a powerful approach for characterizing the effects of environmental stressors on organism health. Environ Sci Technol 37(21):4982–4989
24. Lundström SL et al (2011) Asthmatics exhibit altered oxylipin profiles compared to healthy individuals after subway air exposure. PLoS One 6(8):e23864
25. Pan Z, Raftery D (2007) Comparing and combining NMR spectroscopy and mass spectrometry in metabolomics. Anal Bioanal Chem 387 (2):525–527
26. Favretto D et al (2012) Cord blood metabolomic profiling in intrauterine growth restriction. Anal Bioanal Chem 402(3):1109–1121
27. Ciborowski M et al (2012) Metabolomics with LC-QTOF-MS permits the prediction of disease stage in aortic abdominal aneurysm based on plasma metabolic fingerprint. PLoS One 7 (2):e31982
28. O'Gorman A et al (2017) Identification of a plasma signature of psychotic disorder in children and adolescents from the Avon Longitudinal Study of Parents and Children (ALSPAC) cohort. Transl Psychiatry 7:e1240
29. Luukkonen PK et al (2017) Impaired hepatic lipid synthesis from polyunsaturated fatty acids in TM6SF2 E167K variant carriers with NAFLD. J Hepatol 67(1):128–136
30. Rodrigues CM et al (2007) Metabolic fingerprinting using direct flow injection electrospray ionization tandem mass spectrometry for the characterization of proanthocyanidins from the barks of Hancornia speciosa. Rapid Commun Mass Spectrom 21(12):1907–1914
31. Sarafian MH et al (2014) Objective set of criteria for optimization of sample preparation procedures for ultra-high throughput untargeted blood plasma lipid profiling by ultra performance liquid chromatography–mass spectrometry. Anal Chem 86(12):5766–5774
32. Want EJ et al (2006) Solvent-dependent metabolite distribution, clustering, and protein extraction for serum profiling with mass spectrometry. Anal Chem 78(3):743–752
33. Bruce SJ et al (2008) Evaluation of a protocol for metabolic profiling studies on human blood plasma by combined ultra-performance liquid chromatography/mass spectrometry: from extraction to data analysis. Anal Biochem 372 (2):237–249
34. Tulipani S et al (2013) Comparative analysis of sample preparation methods to handle the complexity of the blood fluid metabolome: when less is more. Anal Chem 85(1):341–348
35. Bruce SJ et al (2009) Investigation of human blood plasma sample preparation for performing metabolomics using ultrahigh performance liquid chromatography/mass spectrometry. Anal Chem 81(9):3285–3296
36. Suvitaival T et al (2016) Serum metabolite profile associates with the development of metabolic co-morbidities in first-episode psychosis. Transl Psychiatry 6:e951
37. Castillo S et al (2011) Data analysis tool for comprehensive two-dimensional gas chromatography/time-of-flight mass spectrometry. Anal Chem 83(8):3058–3067
38. Neuhoff N et al (2004) Mass spectrometry for the detection of differentially expressed proteins: a comparison of surface-enhanced laser desorption/ionization and capillary electrophoresis/mass spectrometry. Rapid Commun Mass Spectrom 18(2):149–156
39. Jantos-Siwy J et al (2009) Quantitative urinary proteome analysis for biomarker evaluation in chronic kidney disease. J Proteome Res 8 (1):268–281
40. Theodorescu D et al (2006) Discovery and validation of new protein biomarkers for urothelial cancer: a prospective analysis. Lancet Oncol 7(3):230–240
41. Dakna M et al (2010) Addressing the challenge of defining valid proteomic biomarkers and classifiers. BMC Bioinformatics 11:594

42. Zurbig P et al (2006) Biomarker discovery by CE-MS enables sequence analysis via MS/MS with platform-independent separation. Electrophoresis 27(11):2111–2125
43. Magalhaes P et al (2017) Association of kidney fibrosis with urinary peptides: a path towards non-invasive liquid biopsies? Sci Rep 7 (1):16915
44. Pejchinovski M et al (2018) Urine peptidomic biomarkers for diagnosis of patients with systematic lupus erythematosus. Lupus 27 (1):6–16
45. Rossing K et al (2016) Urinary proteomics pilot study for biomarker discovery and diagnosis in heart failure with reduced ejection fraction. PLoS One 11(6):e0157167
46. Zhang ZY et al (2017) Novel urinary peptidomic classifier predicts incident heart failure. J Am Heart Assoc 6(8):e005432
47. Albalat A, Mischak H, Mullen W (2011) Clinical application of urinary proteomics/peptidomics. Expert Rev Proteomics 8(5):615–629
48. Klein J et al (2014) Comparison of CE-MS/MS and LC-MS/MS sequencing demonstrates significant complementarity in natural peptide identification in human urine. Electrophoresis 35(7):1060–1064
49. Mischak H et al (2009) Capillary electrophoresis-mass spectrometry as a powerful tool in biomarker discovery and clinical diagnosis: an update of recent developments. Mass Spectrom Rev 28(5):703–724
50. Nkuipou-Kenfack E, Zurbig P, Mischak H (2017) The long path towards implementation of clinical proteomics: exemplified based on CKD273. Proteomics Clin Appl 11(5-6). https://doi.org/10.1002/prca.201600104
51. Zurbig P et al (2012) Urinary proteomics for early diagnosis in diabetic nephropathy. Diabetes 61(12):3304–3313
52. Van JA, Scholey JW, Konvalinka A (2017) Insights into diabetic kidney disease using urinary proteomics and bioinformatics. J Am Soc Nephrol 28(4):1050–1061

Part VI

New Approaches: Gene Editing and Stem Cells to Study Diabetic Kidney Disease

Chapter 19

Formation of Mature Nephrons by Implantation of Human Pluripotent Stem Cell-Derived Progenitors into Mice

Ioannis Bantounas, Edina Silajdžić, Adrian S. Woolf, and Susan J. Kimber

Abstract

In the future, stem cell-based technologies may be harnessed to replace conventional dialysis and transplantation in patients with diabetic nephropathy. Recently, there has been considerable effort to improve methods for the differentiation of human pluripotent stem cells (hPSCs) into kidney cells in culture. Here, we present a protocol for obtaining more advanced kidney structures than have currently been possible in vitro, including vascularized glomeruli and tubular elements. HPSCs are first differentiated in 2D culture to a kidney progenitor stage. These cells are then dissociated and injected subcutaneously into immunocompromised mice. Twelve weeks later, the cells have developed into mature kidney structures and are excised for further characterization. This method constitutes a significant improvement on protocols that involve either exclusively a 2D culture or placing the cells in 3D organoid culture at the air-liquid interface in vitro.

Key words Stem cells, hESC, iPSC, Kidney, Nephron, Organoid, Differentiation, Implant, End-stage kidney disease

1 Introduction

Given that diabetic nephropathy is the leading cause of end-stage kidney disease in adults, stem cell-based technologies may in future usefully be harnessed toward two ends. First, implanted human pluripotent stem cell (hPSC)-derived kidney tissues may be used to complement or even replace conventional dialysis and transplantation, if they were scaled up and fully functional. Second, hPSC-derived "kidneys in a dish" may serve as realistic targets with which to study the detrimental effects of exposure to hyperglycemia and other metabolic derangements associated with the diabetic state.

In recent years, progress has been made in the development of protocols to differentiate hPSCs to kidney tissue. Initially, cells were differentiated in 2D cultures leading to production of a number of different immature kidney-related cell types of both ureteric bud and metanephric mesoderm lineages and patterning of the cells

Luigi Gnudi and David A. Long (eds.), *Diabetic Nephropathy: Methods and Protocols*, Methods in Molecular Biology, vol. 2067, https://doi.org/10.1007/978-1-4939-9841-8_19, © Springer Science+Business Media, LLC, part of Springer Nature 2020

within aggregate structures with distinct domains expressing marker genes corresponding to different parts of the kidney [1, 2]. Although an important first step, these methods had their limitations, as the differentiating kidney structures obtained did not develop beyond a relatively early stage even after prolonged times in culture. In an attempt to remedy this, 3D culture models were developed. In this case, after an initial period of differentiation in 2D, cells were collected, pelleted, and subsequently cultured as 3D organoids on a medium-air interphase for a further 2.5–7.5 weeks [3–5]. This resulted in a marked improvement of differentiation, as the organoids exhibited a higher level of maturity than that obtained in 2D cultures: Developing glomeruli were observed (previously absent in the 2D method), along with most tubular elements of the nephron and also evidence of collecting duct-like structures. Nonetheless, vascularization was still imperfect, as vessel endothelium was only present around the glomeruli and never invading them, as in in vivo kidney development. To overcome these limitations, we decided to differentiate hPSCs to a kidney progenitor stage in 2D cultures, followed by their collection and subcutaneous implantation in immunocompromised mice [4]. Three months later, tissue from the area of implantation was excised and characterized by immunohistochemistry. We observed a further improvement in terms of maturity compared to the in vitro 3D cultures, with the most important difference being that the resulting glomeruli were well vascularized and showed evidence of a mature trilaminar basement membrane. Importantly, the vasculature of the implanted tissue was functionally connected to that of the host, as evidenced by the ability of some hPSC-derived nephrons to filter FITC-labeled 10 KDa dextran injected into the mouse's tail vein. This method advances researchers' ability to study human kidney development from hPSCs and brings nearer the possibility of producing kidney tissue for human transplantation. It will also allow further development of induced pluripotent stem cells (iPSC)-generated kidney rudiments from patients with genetic diseases affecting the kidney, thus facilitating more accurate kidney disease modeling. Here, we describe in detail the method we used to achieve the differentiation of hPSCs to functioning nephrons.

2 Materials

2.1 hPSC Maintenance

1. 6-Well or 24-well cell culture plates (*see* **Note 1**).
2. 50 mL FALCON® tubes.
3. Phosphate-buffered saline (PBS), without calcium and magnesium chloride.

4. 5 μg/mL Human recombinant Vitronectin coating solution (rhVTN-N): Obtained by diluting a 500 μg/mL stock solution 1:100 in PBS.
5. Cells: MAN13 (or other) human embryonic stem cell (hESC) line (*see* **Note 2**).
6. Growth medium: mTeSR1 or TeSR2 medium (*see* **Note 3**).
7. ROCK inhibitor, Y-27632.
8. Cell culture-grade 0.5 mM EDTA solution, pH 8 (diluted in PBS from a 0.5 M stock).

2.2 hPSC Differentiation

1. TrypLE cell dissociation reagent (*see* **Note 4**).
2. Basal medium: "Albumin Polyvinylalcohol Essential Lipids" (APEL) [6]; also commercially available as STEMdiff APEL™2.
3. First-stage differentiation medium (*see* **Note 5**): APEL™2 supplemented with 8 μM CHIR-99021 (a pharmacological GSK3β inhibitor).
4. Second-stage differentiation medium (*see* **Note 5**): APEL™2 supplemented with 200 ng/mL FGF9 and 1 μg/mL heparin.

2.3 Characterization of hPSC-Kidney Progenitor Cultures Prior to Implantation

1. 4% Paraformaldehyde solution.
2. Permeabilization/blocking solution: Dissolve 0.3 mL of Triton-X per 100 mL PBS on a heated block (~40–50 °C) with stirring. Then dissolve 3 g bovine serum albumin (BSA) per 100 mL of the PBS/Triton-X to obtain the final solution.
3. Antibody dilution buffer: Dissolve 3 g BSA per 100 mL PBS.
4. Wash solution: Dissolve 0.1 mL Triton-X per 100 mL PBS.
5. E-cadherin, SIX2, WT1, PAX2, and GATA3 primary antibodies.
6. Alexa-Fluor™-594 anti-mouse and Alexa-Fluor™-488 (goat or donkey) anti-rabbit and anti-goat secondary antibodies.
7. DAPI counterstaining solution: Dilute 5 mg/mL DAPI stock solution, 1:5000 in PBS.

2.4 Cell Implantation

1. Surgical cap.
2. Surgical gown.
3. Face mask.
4. Gloves (sterile, one pair per mouse).
5. Isoflurane.
6. Anesthetizing equipment (clean with 70% ethanol).
7. Scales (clean with 70% ethanol).
8. Heating pad (clean with 70% ethanol).
9. 70% Ethanol spray.

10. Iodine.
11. Water, sterile.
12. Sterile plastic cup for the iodine.
13. Sterile plastic cup for the water.
14. Sterile gauze.
15. Sheet cover for the heating pad (sterile, one per mouse).
16. Sterile 1 mL tuberculin syringes (one per mouse).
17. Sterile 23 G needles (one per mouse).
18. Matrigel, matrix growth factor reduced, phenol red free.
19. APEL™2 medium.
20. Vial cassettes™.
21. TrypLE.
22. 15 mL FALCON® tubes.
23. Box of wet ice containing cells.
24. Female SCID-Beige mice (5–7 weeks of age at implantation).

2.5 Postimplantation Tissue Excision and Characterization

1. CO_2 gas.
2. Phosphate-buffered saline.
3. 10% Formalin.
4. Sterile forceps.
5. Sterile scissors.
6. 20 mL Universals.
7. 1.5 mL Eppendorf tubes.

3 Methods

3.1 hPSC Culture and Passaging

Cells are maintained as a feeder-free culture in a 37 °C/5% CO_2 incubator, in 6-well plates, coated with Vitronectin, with 1.5 mL/well mTeSR1 or TeSR2 medium. The medium is replaced daily. All manipulations involving the cells are performed under sterile conditions in a laminar flow hood. To passage the cells, follow this procedure:

1. Coat 6-well plates with Vitronectin: Add enough Vitronectin coating solution to cover each well (typically 1 mL per well), and then incubate in a 37 °C incubator for at least 30 min (*see* **Note 6**).
2. Remove the medium from the hPSCs in their culture plate and wash briefly and gently with 2 mL PBS; then remove the wash.
3. Add 0.5 mL/well of 0.5 mM EDTA solution and return the cells to the incubator for 3 min.

4. At the end of the incubation, add 2 mL/well of medium (pre-warmed at 37 °C) and dislodge the cells by pipetting the medium up and down using a pipette gun.
5. Collect the cells into a 50 mL FALCON® tube and centrifuge at 700 × *g* for 3 min.
6. Discard the supernatant and flick the tube several times in order to break up the resulting cell pellet and resuspend it into the residual liquid/medium that will have remained in the tube (*see* **Note 7**).
7. Add 2 mL per well of culture medium to the cells and add ROCK inhibitor Y-27632 to a final concentration of 5 nM.
8. Divide the suspension onto the Vitronectin-coated 6-well plates. A 1:4 to 1:6 passaging is typical.
9. After overnight incubation, change the medium with 2 mL fresh medium not containing ROCK inhibitor.

3.2 hPSC Differentiation

Differentiation of cells can be done in either 6-well plates for subsequent implantation (we typically have an approximate yield of between 1.5×10^7 and 2.5×10^7 cells per well) or 24-well plates to characterize differentiating cultures by immunocytochemistry. This is an adaptation of the 2D differentiation protocol described in [1], whereby cells are differentiated in stages, via intermediate mesoderm, to kidney structures. The first stage involves activation of the Wnt pathway by addition of the GSK3β inhibitor CHIR-99021 for 3 days. This is followed by treatment with FGF9 before the cells are collected for implantation on day 12. In the original protocol, this second stage lasts until day 13 and is followed by a third stage where only the basal (APEL™2) medium is used until day 19 [1]. We tried to also implant day-19 cells, but found that these gave much worse results than day-12 cells (the resulting tissue exhibited less mature structures compared to day-12 implants) [4]. This was presumably because, at this more advanced state of differentiation, the cells had lost the necessary plasticity to continue developing in vivo.

1. Coat cell culture plates with Vitronectin as above (*see* Subheading 3.1).
2. Remove the culture medium from the cells and wash once with PBS.
3. Add 0.5 mL TrypLE solution per well of a 6-well plate (*see* **Note 4**) and return cells to the incubator for 1 min.
4. At the end of the incubation add 2 mL of culture medium (mTeSR1 or TeSR2) and collect the cells in a 50 mL FALCON tube as above (*see* Subheading 3.1).
5. Centrifuge the suspension for 3 min at 700 × *g*.

6. Discard the supernatant and resuspend the cell pellet in 1 mL fresh culture medium by pipetting up and down 2–3 times (*see* **Note 8**). Then, you can top up the suspension with additional medium to make subsequent cell counting easier. Typically 2 mL per well of cells (assuming 6-well plates) is required.
7. Determine cell numbers using a hemocytometer or other cell counters.
8. Seed the cells at a density of 18,000 cm^{-2} (typically this is approximately $1.8–2 \times 10^5$ cells per well of a 6-well plate and 3.5×10^4 cells per well of a 24-well plate; also *see* **Note 9**) in culture medium containing 10 nM ROCK inhibitor, Y-27632.
9. The following day (**day 0** of differentiation) start the differentiation by replacing the culture medium with 1 mL/well (for 6-well plates) or 250 μL/well (for 24-well plates) of first-stage differentiation medium (APEL™2 with 8 μM CHIR-99021). Change the medium daily.
10. On **day 3** of differentiation the cells should have acquired a "cobblestone" appearance. Switch to second-stage differentiation medium (APEL™2 with 200 ng mL^{-1} FGF9 and 10 μg mL^{-1} heparin) and keep changing the medium daily.
11. Continue until **day 12**. The cultures should now have begun forming aggregate structures comprising interacting condensations of metanephric mesenchyme and ureteric bud derivatives (which are morphologically much less complex than the ones observed at the end of the 2D protocol; *see* Fig. 1a and **Note 10**).

3.3 Characterization of Cultures Prior to Implantation

An immunocytochemical analysis is advisable to ascertain that the cells are differentiated correctly and are ready for implantation. We have found that this is reliable enough to identify good-quality cultures. However, if desired, the expression of a range of marker genes can be determined by qPCR analysis, as described in [4]. The following double-staining combinations are routinely performed: (1) E-cadherin/SIX2, (2) E-cadherin/WT1, (3) E-cadherin/PAX2, and (4) E-cadherin/GATA3. These diagnostic cultures can run concurrently with the ones to be used for implantation, but initially it may be advisable to start them a few days earlier to allow time for staining before the injections.

1. Wash cells in 24-well plates once with 0.5 mL PBS.
2. Fix the cells by adding 400 μL/well of 4% PFA solution and incubate at room temperature for 20 min.
3. Remove the PFA and wash three times with PBS.
4. Take off the last wash and add 0.5 mL/well of permeabilization/blocking solution (3% BSA/0.3% Triton-X in PBS; *see* **Note 11**). Incubate at room temperature with agitation for 30 min–1 h.

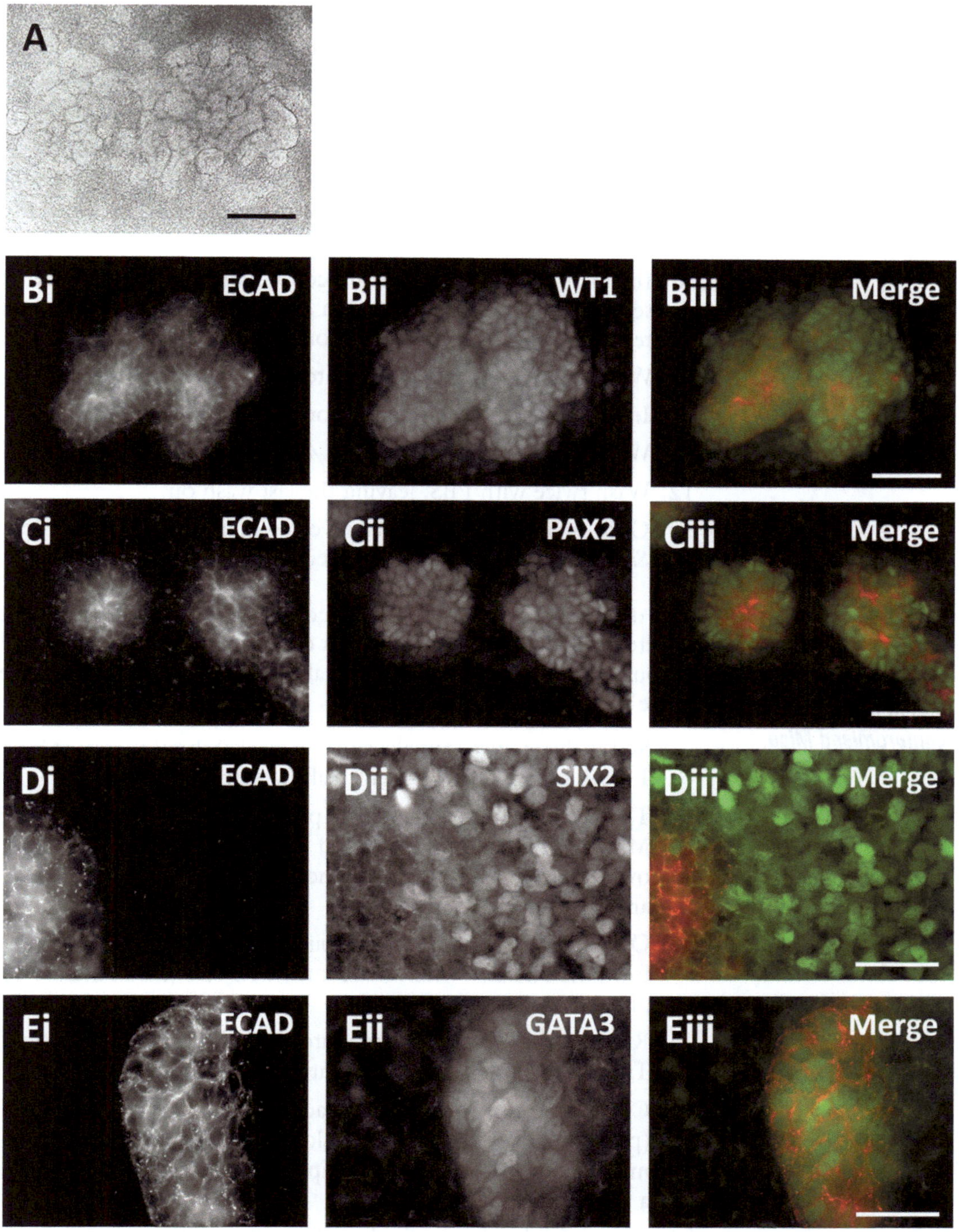

Fig. 1 (**a**) Phase-contrast microscopy image of kidney progenitors (day-12 cultures of differentiating MAN13 cells) prior to collection for implantation. (**b–e**) Examples of immunostained day-12 cultures for various early kidney progenitor markers. E-cadherin (ECAD) marks epithelia; WT1, metanephric mesenchyme; SIX2, nephric progenitors; ECAD/PAX2 or ECAD/GATA3 double-positive staining, collecting duct. Scale bars: A, 240 μm; B–E, 40 μm

5. Take off the permeabilization/blocking solution and incubate with the primary antibodies diluted in 3% BSA/PBS. Both primary antibodies for the double staining are diluted together in the same solution and added on the cells.
6. Incubate with the primary antibodies at 4 °C overnight.
7. Remove the antibody solution and wash three times for 5 min with 0.1% Triton-X/PBS, at room temperature, with gentle agitation.
8. Incubate with the appropriate combination of species-specific secondary antibodies, diluted in 3% BSA/PBS, for 1 h at room temperature with gentle agitation.
9. Wash three times with 0.1% Triton-X/PBS, as above.
10. Incubate with DAPI solution for 5 min.
11. Wash twice with 0.1% Triton-X/PBS, as above.
12. Wash twice with PBS, leaving the last wash on.
13. Cells can be examined on an inverted fluorescence microscope. *See* Fig. 1b–e for typical expected results.

3.4 Implantation of Day-12 Differentiating Cells into Immuno-compromised Mice

The differentiating cells are collected from culture on day 12 and injected subcutaneously on the back of immunocompromised mice at four different locations per animal, at 3×10^6 cells per site (*see* **Note 12**).

1. SCID-Beige mice (female, age 4–6 weeks) should arrive at least 1 week before implantation to allow them to acclimatize.
2. The day before implantation place one 200 μL aliquot of Matrigel for each mouse used in a 4 °C fridge to defrost overnight (*see* **Note 13**). On the day of implantation, transfer and keep on ice until needed.
3. On the day of implantation, aspirate the spent culture medium from the cells and wash with 2 mL/well PBS (assuming 6-well plates).
4. Remove the wash and dissociate the cells with 0.5 mL/well TrypLE for 5 min in the incubator.
5. Carefully remove the TrypLE, add 1 mL of APEL™2 per well (pre-warmed at 37 °C), and dislodge the cells by pipetting the medium up and down using a pipette gun. Collect the cells into a 15 mL FALCON tube.
6. If any visible pieces of cell pellet still remain, wait for a few seconds to let them settle to the bottom of the tube and transfer the rest of the suspension to a fresh tube (*see* **Note 14**).
7. Count the cells (we used Via1-Cassettes™ and a Nucleocounter® NC-200™; alternatively, a hemocytometer may be used) and divide them into 1.5 mL Eppendorf tubes, in aliquots (one

per animal), each containing 1.8×10^7 cells (3.0×10^6 for each of the four injection sites plus 50% more cell suspension per tube to accommodate volume loss during injection).

8. Centrifuge the suspensions at $200 \times g$ at room temperature, discard the supernatant, and resuspend each pellet in 400 μL of APEL™2.
9. Prior to injection, add 200 μL of Matrigel to each tube, quickly mix, and transfer immediately on ice to the animal facility (*see* **Note 13**). This gives a final suspension volume of 600 μL per animal (100 μL per injection site + 200 μL to fill the dead space in the needle and syringe).
10. Meanwhile, sterilize a laminar flow cabinet, scales, heating pad, and anesthetizing equipment using 70% ethanol.
11. Wear sterile scrubs, cap, face mask, and gloves (change gloves between each mouse).
12. In a laminar flow cabinet, anesthetize a mouse using an isoflurane vaporizer with oxygen as a supply gas as follows: Set flow to induction chamber, turn on the oxygen, turn on flow meter to 1000 mL/min, place mouse in induction chamber, seal top, and turn on the vaporizer to 5%. Once the mouse is anesthetized, quickly weigh the mouse, switch flow to nose tube, and place the mouse on the heating pad on top of a sterile sheet with its nose in the nose tube. Reduce supply gas flow to 200 mL/min and vaporizer to 2%. Monitor respiration and response to stimulation during procedure and adjust vaporizer as needed. Clean the injection sites by wiping with gauze soaked in iodine and then sterile water to wash off the iodine and dry with gauze. Mark the ears (for identification).
13. In a laminar flow cabinet, gently fill a tuberculin syringe with 600 μL of the cell suspension plus Matrigel, being careful not to shear the cells in suspension (do not draw cells through the needle) and to avoid creation of bubbles.
14. Place a 23 G needle on the syringe, pointing the syringe needle upward; expel any air in the syringe; and inject the mouse subcutaneously: inject 100 μL (3×10^6 cells) at each of up to four injection sites using the same syringe and needle. The injection sites are on the back on either side of the scapulae (shoulder blades), 1 and 2 cm from the base of the ears. The needle is inserted about 0.5 cm under the skin, almost parallel to the surface in the long axis of the mouse, and the cells are expelled slowly, resulting in the implanted cell plug being deposited approximately 0.5 cm and 1.5 cm away from the base of the ears (*see* Fig. 2a).

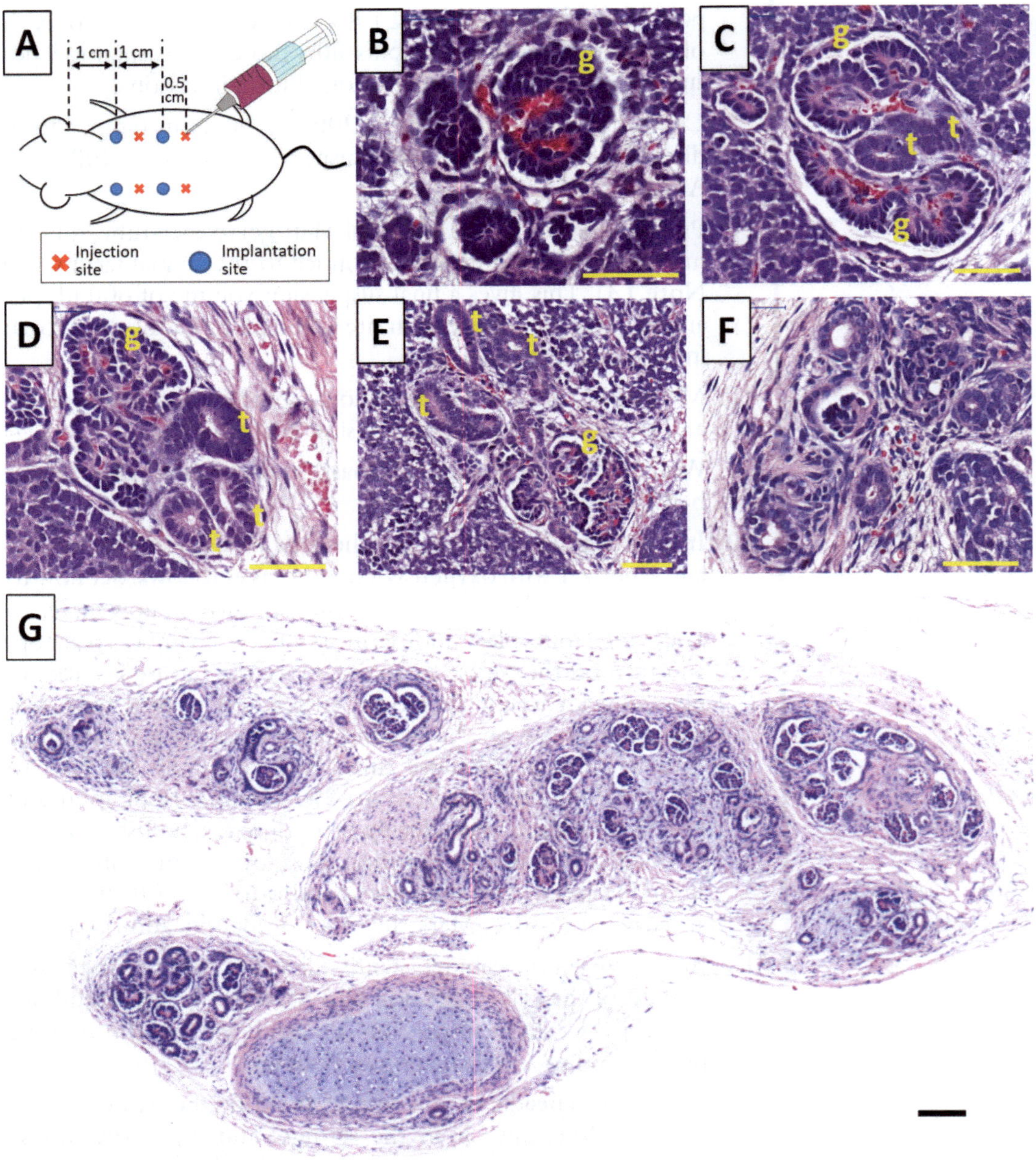

Fig. 2 Implantation of kidney progenitors and histological examination of recovered tissue (hematoxylin and eosin staining). (**a**) Schematic diagram of the location of subcutaneous injections of differentiating kidney progenitor cells into SCID mice. (**b–e**) Examples of tubules (t) and mature glomeruli (g), some with red blood cells in their cores in the excised tissue. (**f**) Example of less mature structures that may be encountered. (**g**) Overview of excised tissue in low magnification (image in **g**, from Bantounas et al. [4]). Scale bars: **b–f**, 50 μm; **g**, 100 μm

15. Very slowly remove the needle and discard, turn vaporizer off, and allow animal to breathe supply gas until it begins to awaken. Once the animal is awake, return it to its cage.
16. Observe the mouse for any adverse reactions and document any leakage of injected material.

3.5 Recovery of Implants

1. Observe mice the day after implantation (to monitor any ill effects of anesthesia), then on a weekly basis. Cellular masses typically form after 6–8 weeks and tend to move slightly from the site of injection.
2. Eleven/twelve weeks postimplantation, the implanted cell mass will have grown to generate a visible lump of tissue under the skin of the mice in many cases (important: *see* **Note 15**, if using this protocol for teratoma assays). Not all injected sites are expected to have macroscopically visible outgrowths. This may mean that the injected cells failed to survive or grow; however, in some cases, despite masses not being macroscopically detectable, we have found that injection sites contained differentiated tissue nonetheless. It is, therefore, recommended that tissue be excised from all injection sites.
3. Mice should be euthanized earlier in the unlikely event that any outgrowth exceeds 1.2 cm in diameter [7].
4. Twelve weeks following implantation, sacrifice the mice by CO_2 asphyxiation.
5. Using sterile surgical scissors and forceps, carefully remove the outgrowths, or the skin surrounding the injection site where no outgrowths are visible by eye.
6. Place the tissue in sterile PBS, and then immediately fix the harvested tissue by placing it in 15 mL universal containing 10% neutral-buffered formalin. These samples can then be used for paraffin embedding for subsequent immunohistochemical analysis. Alternatively, for RNA analysis, either lyse tissue immediately or place into a sterile 1.5 mL Eppendorf and snap-freeze in liquid nitrogen, before transferring the sample to −80 °C for storage. Examples of typical histology of the extracted tissue are shown in Fig. 2b–g and include mature glomeruli with red blood cells in their cores, as well as some less mature structures. On some occasions, cartilage tissue has also been found, reminiscent of what is sometimes observed in dysplastic kidneys.

4 Notes

1. Experiments can be scaled up or down as needed. However, on some occasions we observe an edge effect, whereby there is a preference for organoids to form at the periphery of the well, so we get more organoids per cm^{-2} with smaller wells. Nonetheless, for obtaining progenitors for injection, a 6-well plate gives adequate differentiation.
2. This is the line the original work was performed on. In principle, any hPSC line (hESCs or iPSCs) can be used and, in fact,

we have now successfully differentiated a number of different hESC and iPSC lines. The timing of differentiation can differ slightly from line to line and, while the recommendation to harvest the cells at day 12 for injection (*see* Subheading 3.4) is a good starting point, different lines may require individual optimization.

3. These media work well with MAN13 and other MAN lines adapted for feeder-free culture. The medium in which a particular line is normally cultured is likely to be the preferred option here.
4. The use of EDTA solution to dissociate the cells before differentiation is not recommended, as the aim is to obtain a suspension of fully dissociated (single) cells rather than cell clumps. This is important so as to estimate the number of cells in suspension accurately in order to plate them at the correct density.
5. These media should be stored at 4 °C and used within a week.
6. Alternatively cells can be coated overnight at 4 °C.
7. Do not use a Gilson pipette at this stage, as this may lead to their complete dissociation to single cells, which is not ideal for cell survival and maintenance of their pluripotent state. It also risks damaging the cells.
8. Avoid pipetting more times than this, as there is a risk of damaging the cells.
9. This number is a good starting point and is the optimized density for MAN13 cells. For different lines some optimization of the initial plating density may be required, as they may have different growth properties, and the success/efficiency of differentiation depends sensitively on the initial plating density.
10. Morphology at this stage may differ between cell lines, as stem cells with different genetic backgrounds can differentiate at slightly different rates. There is also some variation between differentiation "runs" with the same line. What is important is that the cells have started expressing "kidney progenitor" markers (*see* Subheading 3.3). Day 12 was chosen after optimization for the MAN13 lines and it is a good starting point for other lines (also *see* **Note 2**).
11. Alternatively, serum from the species in which the secondary antibody was raised may be used for the blocking and antibody binding steps, although we have found that BSA works well with the antibodies listed.
12. In Bantounas et al. [4], we used this number, toward the upper limit specified under our UK Home Office license, in order to maximize our chances of obtaining live, differentiated tissue at the end of the experiment and also to test that unwanted types

of tissue were not produced even at the highest possible number of implanted cells. This number can be further optimized, if needed. Furthermore, it is important to note that the method presented here can be used for implanting undifferentiated stem cells, as a teratoma formation assay, in order to verify their pluripotency. In this case, we typically implant 1×10^6 cells per site and we expect to see the formation of tissues of endo-, meso-, and endodermal origin.

13. The Matrigel should be defrosted in this manner and kept on ice for as long as possible during all subsequent manipulations, as it solidifies quickly at room temperature.
14. Do not over-triturate the cells, as this will lead to cell damage. The cells, at this stage, are more difficult to dissociate than the typical monolayer but it is much preferable to lose some cells that fail to dissociate than to compromise the health of those already in suspension. This is likely to be critical for postimplantation cell survival and proper differentiation.
15. If this protocol is used for a teratoma assay, please note that cell growth is faster, and tissues will require excision after only approximately 5 weeks.

Acknowledgments

We acknowledge grant support as follows: Research Councils UK/Medical Research Council (MRC) MR/K026739/1 UK Regenerative Medicine Platform Hub, Safety and Efficacy of Stem Cells; MRC MICA grant MR/M017344; Kidneys for Life pump priming grant KfL/1/15; Manchester Regenerative Medicine Network strategic funding initiative grant MARMN/1/17; and Kidney Research UK project grant JFS/RP/008/20160916.

References

1. Takasato M, Er PX, Becroft M, Vanslambrouck JM, Stanley EG, Elefanty AG, Little MH (2014) Directing human embryonic stem cell differentiation towards a renal lineage generates a self-organizing kidney. Nat Cell Biol 16(1):118–126
2. Morizane R, Lam AQ, Freedman BS, Kishi S, Valerius MT, Bonventre JV (2015) Nephron organoids derived from human pluripotent stem cells model kidney development and injury. Nat Biotechnol 33(11):1193–1200
3. Takasato M, Er PX, Chiu HS, Maier B, Baillie GJ, Ferguson C, Parton RG, Wolvetang EJ, Roost MS, Chuva de Sousa Lopes SM, Little MH (2015) Kidney organoids from human iPS cells contain multiple lineages and model human nephrogenesis. Nature 526(7574):564–568
4. Bantounas I, Ranjzad P, Tengku F, Silajdzic E, Forster D, Asselin MC, Lewis P, Lennon R, Plagge A, Wang Q, Woolf AS, Kimber SJ (2018) Generation of functioning nephrons by implanting human pluripotent stem cell-derived kidney progenitors. Stem Cell Rep 10 (3):766–779
5. van den Berg CW, Ritsma L, Avramut MC, Wiersma LE, van den Berg BM, Leuning DG, Lievers E, Koning M, Vanslambrouck JM, Koster AJ, Howden SE, Takasato M, Little MH, Rabelink TJ (2018) Renal subcapsular transplantation of PSC-derived kidney organoids

induces neo-vasculogenesis and significant glomerular and tubular maturation in vivo. Stem Cell Rep 10(3):751–765

6. Ng ES, Davis R, Stanley EG, Elefanty AG (2008) A protocol describing the use of a recombinant protein-based, animal product-free medium (APEL) for human embryonic stem cell differentiation as spin embryoid bodies. Nat Protoc 3(5):768–776

7. Gropp M, Shilo V, Vainer G, Gov M, Gil Y, Khaner H, Matzrafi L, Idelson M, Kopolovic J, Zak NB, Reubinoff BE (2012) Standardization of the teratoma assay for analysis of pluripotency of human ES cells and biosafety of their differentiated progeny. PLoS One 7(9):e45532

Chapter 20

Generating Mutant Renal Cell Lines Using CRISPR Technologies

Nuria Perretta-Tejedor, Grace Freke, Marian Seda, David A. Long, and Dagan Jenkins

Abstract

Gene editing using the CRISPR/Cas9 system is an extremely efficient approach for generating mutations within the genomic DNA of immortalized cell lines. This procedure begins with a straightforward cloning step to generate a single plasmid encoding the Cas9 enzyme as well as a synthetic guide RNA (sgRNA) which is selected to target specific sites within the genome. This plasmid is transfected into cells either alone, in order to generate random insertion-deletion alleles ("indels") at the desired locus via the nonhomologous end-joining pathway, or in conjunction with a homology-directed repair template oligonucleotide to generate a specific point mutation. Here we describe a procedure to perform gene editing in IMCD3 and HEK293 cells and to subsequently isolate clonal cell lines carrying mutations of interest.

Key words Gene editing, sgRNA, pX330, IMCD3, HEK293, Transfection, Fluorescence-activated cell sorting

1 Introduction

In recent years, there has been huge growth in the application of gene-editing technologies. The concept of gene editing began in the late 1990s with the development of zinc-finger nucleases (ZFNs) [1] and subsequently with transcription-like effector nucleases (TALENs) [2–4]. However, both of these technologies are limited by their relatively low targeting efficiencies, the relative rarity of suitable ZFN cut sites within the genome, and the need for complex cloning procedures to generate TALEN DNA-binding oligonucleotides. These limitations were circumvented by the development of the clustered regularly interspaced short palindromic repeats/CRISPR-associated endonuclease (CRISPR/Cas9) system [5, 6], following the observation that the type II

Nuria Perretta-Tejedor, Grace Freke, and Marian Seda have contributed equally.

Luigi Gnudi and David A. Long (eds.), *Diabetic Nephropathy: Methods and Protocols*, Methods in Molecular Biology, vol. 2067, https://doi.org/10.1007/978-1-4939-9841-8_20, © The Author(s) 2020

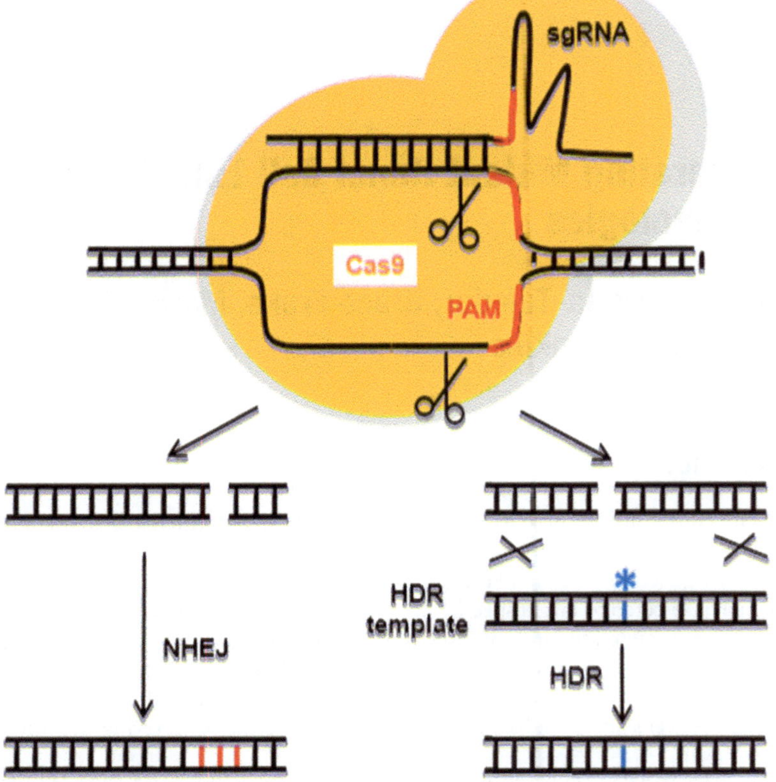

Fig. 1 Gene editing using CRISPR-Cas9. Schematic showing the invasion of a sgRNA into a DNA double helix in concert with Cas9. The sgRNA consists of a short region of homology coupled to a PAM sequence as well as a more complex region with secondary structure. The region of homology is all that is cloned into plasmid pX330 in this protocol. Cas9 cuts the DNA at the PAM sequence causing a double-strand break. This can be repaired either by the NHEJ pathway or, in conjunction with a template oligo, by HDR. These pathways typically result in the introduction of indels (red) or point mutations (blue)

CRISPR system from *Streptococcus pyogenes* (SpCas) could be engineered to edit mammalian genomes [7, 8]. This editing system combines the Cas9 endonuclease with a synthetic guide RNA (sgRNA) that acts as a signal to deliver Cas9 to a specific genomic target sequence where it can induce a double-strand break (DSB; Fig. 1). Cas9 recognizes a protospacer adjacent motif (PAM) located immediately downstream of its sgRNA in order to elicit its function. DSBs can be repaired by one of the two mechanisms which act according to the presence or absence of a donor DNA template: nonhomologous end-joining (NHEJ) or homology-directed repair (HDR). NHEJ is error-prone, often introducing base insertions or deletions (indels), typically leading to a frameshift mutation. On the other hand, HDR employs a repair template with homology to the target site [9, 10]. To verify the efficiency of Cas9 cleavage at the target site we employ the T7 endonuclease (T7EI) assay. T7EI recognizes and cleaves DNA heteroduplexes containing mutant DNA sequences following PCR amplification of the targeted site and reannealing, and serves as a simple means of gauging targeting efficiency and screening for clonal cell lines that carry mutations [11–13].

Here we describe a procedure which we have adapted from the Zhang Lab at the Broad Institute [9], in order to generate frameshift and point mutations in renal cell lines. Key features of this protocol include the following: (1) sorting of cells co-transfected with GFP together with the Cas9/sgRNA-expressing plasmid enhances the overall targeting efficiency. (2) We culture cells for at least 2 weeks following transfection of these plasmids before sorting single cells into clonal cell cultures, as we have found that shorter periods of time post-transfection are associated with a higher level of mosaic mutations, presumably owing to continued expression of Cas9/sgRNA. (3) For introduction of point mutations via HDR, we have found that a template oligo consisting of 60 nucleotides on either side of the DNA mismatch has good targeting efficiency (*see* **Note 1**).

To date, our lab has successfully employed these methods to produce immortalized renal cells carrying desired mutations (and defined genotypes) at over 60 genomic loci. We have predominantly used inner medullary collecting duct (IMDC3) cells, which are mouse epithelial cells allowing us to study the genes involved in cilia function, and human embryonic kidney (HEK293) cells, which have enabled us to model features of human renal diseases including polycystic kidney disease. We have also used this protocol successfully in other cell lines, including Chinese hamster ovary (CHO) cells, and the techniques could be used to edit genes in glomerular podocytes and endothelium, cells particularly affected in diabetic nephropathy. In other works, we have found that analysis of multiple clonal IMCD3 or HEK293 cell lines carrying biallelic mutations in genes of interest can have the advantage of reducing phenotypic variability, as compared to results generated using primary cell lines or transient gene-knockdown approaches, thereby revealing novel cellular phenotypes [14, 15]. The improved phenotypic consistency of these cellular models means that the CRISPR/Cas9 system is invaluable for studies of disease mechanisms and for drug screening approaches.

2 Materials

2.1 Cloning of sgRNA into Plasmid pX330

1. Oligos 1 and 2 (designed in Subheading 3.1).
2. PCR primers (designed in Subheading 3.1).

3. pX330-U6-Chimeric_BB-CBh-hSpCas9 (Addgene plasmid ID: 42230).
4. BbsI enzyme (5000 U/mL; NEB).
5. 10× T4 ligase buffer (NEB).
6. T4 ligase enzyme (NEB).
7. *E. coli* JM109 competent cells (Promega).
8. Super Optimal broth with Catabolite repression (SOC) medium.
9. Luria Broth (LB) agar Amp plate: LB agar plate containing 100 μg/mL ampicillin.
10. LB Amp medium: LB medium containing 100 μg/mL ampicillin.
11. QIAprep Spin Miniprep kit (QIAGEN).
12. pX330 sequencing primer: 5′-CGTAACTTGAAAGTATTT CGATTTCTTGGC-3′.

2.2 Cell Culture and FACS

1. HEK293 cells (ATCC CRL-1573).
2. IMCD3 cells (ATCC CRL-2123).
3. Dulbecco PBS, no calcium, no magnesium (Gibco).
4. Medium for HEK293 cells: DMEM with GlutaMAX (Gibco) supplemented with 10% FBS (and 1% penicillin-streptomycin if desired).
5. Media for IMCD3 cells: DMEM/F-12 with GlutaMAX media (Gibco) supplemented with 10% FBS (and 1% penicillin-streptomycin if desired).
6. Trypsin for HEK293 cells: Trypsin-EDTA 0.05% (Gibco).
7. Trypsin for IMCD3 cells: Trypsin-EDTA 0.25% (Gibco).
8. FuGENE 6 (Promega).
9. Opti-MEM reduced-serum medium (Gibco).
10. pAcGFP1-C1 (Clontech).
11. Lipofectamine 2000 transfection reagent (Thermo Fisher).
12. MoFlo XDP (Beckman Coulter).

2.3 Genotyping Analysis

1. Molecular kit to extract genomic DNA (e.g., DNeasy Blood and Tissue Kit from Qiagen).
2. Pwo Master (Sigma-Aldrich).
3. 10× NEBuffer 2 (NEB).
4. T7 endonuclease I (NEB).
5. Agarose.
6. 1× TAE buffer (Invitrogen).
7. 1 kb DNA ladder (NEB).

3 Methods

The methods presented below should be used to generate random indels by NHEJ. A variation of this protocol can be used to generate a defined single base change mutation (or if required, substitution, insertion, or deletion of a few nucleotides) by HDR (*see* **Note 1**). For simplicity, the following methods describe the design and use of one sgRNA (*see* **Note 2**; Fig. 2).

3.1 sgRNA Design

1. Find your gene of interest within the relevant species on the Ensembl genome browser (www.ensembl.org). For HEK293 search the human genome, and for IMCD3 search the mouse genome.
2. Select a 23–500-nucleotide (nt) genomic region that you wish to edit (*see* **Note 3**).

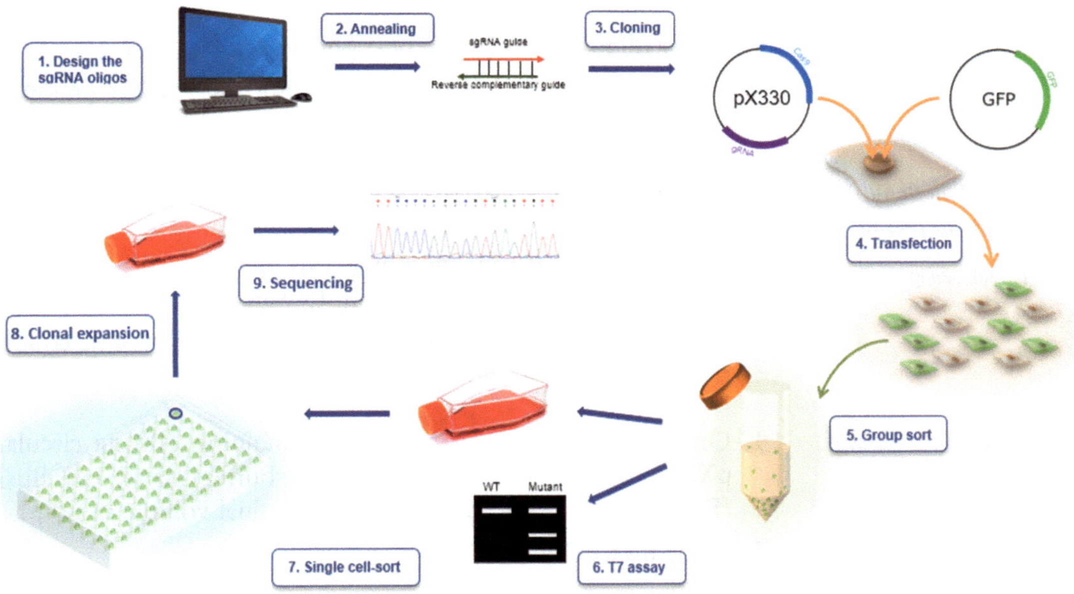

Fig. 2 Overview of methodology. A sgRNA is designed and ordered as two oligos (1), which are annealed (2) and cloned into plasmid pX330 to yield plasmid pX330-sgRNA (3), which contains a Cas9 expression cassette and a sgRNA expression cassette. IMCD3 or HEK293 cells are transfected with pX330-sgRNA and pAcGFP1-C1, a GFP expression vector used as a positive marker of transfection (4). Fluorescence-activated cell sorting (FACS) is used for enrichment of GFP-positive cells in a step we term the "group sort" (5); these cells are presumed to have also successfully been transfected with pX330-sgRNA. Half of the group-sorted cells are reseeded and subcultured for 2 weeks (*see* **Note 15**). gDNA is extracted from the remaining cells and analyzed by T7 endonuclease I (T7EI) assay (6), to detect indels at the genomic target site within the cell population. After 2 weeks of subculture, the reseeded CRISPR cells are subjected to FACS again, and a single cell is seeded into each well of a 96-well plate, in a step that we call the "single-cell sort" (7) which is followed by clonal expansion (8). Each single cell has the propensity to establish a clonal colony, if it proliferates. Colonies are genotyped by PCR and Sanger sequencing to confirm the presence and nature of mutations in each (9)

3. Open the CRISPOR design tool (crispor.tefor.net). Select the appropriate target genome and paste your sequence into the search box. Submit the search. The online tool will produce a ranked list of all possible sgRNAs within the genomic sequence (*see* **Note 4**).
4. Identify a suitable sgRNA sequence from the displayed list (*see* **Note 5**).
5. Take the 20 nt sgRNA sequence (without the PAM). If its first nucleotide is not a "G," then add a "G" at the 5′ end. This sequence will form the foundations of oligo 1.
6. Find the reverse complement of the sgRNA sequence (including the extra "G" nucleotide, if added). This will form the foundations of oligo 2.
7. To the 5′ end of oligo 1, insert nucleotides "CACC." Design of oligo 1 is now complete.
8. To the 5′ end of oligo 2, insert nucleotides "AAAC." Design of oligo 2 is now complete.
9. Order oligos 1 and 2 as 5′ phosphorylated oligos.
10. Design a pair of PCR primers flanking the sgRNA genomic target site (*see* **Note 6**).

3.2 Cloning of sgRNA Into Plasmid pX330

3.2.1 Annealing of Oligos 1 and 2

1. Resuspend each oligo (ordered in Subheading 3.1, **step 9**) to a concentration of 100 μM in Milli-Q water.
2. In a 0.2 mL PCR tube, combine 1 μL oligo 1 (100 μM), 1 μL oligo 2 (100 μM), and 8 μL Milli-Q water.
3. Anneal in a thermocycler using the following cycling conditions: 95 °C for 5 min, ramp down to 25 °C at 5 °C/min.

3.2.2 pX330 Linearization

1. On ice, prepare a 50 μL reaction containing 100 ng circular pX330 vector, 5 μL restriction enzyme buffer (10×), 4 μL BbsI (5000 U/mL), and Milli-Q water to a final volume of 50 μL.
2. Incubate for 2 h at 37 °C.

3.2.3 Ligation of Annealed Oligos into pX330

1. Dilute annealed oligos (from Subheading 3.2.1) 1:200 in Milli-Q water.
2. Prepare a 10 μL reaction mix containing 50 ng of linear pX330 (from Subheading 3.2.2), 1 μL diluted oligos, 1 μL 10× T4 ligase buffer, 1 μL T4 ligase enzyme, and Milli-Q water to a final volume of 10 μL.
3. Incubate for at least 1 h at room temperature, or overnight at 4 °C.

3.2.4 Transformation of Competent Cells with the Ligation Mix and Isolation of Plasmid DNA

1. Thaw *E. coli* JM109 competent cells on ice until just thawed.
2. Add 5 μL of the ligation reaction (from Subheading 3.2.3) to the tube of competent cells. Mix by flicking the tube 4–5 times (do *not* mix by pipetting) and incubate cells for 30 min on ice.
3. Heat shock the cells for 45 s in a water bath at exactly 42 °C; do not shake. Immediately return the tube to ice for 2 min.
4. Add 450 μL room-temperature SOC medium to the tube and incubate for 1 h at 37 °C with shaking.
5. Plate 100 μL of the transformation mix onto an LB agar Amp plate.
6. Incubate plate overnight at 37 °C.
7. The next day, inspect the plate for colony growth. Pick two or three colonies to check for correct insertion of the sgRNA. Inoculate a single colony into a 5 mL culture of LB Amp medium. Incubate cultures overnight at 37 °C with shaking.
8. Isolate plasmid DNA from the cultures using a QIAprep Spin Miniprep kit, according to the manufacturer's instructions.
9. Verify the sequence of each plasmid by Sanger sequencing using the pX330 sequencing primer. We will call this plasmid pX330-sgRNA.

3.3 Transfection of HEK293 or IMCD3 Cells

A different transfection reagent is used depending on the cell line (*see* **Note** 7). Choose Subheading 3.3.2 for transfection of HEK293 cells and Subheading 3.3.3 for transfection of IMCD3 cells. Regardless of transfection reagent, three transfection conditions will be used: (1) a co-transfection with pX330-sgRNA and pAcGFP1-C1 ("CRISPR" transfection); (2) a transfection with pAcGFP1-C1 ("GFP-only" transfection); (3) a mock transfection without plasmid DNA ("non-transfected" condition). The latter two conditions act as positive and negative controls of transfection, respectively.

3.3.1 Seeding of Cells for Transfection

1. The day before transfection, seed cells into three wells of a 6-well plate (*see* **Note 8**). Plate 1×10^5 to 3×10^5 cells/well in 2 mL/well complete medium. Leave overnight to achieve a desired confluence of 50–80%, appropriate for transfection.

3.3.2 Transfection of HEK293 Cells

1. Label three sterile microcentrifuge tubes, one for each transfection condition.
2. In each tube, mix 3 μL FuGENE with 97 μL Opti-MEM reduced-serum media and incubate for 5 min at room temperature.
3. Add the appropriate plasmid DNA to each tube and mix. For the CRISPR transfection, add 500 ng pX330-sgRNA and 500 ng pAcGFP1-C1. For the GFP-only transfection, add

1 µg pAcGFP1-C1. No plasmid DNA is added for the non-transfected condition. Incubate for 15 min at room temperature.

4. To each well of plated cells, add 100 µL of transfection mixture in a dropwise manner.
5. Return cells to the incubator for 48 h, prior to cell sorting (*see* **Note 9**).

3.3.3 Transfection of IMCD3 Cells

1. Label six sterile microcentrifuge tubes. For each transfection condition, there will be one tube for Lipofectamine and one tube for plasmid DNA.
2. In each of the three tubes, mix 8.5 µL Lipofectamine 2000 transfection reagent with 150 µL Opti-MEM and incubate for 5 min at room temperature.
3. In the remaining three tubes, mix 150 µL Opti-MEM with the appropriate plasmid DNA. For the CRISPR transfection, add 1.25 µg pX330-sgRNA (obtained in step 3.2.7) and 1.25 µg pAcGFP1-C1. For the GFP-only transfection, add 2.5 µg pAcGFP1-C1. No plasmid DNA is added for the non-transfected condition.
4. Add each plasmid mixture to a separate tube of Lipofectamine and mix well. Incubate for 30 min at room temperature.
5. To each well of plated cells, add 300 µL of transfection mixture in a dropwise manner.
6. Return the cells to the incubator for 48 h, prior to cell sorting (*see* **Note 9**).

3.4 Group Sort by Fluorescence-Activated Cell Sorting (FACS)

1. Label a 15 mL centrifuge tube for use as a CRISPR sample collection tube. Add 500 µL fresh medium to the tube, put it on ice, and set aside.
2. Wash the CRISPR and non-transfected wells of cells twice each with 1 mL/well sterile DPBS (*see* **Note 10**).
3. Add 1 mL/well trypsin-EDTA and incubate at 37 °C until cells dissociate.
4. Add 2 mL/well complete media and transfer each 3 mL cell suspension to a 15 mL centrifuge tube.
5. Pellet cells by centrifugation at 200 × *g* for 5 min.
6. Discard the supernatant and resuspend cells in 300 µL Opti-MEM reduced-serum media (*see* **Note 11**).
7. Pass cells through a 70 µm cell strainer to remove clumps (*see* **Note 12**).
8. Put the tubes directly on ice.
9. Proceed directly to FACS (*see* **Note 13**). Use non-transfected cells to discern single cells from cell clumps when setting up the

cell sorter. Isolate GFP-positive cells from the CRISPR sample and collect these in the collection tube (prepared in Subheading 3.4, **step 1**). Run the entirety of the sample or collect at least 5×10^5 cells per sample (*see* **Note 14**). Keep collected cells on ice.

10. In a sterile safety cabinet, take one-half of the GFP-positive CRISPR sample and seed them in a 25 cm^2 tissue culture-treated flask containing 5 mL complete medium. Return the cells to the incubator and continue to grow them for 2 weeks, passaging as and when necessary (*see* **Note 15**).
11. Separately pellet the remaining GFP-positive CRISPR cells and the non-transfected cells for gDNA extraction, by centrifugation at $300 \times g$ for 5 min. Discard the supernatant. Proceed directly to the next step, or store the cell pellets at −20 °C.

3.5 T7 Endonuclease I (T7EI) Assay

1. Extract genomic DNA (gDNA) with the DNeasy Blood and Tissue kit, following the manufacturer's instructions.
2. Use the extracted gDNA as template to perform a 50 μL PCR reaction using the genotyping primers (designed in Subheading 3.1, **step 10**) and Pwo Master (*see* **Note 16**).
3. Run 25 μL of the PCR in an agarose gel (adjusting the agarose percentage depending on the expected size of the PCR product) against a 1 kb DNA ladder to check whether there is a single product (*see* **Note 17**).
4. In a 0.2 mL PCR tube, prepare a 19 μL reaction containing 10 μL PCR reaction, 2 μL 10× NEBuffer 2, and 7 μL Milli-Q H_2O.
5. Melt the PCR products in a thermocycler using the following conditions: 95 °C for 5 min, ramp down to 85 °C at −2 °C/s, ramp down to 25 °C at −0.1 °C/s, and hold at 4 °C.
6. Add 1 μL T7 endonuclease I to the melted PCR products and incubate at 37 °C for 1 h.
7. Run the T7 cleavage products in an agarose gel and look for cleavage of the PCR product (*see* **Notes 17** and **Note 18**; Fig. 3).

3.6 Single-Cell Sorting of CRISPR Cells to Establish Clonal Cell Lines

3.6.1 Preparation of Conditioned Media

1. In a 50 mL centrifuge tube, make up 16 mL of conditioned medium per 96-well plate (*see* **Note 19**), by mixing 8 mL fresh medium with 8 mL medium removed from a 75 cm^2 flask of cells at ~70% confluence (*see* **Note 20**).
2. Sterile-filter the conditioned medium with a 0.2 μm filter (*see* **Note 21**).
3. Fill a 96-well plate with 150 μL/well. Place the 96-well plate in the 37 °C incubator.

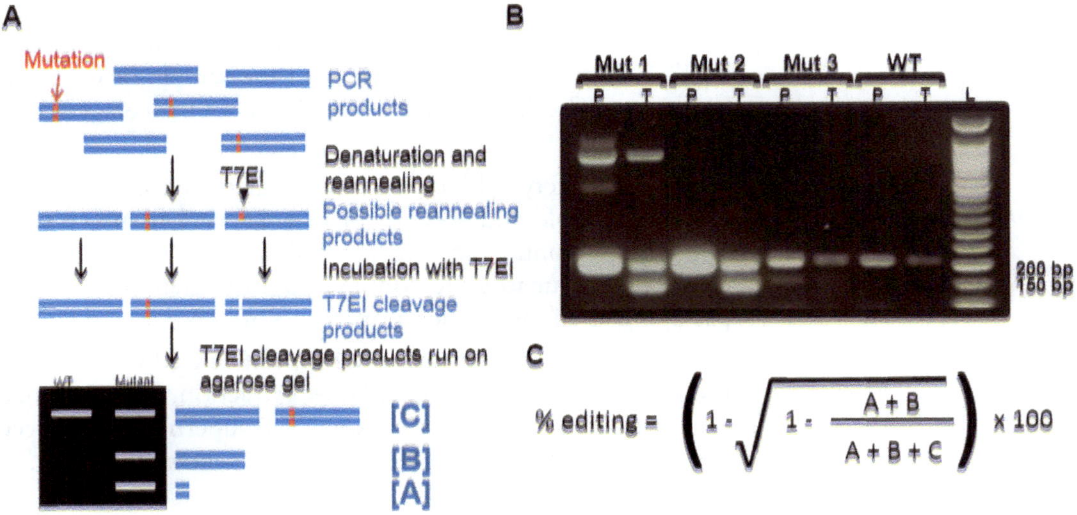

$$\%\ \text{editing} = \left(1 - \sqrt{1 - \frac{A+B}{A+B+C}}\right) \times 100$$

Fig. 3 T7EI assay. (**a**) Overview of the T7EI assay: The T7EI assay is used to detect indels at the genomic target site. The target site is first PCR-amplified and the PCR products denatured and reannealed. If a mutation is present, reannealing products include WT homoduplex DNA, mutant homoduplex DNA, and WT/DNA heteroduplex DNA. The T7EI enzyme identifies and cleaves DNA mismatches. Incubation of reannealing products with T7EI therefore results in cleavage of heteroduplex DNA, whereas homoduplex DNA is left intact. When run on an agarose gel, T7EI cleavage products can be detected. (**b**) Example PCR and T7EI assay results. PCR (P) and T7EI assay (T) products of three group-sorted CRISPR populations (Mut 1, 2, 3) and a wild-type (WT) were run alongside a DNA ladder (L) in an agarose gel. The expected PCR amplicon size was 204 bp. In the WT sample, the 204 bp amplicon was not cleaved by the T7EI. Mutant 1 was a heterogeneous population, revealed by the presence of more than two PCR amplicons. Mutant 2 had small indels at the target site, revealed by a single PCR amplicon that is cleaved by the T7EI. Mutant 3 possessed an allele with a large deletion, revealed by the presence of an additional, smaller PCR amplicon. (**c**) Calculation of targeting efficiency. Assuming that all indels are not identical, the equation approximates the targeting efficiency, where A, B, and C refer to band intensities labeled in (A)

3.6.2 Preparation of CRISPR Cells for FACS

1. Wash cells in 25 cm^2 flask twice with 5 mL sterile DPBS.
2. Add 1 mL trypsin-EDTA and incubate at 37 °C until cells dissociate.
3. Add 4 mL complete media and transfer cell suspension to a 15 mL centrifuge tube.
4. Pellet cells by centrifugation at 200 × *g* for 5 min.
5. Discard the supernatant and resuspend cells in 300 μL Opti-MEM reduced-serum media (*see* **Note 11**).
6. Pass cells through a 70 μm cell strainer to remove clumps (*see* **Note 12**).
7. Put the tubes directly on ice.
8. Proceed directly to FACS with the cell suspension and the 96-well plate containing conditioned media. Sort a single cell into each well of the 96-well plate (*see* **Note 22**).
9. Spin the 96-well plate at 200 × *g* for 2 min and immediately return them to the incubator (*see* **Note 23**).

3.6.3 Expansion of Cell Colonies

1. Incubate the cells for 2 weeks, to allow colonies to establish (*see* **Note 24**).
2. After 2 weeks, check individual wells under the microscope to identify those that contain a cell colony. Monitor cell confluence in these wells over the ensuing days.
3. When a well is confluent (*see* **Note 25**), wash the cells twice in 200 μL sterile DPBS. Then dissociate cells in 30 μL trypsin-EDTA and transfer them directly into 1 mL medium in a well of a 12-well plate (*see* **Note 26**). Return the cells to the incubator and monitor their growth over the following days.
4. When a well of a 12-well plate is confluent, wash the cells twice with 1 mL sterile DPBS. Then dissociate cells in 150 μL trypsin-EDTA and transfer directly to a 25 cm^2 flask containing 5 mL medium. Return the cells to the incubator and monitor their growth over the following days.
5. When a 25 cm^2 flask is confluent, passage the cells into two new 25 cm^2 flasks. Return these flasks to the incubator.
6. When the two 25 cm^2 flasks have reached ~70% confluence, freeze down and store the cells from one of the flasks.
7. With the remaining flask, wash cells twice with 5 mL DPBS, and then dissociate in 1 mL trypsin-EDTA. Add 4 mL complete media and transfer the 5 mL cell suspension to a 15 mL centrifuge tube. Pellet the cells for 5 min at 300 × *g* and discard the supernatant. Proceed directly to the next step, or store the cell pellet at −20 °C.

3.7 Genotyping of Clones

This method describes the genotyping of a single-cell colony.

1. Extract genomic (g) DNA with the DNeasy Blood and Tissue kit, following the manufacturer's instructions.
2. Use the extracted gDNA as template to perform a 50 μL PCR reaction with the genotyping primers (designed in Subheading 3.1, **step 10**).
3. Run the 50 μL PCR in an agarose gel against a 1 kb DNA ladder. If there are multiple amplicons present, ensure that they are well resolved (*see* **Notes 27** and **28**).
4. Gel-purify the PCR products.
5. Sanger sequence the extracted amplicon(s) to identify the presence and nature of mutations generated by CRISPR (*see* **Note 29**; Fig. 4).

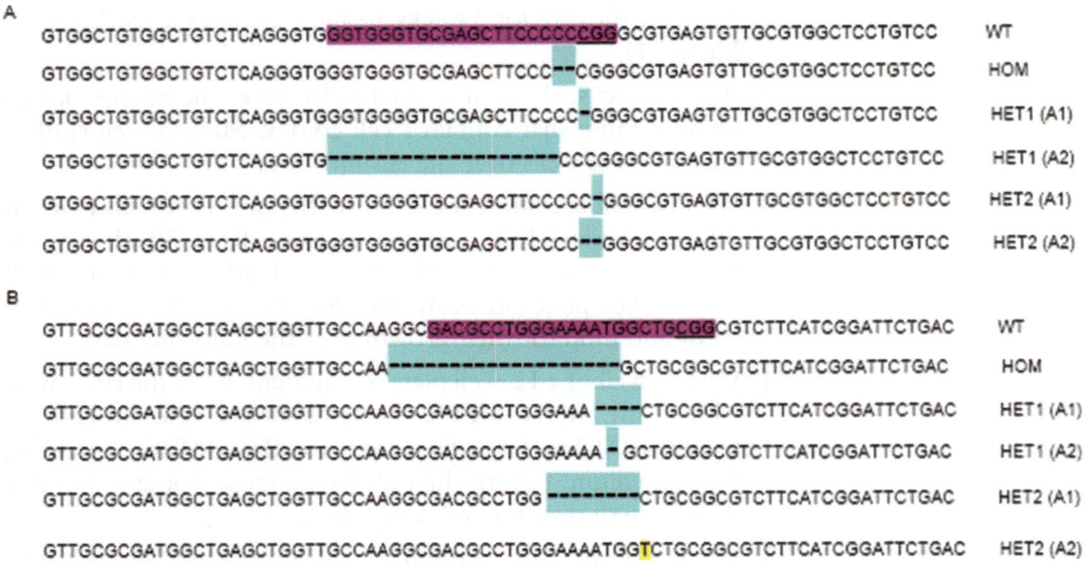

Fig. 4 Different mutations found in each cell line after sequencing. Homozygotes and compound heterozygotes have been found in both HEK 293 and IMCD3 cells. (**a**) Mutations found in single clones in HEK 293 cells after Sanger sequencing. (**b**) Mutations found in single clones in IMCD3 cells after Sanger sequencing. The sgRNA is highlighted in purple and the PAM sequence is underlined in WT samples. Note that the cyan color shows deleted bases and yellow indicates inserted bases

4 Notes

1. The given methods describe the use of the NHEJ pathway to knock out a gene by generating random indels. We have adapted these methods to knock in a specific point mutation in IMCD3 cells using the HDR pathway, by integrating methods from the literature [9, 10, 16]. The basic protocol presented in this chapter can be followed, making the following three changes:
   (a) In Subheading 3.1, the sgRNA must be designed to target the Cas9 to cut as close to the point at which the single base change is to be introduced, ideally within 10 bp. The necessity of a PAM site being proximal to the desired mutation site is a constraint of the HDR method.
   (b) A repair template (single-stranded oligodeoxynucleotide, ssODN) is required. This must contain the desired base change flanked by 60 nt homology arms, as well as a silent PAM mutation. Mutation of the PAM site prevents further Cas9 cleavage after mutation generation. It is important that the PAM mutation is silent to avoid introduction of an unwanted missense mutation. The ssODN should be ordered as an oligonucleotide and resuspended in

Milli-Q water to a concentration of 10 μM, prior to proceeding to Subheading 3.3.

(c) The CRISPR transfection of IMCD3 cells (in Subheading 3.3) must accommodate the ssODN. For the CRISPR transfection, add 1.2 μg pX330-sgRNA (obtained in step 3.2.7), 1.2 μg pAcGFP1-C1, and 1 μl ssODN (10 μM).

2. We have found that HEK293 cells can be transfected with high efficiency using the FuGENE 6 reagent (Promega). In IMCD3 cells, higher transfection efficiency was achieved with the Lipofectamine 2000 transfection reagent (Thermo Fisher) than with FuGENE.

3. If you are not interested in editing a specific locus, the chance of gene knockout will be improved by choosing a sgRNA target site that is in an early exon of the gene. However, it is also worth assessing whether internal translation initiation codons are present within the gene, as these could generate transcripts not affected by a frameshift mutation.

4. Several online sgRNA design tools are now available. We have successfully used CRISPOR (crispor.tefor.net), Chopchop (chopchop.cbu.uib.no), and Benchling (benchling.com) to design sgRNAs. Chopchop does not require the genomic region of interest to be pasted into the search box; instead, the gene of interest can be searched for within the appropriate genome, and all possible sgRNA options spanning the entire gene are presented.

5. When choosing a sgRNA it is important to consider its score (out of 100). A high score indicates a faithful sgRNA. A low score indicates a sgRNA with predicted off-target activity. For each sgRNA, off-target loci (including those with mismatches) are predicted, which are listed when the sgRNA is selected. The number of off-target sites within genes is also listed. Select a high-scoring sgRNA that does not have any predicted off-target sites in genes.

6. Design primers to generate an amplicon of 200–500 bp. The expected Cas9 cut site (~3 bp upstream of the "NGG" PAM) should not lie centrally within the amplicon, or else two products of roughly equal size will be produced by the T7EI assay and it will not be possible to resolve these by gel electrophoresis. It is recommended that the target genomic region, including the primer-binding sites, is Sanger sequenced within the cell line of choice. Primers should be designed to generate an amplicon that does not contain monoallelic mutations; these will give false positives in the T7EI assay and may bias primer binding (if they fall within primer-binding sites).

7. In a variation of the method presented here, two sgRNAs can be used in combination to excise a genomic region. In this case,

two sgRNAs should be designed in Subheading 3.1. Each can be independently cloned into a pX330 vector, to generate two separate pX330-sgRNA plasmids, one for each sgRNA. Transfection conditions can be adapted (in Subheading 3.3), to accommodate transfection of two pX330-sgRNA plasmids with the pAcGFP1-C1 plasmid. Larger deletions can be detected by running PCR products on an agarose gel (Fig. 5).

8. The procedure can be adjusted for other culture vessel sizes; scale reagents as necessary.
9. Confirm GFP expression in CRISPR and GFP-only cells by fluorescence microscopy 18–24 h post-transfection. The GFP-only cells are used purely as a control for transfection, and can be discarded prior to the group sort.
10. When preparing cells for FACS, take extra care not to cross-contaminate the different samples. The GFP-only cells do not need to be prepared for FACS (*see* **Note 9**).

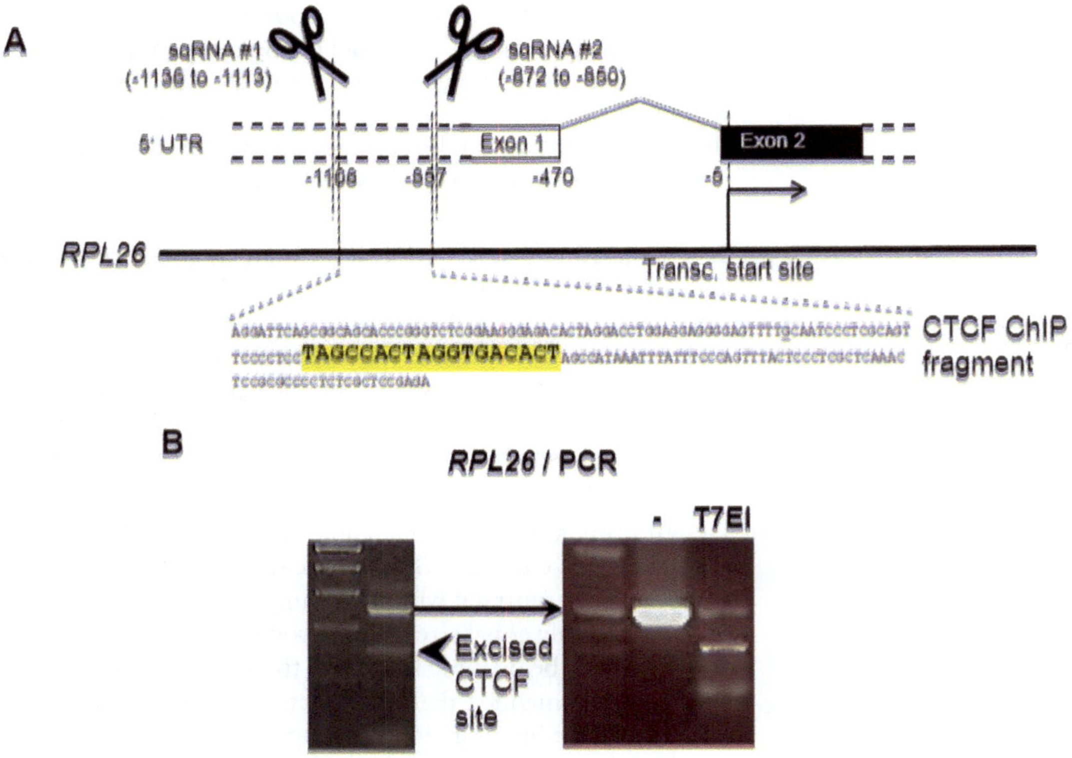

Fig. 5 Example of using pairs of sgRNAs for efficient excision of a DNA fragment. (**a**) In this example, a predicted CTCF-binding site (highlighted in yellow) within a CTCF ChIP fragment was excised using two sgRNAs located 239 nt apart. (**b**) PCR products were used to amplify the region surrounding these sgRNA-binding sites leading to a significant level of successful targeting, with excision of the desired sequence (arrowhead, left). The undigested fragment (indicated by the arrow) contained a high level of likely indels, as demonstrated by T7EI digestion of this product (right)

11. It is important to use serum-free medium so as not to clog the FACS apparatus with sera.
12. Cell straining is optional, although it is advised, particularly for IMCD3 cells. This will reduce cell clumps.
13. We use a MoFlo XDP (Beckman Coulter) equipped with three air-cooled lasers: a 150 mW 488 nm argon laser, a 100 mW 643 nm red laser, and a 100 mW 355 nm UV laser. A 100 nm nozzle tip is used with 30 PSI sheath pressure. eGFP signal is collected in FL1 channel through a 530/40 band-pass filter and FL3 channel with a 613/20 band-pass filter is used to separate true GFP-positive cells from autofluorescence background. A light scatter gate drawn in the FSC versus SSC plot is used to exclude debris and clumps and include viable cells. Cells in this gate are displayed in a SSC versus SSC-W to further target single cells. Single and viable cells are then analyzed in a FL3 versus FL1 plot and a final gate is drawn on green cells for cell sorting.
14. It is possible to complete the protocol if less than 5×10^5 cells are collected. In this case, prioritize cells for seeding into a culture vessel (Subheading 3.4, **step 10**); use a vessel of a size appropriate to the number of cells being seeded. If too few cells remain for gDNA extraction (Subheading 3.4, **step 11**, to Subheading 3.5, **step 1**), split some of the reseeded cells for gDNA extraction once they have begun to proliferate.
15. We have observed that single-cell sorting cells 2–3 days post-transfection tends to give rise to heterogeneous populations of cells, rather than clonal colonies (they possess more than two alleles when genotyped). We hypothesize that this is due to continued expression of the sgRNA and Cas9 in daughter cells, after division of the single-cell sorted cell. We passage cells for 2 weeks, to await loss of pX330 plasmid from the cells.
16. Optimize PCR conditions according to your needs. Pwo polymerase may be substituted for another polymerase of your choice. Ensure that the polymerase is of high fidelity and/or possesses proofreading ability (3′ to 5′ exonuclease activity); errors during PCR amplification will give false positives in the T7EI assay.
17. Use non-transfected cells as a control; these should behave as WT to give a single PCR product which is not cut by the T7EI assay. Multiple PCR products may be resolved from the CRISPR sample if it contains alleles with large indels. If there is a significant size difference between these PCR products, the T7EI assay may produce more than three bands on the gel.
18. sgRNA efficiency can be determined from the intensity of the products resulting from T7EI assay of the CRISPR sample: compare the intensity of the uncut product to that of the

cleavage products; the brighter the cleavage products (relative to the uncut product), the more efficient the sgRNA. If T7EI assay of the CRISPR sample does not result in cleavage products, sgRNA activity may be inefficient, and design of a new sgRNA should be considered.

19. Use as many 96-well plates as needed. We typically use 2–3 plates to maximize the number of colonies obtained.
20. It is necessary to passage some cells (of the same line) 24–48 h before preparing transfected cells for FACS, in order to formulate conditioned medium. Conditioned medium is used to improve the likelihood of cell survival after the single-cell sort. It comprises fresh medium (containing necessary nutrients) and medium taken from cells at ~70% confluence. The latter contains signaling components secreted by healthy cells in exponential growth phase, to encourage the sorted single cells to grow.
21. Conditioned medium must be sterile-filtered to remove contaminating cells, which may derive from media taken from cells at ~70% confluence. Contaminating cells will obstruct the establishment of clonal cell lines.
22. The majority of cells will no longer be GFP positive. Isolate any single cells, regardless of GFP expression.
23. Centrifugation of the 96-well plate improves chances of cell adhesion, by moving cells to the bottom of the plate. It is important to get the single-cell sorted cells into the incubator as quickly as possible after FACS, to maximize viability.
24. Changing medium is not necessary; this risks loss of cells from the wells.
25. It may be necessary to passage the cells before the entire well is confluent, if cells become dense but do not spread across the well, and media become orange/yellow in color.
26. Confirm cell detachment under the microscope prior to transferring cells to the new culture vessel. Transfer the full volume of cell suspension to the 12-well plate without pelleting cells. Then check the (empty) well of the 96-well plate under the microscope again, to ensure that all cells have been transferred. Loss of cells during passage will result in reduced cell density in the 12-well plate, which may decrease cell viability.
27. Presence of more than two PCR products indicates that the colony is a clone with aneuploidy, or that it is not clonal (it is a heterogeneous population).
28. It is possible to perform the T7EI assay to genotype clones. However, note that T7EI will not cleave PCR products derived from homozygous mutants. T7EI will only give a positive result (cleavage) in PCR products derived from heterozygotes or compound heterozygotes.

29. If Sanger sequencing produces two overlapping traces, the clone is a heterozygote or a compound heterozygote. Cloning of PCR products in pGEM-T Easy vector systems (Promega) can be used to isolate allelic sequences. If more than two overlapping traces are seen, the colony is a clone with aneuploidy, or it is not clonal (it is a heterogeneous population).

Acknowledgments

This work was funded by a Medical Research Council New Investigator Research Grant (MR/L009978/1), Action Medical Research Project Grant (GN2595), Biotechnology and Biological Sciences Research Council Doctoral Training Grant (STU100044631), and Wellcome Trust Collaborative Award in Science to DJ (210585/Z/18/Z). This research was also supported by the National Institute for Health Research Biomedical Research Centre at Great Ormond Street Hospital for Children NHS Foundation Trust and University College London. Nuria Perretta Tejedor, Grace M. Freke, and Marian Seda contributed equally to this work.

References

1. Beerli RR, Segal DJ, Dreier B, Barbas CF 3rd (1998) Toward controlling gene expression at will: specific regulation of the erbB-2/HER-2 promoter by using polydactyl zinc finger proteins constructed from modular building blocks. Proc Natl Acad Sci U S A 95 (25):14628–14633
2. Boch J, Scholze H, Schornack S, Landgraf A, Hahn S, Kay S, Lahaye T, Nickstadt A, Bonas U (2009) Breaking the code of DNA binding specificity of TAL-type III effectors. Science 326(5959):1509–1512. https://doi.org/10.1126/science.1178811
3. Moscou MJ, Bogdanove AJ (2009) A simple cipher governs DNA recognition by TAL effectors. Science 326(5959):1501. https://doi.org/10.1126/science.1178817
4. Gaj T, Gersbach CA, Barbas CF 3rd (2013) ZFN, TALEN, and CRISPR/Cas-based methods for genome engineering. Trends Biotechnol 31(7):397–405. https://doi.org/10.1016/j.tibtech.2013.04.004
5. Zhang F, Wen Y, Guo X (2014) CRISPR/Cas9 for genome editing: progress, implications and challenges. Hum Mol Genet 23(R1): R40–R46. https://doi.org/10.1093/hmg/ddu125
6. Maeder ML, Gersbach CA (2016) Genome-editing technologies for gene and cell therapy. Mol Ther 24(3):430–446. https://doi.org/10.1038/mt.2016.10
7. Cong L, Ran FA, Cox D, Lin S, Barretto R, Habib N, Hsu PD, Wu X, Jiang W, Marraffini LA, Zhang F (2013) Multiplex genome engineering using CRISPR/Cas systems. Science 339(6121):819–823. https://doi.org/10.1126/science.1231143
8. Mali P, Yang L, Esvelt KM, Aach J, Guell M, DiCarlo JE, Norville JE, Church GM (2013) RNA-guided human genome engineering via Cas9. Science 339(6121):823–826. https://doi.org/10.1126/science.1232033
9. Ran FA, Hsu PD, Wright J, Agarwala V, Scott DA, Zhang F (2013) Genome engineering using the CRISPR-Cas9 system. Nat Protoc 8 (11):2281–2308. https://doi.org/10.1038/nprot.2013.143
10. Paquet D, Kwart D, Chen A, Sproul A, Jacob S, Teo S, Olsen KM, Gregg A, Noggle S, Tessier-Lavigne M (2016) Efficient introduction of specific homozygous and heterozygous mutations using CRISPR/Cas9. Nature 533(7601):125–129. https://doi.org/10.1038/nature17664

11. Guschin DY, Waite AJ, Katibah GE, Miller JC, Holmes MC, Rebar EJ (2010) A rapid and general assay for monitoring endogenous gene modification. Methods Mol Biol 649:247–256. https://doi.org/10.1007/978-1-60761-753-2_15
12. Vouillot L, Thelie A, Pollet N (2015) Comparison of T7E1 and surveyor mismatch cleavage assays to detect mutations triggered by engineered nucleases. G3 (Bethesda) 5 (3):407–415. https://doi.org/10.1534/g3.114.015834
13. Zischewski J, Fischer R, Bortesi L (2017) Detection of on-target and off-target mutations generated by CRISPR/Cas9 and other sequence-specific nucleases. Biotechnol Adv 35(1):95–104. https://doi.org/10.1016/j.biotechadv.2016.12.003
14. Bryant D, Liu Y, Datta S, Hariri H, Seda M, Anderson G, Peskett E, Demetriou C, Sousa S, Jenkins D, Clayton P, Bitner-Glindzicz M, Moore GE, Henne WM, Stanier P (2018) SNX14 mutations affect endoplasmic reticulum-associated neutral lipid metabolism in autosomal recessive spinocerebellar ataxia 20. Hum Mol Genet 27(11):1927–1940. https://doi.org/10.1093/hmg/ddy101
15. Taschner M, Lorentzen A, Mourao A, Collins T, Freke GM, Moulding D, Basquin J, Jenkins D, Lorentzen E (2018) Crystal structure of intraflagellar transport protein 80 reveals a homo-dimer required for ciliogenesis. elife 7:e33067. https://doi.org/10.7554/eLife.33067
16. Mianne J, Codner GF, Caulder A, Fell R, Hutchison M, King R, Stewart ME, Wells S, Teboul L (2017) Analysing the outcome of CRISPR-aided genome editing in embryos: screening, genotyping and quality control. Methods 121-122:68–76. https://doi.org/10.1016/j.ymeth.2017.03.016

Index

Luigi Gnudi and David A. Long (eds.), *Diabetic Nephropathy: Methods and Protocols*, Methods in Molecular Biology, vol. 2067, https://doi.org/10.1007/978-1-4939-9841-8, © Springer Science+Business Media, LLC, part of Springer Nature 2020

MIX
Papier aus verantwortungsvollen Quellen
Paper from responsible sources
FSC® C105338

If you have any concerns about our products,
you can contact us on
ProductSafety@springernature.com

In case Publisher is established outside the EU,
the EU authorized representative is:
Springer Nature Customer Service Center GmbH
Europaplatz 3, 69115 Heidelberg, Germany

Printed by Libri Plureos GmbH
in Hamburg, Germany